Birthing

Women's Experiences of Planning Home Births

Is home birth dangerous for women and babies?
Shouldn't women decide where to have their babies?

Home birth is a highly contentious issue in a number of countries, including Britain. The UK Government appears to support a policy of more home births, while mainstream medical opinion remains firmly opposed to it and a growing number of women and midwives struggle to make it a realistic option. Research suggests that for healthy women and babies home birth is safe and has certain benefits for those who plan it, yet women planning home births are sometimes accused of being reckless and of taking risks with their babies' and their own lives.

Birthing Autonomy brings some balance to these difficult arguments by focusing on women's views and their experiences of planning home births. It is the first in-depth exploration of how women make decisions about home births and what aspects matter most to them. The book compares how differently the pros and cons of home births are constructed and contemplated by mothers and by the medical profession, and looks at how current obstetric thinking and practices can disempower and harm women emotionally and spiritually as well as physically.

The book is written in an accessible way and will be enlightening for student and practising midwives and obstetricians, as well as researchers and students of nursing, medical sociology, health studies, gender studies, feminist practitioners and theorists. It will also be invaluable to expectant mothers who want to be more informed about the choices they are facing and the wider context within which their birth options are considered.

Nadine Pilley Edwards has worked with AIMS since 1980. She is a part-time research associate at the University of Sheffield, and lectures and writes on maternity issues in the UK and overseas. She has written numerous articles and chapters on relationships between women and midwives, informed choice, safety and risk, and research methods.

Birthing Autonomy
Women's Experiences of Planning Home Births

Nadine Pilley Edwards

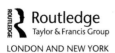

Routledge
Taylor & Francis Group

LONDON AND NEW YORK

First published 2005
by Routledge
2 Park Square, Milton Park, Abingdon, Oxon OX14 4RN

Simultaneously published in the USA and Canada
by Routledge
270 Madison Ave. New York, NY 10016

Routledge is an imprint of the Taylor & Francis Group

© Nadine Pilley Edwards, 2005

Typeset in Sabon by J&L Composition, Filey, North Yorkshire
Printed and bound in Great Britain by Antony Rowe Ltd.,
Chippenham, Wiltshire

British Library Cataloguing in Publication Data
A catalogue record for this book is available from the British
Library

Library of Congress Cataloging in Publication Data
Edwards, Nadine Pilley, 1957–
Birthing autonomy: women's experiences of planning home births/
    Nadine Pilley Edwards.
        p. ; cm
Includes bibliographical references and index.
ISBN 0–415–35408–0 (hbk: alk. paper)
ISBN 0–415–35409–9 (pbk: alk. paper)
Childbirth at home—Great Britain.
[DNLM: 1. Home Childbirth—England. 2. Feminism—England. 3. Health
Knowledge Attitudes, Practice—England. 4. Midwifery—England. 5. Women's
Rights—England.] I. Title.
RG661.5.E39 2005
618.2—dc22   2005002812

Contents

Foreword

Home births are important because their existence within the NHS keeps options open and demonstrates an alternative to the industrialised model of birth within increasingly large, centralised and uniform hospitals. The women who seek home births are important because they take the rhetoric of maternity care seriously. They seek to engage with it rather than take the more passive role of service consumer. These women seek choice, control and continuity of carer when most midwives and women accept this as impractical or even impossible.

The experiences of 30 women who booked home births are presented here with clarity and integrity. Each woman was interviewed four times and trust grew as her story developed, was heard and was respected. In good research, as in good midwifery, listening to women demonstrates that their thoughts are worth hearing and such valuing attention fosters growth. Here insightful stories grew, together with confidence and babies. These stories are presented in dialogue with a wide and diverse literature from many disciplines.

Nadine Edwards presents food for thought for women and for midwives. Issues such as safety, risk and ethics are explored within the experience of childbearing women, rather than the received guidelines of professions.

The importance of this book goes beyond home birth. It explores the potential for dialogue between the woman undergoing life transition and her professional companions. It challenges the defensive reactions of professionalism and of bureaucracy and shows that dialogue is both possible and fruitful.

As a midwife, this book gives me hope, as it demonstrates the strength and insight of childbearing women. The generosity of spirit with which this book is structured ensures that many issues are explored and many voices are heard and that it ends with women speaking of the power of birth and the potential of midwifery. To achieve that potential we must challenge both the preconceptions and the structures of NHS maternity care. The book shows the sacrifices women find they have to make if midwives do not make those challenges. This is therefore a book of considerable political importance for mothers and midwives.

Mavis Kirkham

Acknowledgements

Many, many people have contributed to this book in many different ways and I sincerely thank all those who have contributed. I am sorry I cannot name them all.

This work was inspired by the many women who have talked to me about their experiences of pregnancy, birth and motherhood. I have learnt most of what I know from them, especially the thirty women who took part in the study on which this book is based. I am deeply grateful to them for their honesty, clarity and willingness to share.

This work became a possibility due to the initial support of Rosemary Mander and Steve Tilley. Rosemary's support over the years has been generous and consistent.

Its execution was made possible by my family, Peter, Mike, Rowenna and Martin Edwards, and my parents, Bruce and Ginette Pilley. They provided an endless combination of emotional, intellectual, practical and financial support. My gratitude is beyond words. My friends, Nicky, Rod, Sophie and Maddi Macphail frequently provided food, laughter and the sustaining joy of friendship way beyond the call of duty. MB provided me with a nourishing haven when I was away from home as well as incisive comments throughout the process. Support from Anne Till and Caroline Weddell was invaluable. Margaret Hilton was a key person during my secondary education. Her ability to broaden minds developed critical thinking at a young age.

Mavis Kirkham's close involvement had a profound effect on the depth of this work. Her trust, wisdom and patience encouraged me to follow my instincts and intellect. If pregnant and birthing women could be midwifed in the way that she has midwifed this project, many more women would feel genuinely empowered. I cannot thank her enough for her consistent and continuing support and time.

Jan Webb's insightful and intellectual contributions enabled me to bring birth, midwifery and sociology into a more open dialogue. Jo Murphy-Lawless' knowledge, integrity and clarity encourages my thinking to be ever more sensitive to women, deeply reflective, rigorous and global. I hope I have done her teaching some justice.

Helen Shallow has had a profound influence on me for many years. Her courage and willingness to listen, speak out and really be with women, never fail to inspire me. Many other exceptional midwives have contributed to my understanding about birth and midwifery. Wendy Ashcroft, Linda Bryce, Mary Cronk, Jane Evans, Helen Stapleton and Sara Wickham have been particularly influential.

Members of the Association for Improvements in the Maternity Services have provided me with a rich education over the years since 1980, especially Beverley Beech, Tracey Black, Lyssa Clayton, Erin McNeill, Jean Robinson, Christine Rodgers, Lee Seekings Norman, Cathleen Sullivan, Pat Thomas and Sandar Warshal. Those involved in the Birth Resource Centre in Edinburgh and the Scottish Birth Teachers Association have provided endless insight, support, interest and enthusiasm.

I thank those whose comments on drafts of this book improved it beyond measure – Beverley Beech, Alice Charlwood, Diana Green, Mavis Kirkham, Jo Murphy-Lawless, Jean Robinson, Andrea St Clair, Lee Seekings Norman and Sara Wickham.

I would like to thank Jane Durell for her excellent technical support, which has always been reliably and willingly provided, Margaret Ford, Shamlah Husain and Ann Rennie, who assisted in the transcriptions of my interviews, and Clare Brady for her help with the references. Finally, I thank the University of Edinburgh for enabling me to start this work and the University of Sheffield for the bursary I was awarded. Without it, I would have been unable to devote the time I needed to carry out and complete the research on which this book is based.

I thank all those at Routlege (Karen Bowler, Claire Gauler, Christine Firth and Manjula Goonawardena) who have been so supportive and encouraging since receiving the first early manuscript. Finally, my inspired and inspiring yoga teacher, John Stirk, who reminds me that good health depends on nurturing our bodies and spirits, as well as our minds.

Introducing the women

Who are these women?

I wanted to write this book because birth has such a profound impact on women's lives and those of their babies and families. Women describe being affected both positively and negatively for months and years after the births of their babies.[1] I wanted to focus on home birth because we know relatively little about the detailed experiences of those women who plan them. Most of what we know is based on single interviews, or surveys after the baby's birth.[2] We do know that women who have experienced home birth almost always want home births again.[3] The women in this book felt the same. This suggests that women experience benefits that might be useful to know more about. We know little about whether women planning home births are different from those planning hospital births. Some studies show little difference, others suggest that these women are more likely to have previous knowledge about home birth, be professional, well-educated, openly feminist and believe that home birth is safer than hospital birth.[4] Perhaps the most significant knowledge we have is that if home birth is marginalized it becomes an option limited by and reflecting socio-economic status. When midwives make it easily available, social status of any kind ceases to be a barrier to it.[5]

Research in Australia, Canada, England, Finland, Ireland, New Zealand and North America, where home birth is generally marginalized and obstetric hospital birth the norm, discusses some of the views and beliefs that women planning home births may have. While not all women share the same views, many believe that home birth is safe, that hospital birth can be risky and that home birth offers benefits to them, their babies and their families. They often want to avoid negative experiences of hospital birth, make birth as normal as possible, feel relaxed, private and secure enough to give birth, maintain their personal autonomy and integrity as well as the well-being of the family unit, receive supportive, non-interventionist care from a known midwife and maintain a sense of ownership over their births. They particularly appreciate support for their plans from family, friends and professionals. They are generally positive about home birth and its contribution to their confidence in themselves as birth givers and mothers. Some describe how home birth healed negative, past experiences of birth. Overall women's hopes and concerns around birth are much broader than those of obstetric medicine.[6] I hoped to learn more about these.

To do this I followed thirty women planning home births through their pregnancies until six to eight months after their babies' births, in the late 1990s. To help me contact these women, community midwives in several areas of Scotland kindly agreed to give information about my study to any woman who booked a home birth with them. Women then contacted me if they wanted to take part in the study. I interviewed each woman who contacted me twice before her baby's birth and twice following the birth, usually spending two to three hours at each visit.

Like women in the studies mentioned above, these women shared both similarities and differences. The youngest woman I interviewed was in her early twenties and the oldest woman in her early forties. Some of the women were well-off financially, others not so. Most women were white, but came from a variety of European and North American countries. Most had some form of further education and most were living in nuclear families in urban or semi-rural situations.

Thirteen women were expecting their first babies, others were expecting second, third and fifth babies. For some this was their first experience of home birth, for others it was their second or third home birth. Seven of the women gave birth in hospital. Three of these women had normal births after transferring to hospital because their babies passed meconium during labour. One woman had an induction with no further interventions, another had a caesarean section following an induction which led to her baby moving into a transverse position, another had a caesarean section after a long labour and one woman had a forceps birth following a long labour. All the fathers were present at their babies' births and half the women planned to have their mother, mother-in-law, sister, friend or birth supporter present, though one or two babies arrived before supporters arrived. Most women were attended by two community midwives; a few had independent midwives in this or previous births. Eleven women planned to use birth pools, though two were unable to do so because of complications during labour. Of the seventeen women with children, some planned to have their children present, some children were asleep and five women planned to have their children looked after elsewhere.

Each woman made a unique contribution to this book and to the coexisting puzzles and possibilities of birth. I have tried to maintain the integrity of the 120 interviews with the thirty women and the conversations I have had with other women, by weaving in the similarities and differences between them and reflecting the complexities of their lives. I have tried to let their stories about birth and how they dreamt of its possibilities be told – stories that deeply challenge accepted knowledge about birth and its practices.

Often, neither I nor they had the knowledge, imagination or words to move beyond the powerful norms of our times and cultures. Yet among the medical terms and concepts that commonly define our bodies in birth, our language of possibilities created fractures and fissures. We stumbled across ideas and meanings, sometimes in a flash of insight, often beginning as seedling notions. As we talked, I understood more about how birth is an integral part of women's life journeys. Others have referred to the idea of journeying through birth,[7] but talking to women before and after birth connected the birth journey to women's life journeys and brought out the sense of transition through birth. This was captured by one of the women who initially planned a hospital birth but changed to planning a home birth during her first pregnancy:

I mean, once you see it from the other point of view, you realize that it makes a lot more sense in a way, not to go away from your home to have a baby.

Her thinking changed further over the course of two pregnancies. She had previously stated that she would always think of hospital birth first as this is the norm, but now no longer felt this:

No, I don't feel that way anymore. It wouldn't even occur to me really. I suppose that has been expiated by the births that I've had at home. No, I don't feel that I have to relate everything to what happens in hospital.

How birth and life journeys interact is complex but birth journeys were sometimes part of a more sustained journey of re-examining other cultural beliefs about nutrition, vaccination and schooling for example. Robbie Davis-Floyd (1992) found that the women in her study who planned home births after previous hospital births became interested in natural therapies, recycling, wholewheat bread and so on. 'It seemed, in fact, that they were actually using their births as a means to change their personal belief systems – undergoing on an individual level what Thomas Kuhn, speaking of changes in scientific models of reality has called a paradigm shift.'[8] Women's birth journeys could reconnect them with different parts of themselves and their histories, and enable them to create new identities and lifestyles for themselves and their families. The idea of journey could even extend across generations, as one woman explained:

> *Somehow I had a very strong feeling that because she's a girl and she might one day have babies of her own, that maybe I'd set her one stage freer than I'd been myself. Because I knew my own birth was not anything like her birth was. And I kind of got the feeling that I'd achieved something on that level too, especially because she's a girl. That maybe I'd broken something, a long cycle of family history of difficult labours and babies being born in traumatic ways, and maybe I'd left her with something to go on in her life with, and that was a very good feeling.*

Of course women approached pregnancy, birth and motherhood from very different places. For example, for some, home birth was a first choice. Other women had thought about home births but were put off by health practitioners or partners during previous pregnancies. Others chose home births due to an erosion of trust in obstetric ideology following unsatisfactory or traumatic births in hospital and some because of growing confidence in their abilities to birth their babies following straightforward births in hospital. Some women initially went along with hospital bookings until they had the information and confidence they needed to book the home birth they wanted. Some changed from a hospital booking they had previously chosen, sometimes just before giving birth. Having a previous home birth made the decision about where to have a subsequent baby a 'foregone conclusion' for one woman, another felt anxious about 'pushing her luck'. Like women in other studies they focused on a peaceful environment in which they could birth their babies in their own time and way.[9]

Women planning home births are not all 'earth mothers'

While women gave similar reasons for planning home births, their priorities varied. A number of women talked about previous traumatic, violating births in hospital which they did not wish to repeat. For these women home birth offered protection. Several women held spiritual beliefs, which they felt could best be maintained in their own homes. Some believed that their lives would be enriched by living them through their families and homes rather than through formal institutions. Some women focused on the baby as a fully conscious, highly sensitive individual. In line with work by obstetricians Frederic Leboyer (1977) and Michel Odent (1999) and psychologist David Chamberlain (1998), they saw the experience of birth as formative and home birth as providing the gentlest, most protective circumstances for their babies. Another woman described home birth as being part of a journey of self-discovery and reclaiming her self-esteem and power, which she felt had been lost during her life and experiences of earlier births. These are some of the comments they made:

> *My God, the idea of trying to have any sort of spiritual experience in a hospital ward, or even in a labour suite with a bunch of doctors and nurses who I don't know, and not in my own space. You know, I just can't think of anything more offputting to my kind of sense of what's essential and what's important in life than a hospital really.*

> *Another point which drew me towards home birth had a lot to do with my faith. And for me not to go through something as huge as childbirth in this light would be a denial of how I live my life. I felt I could express much more of that in my own environment. It might seem out of place in hospital, whereas here, this is where so much of my faith is lived out. You know, I feel very happy expressing it here.*

> *It seems unnatural to me to split up the family when there's something so important happening and such a natural event happening.*

> *I think it [home birth] was largely for the baby. That was always largely my concern. I just saw how it [birth] was such a crucial part of our beings – how you come into the world and I just thought, the smoother and more gentle the passage could be.*

There were women in the study who valued birth as a powerful experience in itself, and saw home birth as offering the potential for birth to be a sacred, spiritual, sensual and empowering process. These women expected the transition from pregnancy to motherhood to provide opportunities for positive growth and transformation.

> *I always thought that it would be a total thing that's about your femininity and the way you feel and everything, cos it's like your transition from maiden to mother. You can't be you and worried about your normal things of life when you're giving birth. So through that you're opening to something far wider than our usual ego little lives and also the connection with all the woman who've ever given birth from the beginning of time.*

> *I imagine a nice lively, colourful kind of event – more like a celebration really. In hospital it felt more like a chore going through labour – but at home I'd like it to be a joyful celebration really.*

> *One of the reasons I wanted a home birth was so that it could feel kind of earthy and quite sexual.*

A few women, like some of those in Marie O'Connor's (1992) study, saw birth as a necessary, but painful and traumatic transition from pregnancy to having a baby. They did not necessarily value birth as a positive experience in itself, but thought that home birth might minimize the pain and trauma they expected. For some of these women, the loss of control that might result from being in hospital was more troubling than the pain of labour. Some stressed their ordinary-ness, stating that they were not 'radical', and did not want to be perceived as 'different', 'difficult' or 'making a fuss':

> *What gets me is that I'm not very radical. I'm not radical at all. I just didn't want drugs. I didn't want monitoring. I just wanted to give birth.*

> *I think in a lot of ways my lifestyle's very conventional, so you might not have predicted that I was the sort of person that would have my baby at home.*

> *Nadine: What sort of person might that be?*

> *Well, I think the people that I've spoken to that have had their babies at home – their questioning of the medical profession goes a lot wider than mine. On the whole I'm reasonably per-*

*suaded by modern medicine, but I just don't think that's really
got anything to do with having babies.*

Some women wanted antenatal screening and were prepared to ter-
minate their pregnancies in the event of serious abnormalities, others
did not and would not have terminated a pregnancy. Some wanted to
avoid pain relief, while others wanted pethidine available in case they
needed it. There were different views about water labour, water birth,
entonox, TENS machines, syntometrine and vitamin K, to mention
but some of the issues on which opinions differed. For some women,
hospital and home birth did appear to represent a set of more general
beliefs in other parts of their lives. These included a general trust in
and affinity with what they conceptualized as nature and natural
home-based processes and a general distrust of and unease with technology and institutions. Some women felt that the potentially oppressive impact of living our lives through formal institutions contributes
to the destruction of communities. Of course this is a contested area,
as communities are a form of institution and can be as oppressive as
formal institutions:[10]

*I feel very strongly that we sterilize our lives now. That all those
things that are really important to us – birth and death – are
shoved away. They're taken away and everything's made clean
and neat and tidy and somehow unnatural. We put our grannies
in homes and we send our labouring women alone to places
where they don't feel comfortable. And it seems to me that
these things are part of our natural lives and part of our natural
experience. It worries me that we do that and I'm not quite sure
why we do it. Are we so busy that we can't fit these important
parts of life that are common to us all into the pattern of our
lives?*

For some women home birth was a means for achieving particular
needs – avoiding a caesarean section or other interventions for example. Many women held varying combinations of beliefs about birth,
and overall aligned themselves with natural rather than technological
birth. But they challenged any notion of discrete boundaries between
belief systems by moving between them and describing them in terms
of unhelpful stereotyping. So while women planning home births are
often stereotyped as 'earth mothers' or 'radical', each woman was
unique.

Why were they thinking about home births?

We do not really know how women come to be thinking about home births. Experiences throughout our lives are likely to impact on decisions about birth,[11] and women may have specific reasons for planning home births.[12] My interviews suggest that women approach planning home births from multifaceted positions to do with what they believe and how they live their lives, and that these positions are influenced by significant experiences and relationships.[13] But it is difficult to really know how their own experiences and the marginalization of home birth interact and impact on their decisions. All the women I interviewed had had contact with home birth, through being born at home, or through family members, friends, communities both in Britain and abroad and antenatal groups. For many women this was a close connection, through mothers, sisters and close friends, and was part of their life stories and, for two women, videos seen in other contexts seemed influential. Interestingly, Banyana Madi (2003) found that women planning hospital births often reported not knowing other women who had had home births and not knowing that it was a possibility.[14] For some women growing up with knowledge of home birth, knowing others who had had home births and having contact with home birth support groups was important:

> *The feeling of my mum having been born at home and my grannie having been born at home. It means something to me to have that continuity. I think my mum must have given me a very positive message about it, in a way that I don't really remember. But it was never a question for me, it was an assumption that I would have a home birth.*

> *Quite a lot of my friends have had babies at home, and their friends had had their babies at home, so I think probably because of that culture being around, in my friends, it certainly makes me more positive about it.*

Some women suggested that support for home birth interacts with the pull towards hospital birth in complex ways. Even if obstetric ideology contradicts their own views, and they have support for home birth, few women plan them. As one woman remarked recently in one of my antenatal groups:

> *Even though I was born at home and my brother was born at home, and my mother said, 'Oh, no problem,' I couldn't do it*

the first time. And now of course I realize I could. But I didn't know.

Another woman made a similar comment:

> *My mum had me at home and my brother at home so I'd always thought of home birth as being like something that was normal. But being a nurse I then had the other side where I knew a bit too much, and with my first child I just thought that I felt safer myself going into hospital to have her.*

But half-way through her second pregnancy, this woman visited a close friend a few hours after the friend's home birth and decided to plan a home birth herself:

> *This time round I was thinking of doing pretty much the same thing, just going in [to hospital] and staying overnight and coming back out again, until I went to visit a friend who was planning on a home delivery. And it was just I think the whole atmosphere. We were there the day she actually had the baby and it just felt so normal and part of everyday life, and their other wee girl was there and everything felt like that's how it should have been. Nothing was taken out of place, you didn't have to be going out travelling somewhere and taking children out, you know, upsetting other children in the family, so that's really what made me change my mind.*

Because of the widely held obstetric beliefs about birth, it was exceptional for women not to seek support for their decisions from their partners as well as health practitioners. Given the prevalence of the nuclear family and that twenty of the thirty women were geographically distant from their families of origin or had lost their own mothers, their partners' support was almost always crucial. All but two woman stressed that they would not have gone ahead with their plans to have home births without their partner's agreement – though it was frequently the women themselves who changed the views of those in their own circle of family and friends, as women often do.[15]

What did their family and friends think?

Women's partners

Some of the women's partners were keen to have a home birth and initiated or encouraged plans for this. As midwife Maggie Banks, describes, men can be equally traumatized following hospital births in which they felt unable to protect their partners.[16] Others were not opposed to home birth but expected the woman to be the main decision-maker about this:

> *He was determined I was having it at home, because he hated what I went through in hospital, and he just said, I don't want you having all that interference and everything again, and, I'd rather you had it at home.*

> *My partner thought it was a good idea. I think his main concern was that I felt confident. He was happy with it from the start. I mean, he was as far as I know. It was basically what I wanted, since I was the one giving birth.*

A number of partners however, were apprehensive until they experienced impersonal hospital services themselves, found out about the research on home birth, realized that there was a community service and discovered that similar others had planned home births:

> *He instantly said, oh no, cos he's very working class and just said, we need men in white coats there for it to be a proper – sort of half-joking. And then he's also very tidy, so he said, what about the mess. So that was his concerns. Well, I got the feeling that he wanted some sort of facts and figures about what are the risks and all that sort of thing. But actually he's come round very quickly. I think, just going on these hospital visits, he just has felt so marginalized and really not respected.*

> *Speaking to my partner about it, he started off from a very sceptical sort of position. I think his belief was that all hospitals are good things and doctors are good things. So I think having to be clear about what I was saying to him so that he knew what I was thinking was very useful. And he's come to fully support me and think that it's definitely the right place to give birth, at home.*

> *When I first suggested it to my partner he was like – a home birth? Oh! You know, it wasn't until he realized that they bring*

equipment and the midwife's here. Until he realized all this, he was a bit unsure himself.

I then started thinking about home birth. My husband wasn't terribly keen. I think he thought I was a bit mad, and he obviously thought it was dangerous and things. And then we started going to antenatal classes and there was one couple there who had planned a home birth and they were both nurses, and I think that was what convinced my husband that it's not weird people with sandals and joss-sticks in the corner who had home birth but actually people who could actually assess the risk.

For one or two women who had had traumatic experiences of hospital births, avoiding a similar experience was so crucial that the plan to have a home birth was negotiated before the woman felt able to have another child:

I think when my husband and I started talking about having another baby, the first thing that came in to my mind was, I can't bear going through all that antenatal care. It made me angry, and going into a labour ward. And, okay, I might not know what's going to happen, but I'm still going to feel very disempowered and suspicious that nobody's listened to me. And that was even before I got pregnant. I really felt that had to be sorted out and I was voicing lots of doubts about being in hospital to my husband and he just said, out of the blue one night, why don't you have the baby at home then? And I thought, hurrah, because I had been really scared to mention that to him, cos I thought he'd just go, oh no way, I couldn't possibly cope with that.

Women's close family

For some women, the views of parents and parents-in-law were important. This was often the case when parents planned to provide practical help and support around the time of birth. Responses from them were as varied and as open to change as those from partners. Some of the women's mothers were positive:

My mum was great. She said, oh you'll enjoy it. She said, I had you at home, you'll enjoy it. She didn't like hospitals.

For others it raised mixed feelings:

I mean my mother, in some way I would say that she's delighted at what I'm doing, but I think tinged with – not jealousy – but because her births were just awful, you know.

And yet others were against the idea altogether:

My own mother, despite two particularly unpleasant births in hospital for myself and my sister, is not happy about my decision.

A number of women were troubled by the lack of support from their mothers. But, like partners, most parents became positive over time:

You see, she's been against it from the start. I think she thought initially that it was me that was wanting to go ahead and that my partner wouldn't be interested, so she took him aside one day and she was at him, and he put her straight. He said, 'Look, it's both of us – we've talked about it.' You know, we've discussed it at length for months now, before I was even pregnant and she's still not coming round to the idea at all. I mean obviously I've got a lot of books out on home birth and my partner and I did quite a lot of reading before I was even pregnant, so I said to my mum, well look, have a look at this. But she wouldn't even read one of the books. You know, it's her granddaughter or grandson I'm going to bring into the world and she wouldn't even read a book.

Some weeks later her mother's view had changed:

She's read the books and she's changed her mind quite a bit. She also got speaking to some lady in her office who thought it was a wonderful idea. So I think that's helped my mum, and reading the books. And I think as well, seeing how happy and healthy I've been. I think reading the books she's said to me that she was quite surprised. I think she'd never heard of it before. I think this is what the problem was – she'd never heard of home births. She'd never heard of anybody who'd had

*a home birth and she just got it into her head, you know, my
daughter's being stupid, she's just taking silly chances here. And
it wasn't till she started reading the books and started talking
to other people about it – and then they would say, oh I think
that's great, or, oh I know somebody that did that – and I
think that's all helped. So yeh, she thinks it's a great idea now
so she's completely come round, which helps me because she
was a wee bit stressing me out, cos I was so keen on it and I
wanted her to be really keen on it, you know, and she's like,
oh, I've got my doubts. But na, she's great actually.*

Women's friends and colleagues

Responses from friends, colleagues and acquaintances were equally
mixed, but positive responses were experienced as supportive and
encouraging:

*There was this very positive encouragement from my best friend
who had a home birth and I mean, when hers went well – she
was three months ahead of me – anyway, when hers went well
and I got her account first hand, I mean it certainly increased my
confidence and I was looking forward to it.*

Negative responses were disappointing:

*They [friends] think it's shocking that I'm even considering hav-
ing a home birth, you know. What if anything goes wrong? And,
you're putting your baby at risk. And, I think it's terrible. So
we've decided to drop the subject. But I'm a bit disappointed in
everybody's attitude.*

But women educated their friends in the same way that they educated
their families:

*They're all coming round. It was like she's having a home
birth, you know, and folk were like – well what's that? What
does that involve and is she taking risks? And I think everybody thought it was a risk to the baby and maybe to myself.
And obviously the more I read, the more I was able to tell
them – well look, there's the proof that there's less this and less
this or whatever when you have a home birth, and I was*

actually able to show them the statistics and things. I think that slowly but surely brought them round.

When family and friends were unsupportive of home births, it was often through lack of knowledge and experience of home birth. Most people, as Charlotte Williamson (1988, 1992) pointed out, tend to reflect commonly held beliefs about health. Many had unquestioningly accepted the view that hospitals are safer for birth. But when this was challenged by women they knew well, most were prepared to question their own assumptions and listen to other views.

What did women hope for?

The women's hopes were often shaped by their concerns about hospital birth. Whether or not the advantages of home birth and the disadvantages of hospital birth are intrinsic to place of birth is somewhat equivocal. Accounts of births in birth centres,[17] one-to-one care schemes,[18] and 'home-from-home' settings[19] disrupt any clear boundary, yet, as Ruth Wilkins (2000) found, the women I talked to suggested that there are aspects of home birth that cannot be transferred to hospital. Obvious examples include the stress of moving during labour, not being surrounded by their own environment and belonging, and the association of hospitals with sickness, dying and death.

Women hoped to reduce the likelihood of invasive interventions and routine practices such as vaginal examinations. They hoped to reduce the likelihood of being attended by strangers who may not appreciate their beliefs, hopes and concerns. They wanted to avoid feeling anxious, intimidated or embarrassed, and to avoid being separated from their babies and partners. The following quotations express some of their concerns about not being listened to, being separated from their partners, lack of privacy, or having things done to them and feeling disempowered. There was a sense from many of the women that in hospital they had been or would be captives of obstetric policies and practices and that any control would lie in the hands of those in the institution:

Just being afraid of surrendering myself to other people who might not know what's good for me actually. Also because I didn't feel they knew me very well or that they were in touch with my body. In hospital you're just one of a crowd.

And then it's – we've sent your husband home, you're going to have a long labour, it's going to be through the night, we're going to put the television off, put the lights off and we want you to lie down and try and get some sleep. And how am I going to sleep, you know? So he got sent home [said incredulously] and it wasn't until a few hours later I said, look, no, I'm not happy with this, you know, go and phone him, I want him back here. I think as well, at the time when she said to me, you have to rest, I thought, well, they're midwives and they deliver babies all the time. They know what they're talking about. And it wasn't until I'd lain there for an hour and tried to suffer these pains in the darkness and I thought, no. I don't want this. And then you think, oh, I don't want to be a burden. I don't want to be a pest to these nurses [midwives]. But then it's your birth – you want your birth to be the way you want it, you know.

The main thing is the lack of control and respect that I feel and the number of people you have to relate to over and over again – and say the same things. It's just so tiring when you feel – like I was really distressed and they're just not trained to address that part of what's going on at all.

I mean it's those things – noise and lack of privacy – and also that you become an object and people feel it's much more difficult to say no to things that you don't want. I get very disempowered around doctors generally, because they start treating my body as if it belonged to them instead of me. Or that's how I feel. I hate the idea of going into hospital for a birth.

Freedom from technology in hospitals I think is another reason.

Well, being strapped down you're not in control. I can't even remember if you were physically strapped at the birth. I think I was cos I think I'd have fallen out otherwise but I had a definite feeling of being strapped down. And if somebody's got you sitting in some seat that you can't get out of, then you have no control at all.

Women wanted to avoid practices which they felt could not support or respond to their individual and unique ways of giving birth. When they talked about their expectations of home birth they hoped to have control over decision-making, privacy, time, and personalized care from known attendants. They hoped to feel listened to, relaxed, free to respond to their own needs, confident, safe, uninhibited, comfortable and at ease. They hoped to avoid separation from their babies

and families, interventions, invasive practices and routines. They wanted to create a loving and nurturing environment for birth, get to know their babies, establish breastfeeding and enjoy the advantages of being at home after birth (cleanliness, good food, rest and quiet):

I felt that the care that there would be at home would be more personal and more concerned with me and that at home, people would be more willing to listen to my point of view.

I'll be so much more relaxed and comfortable in my own environment. I'll have my own things around me. I won't have to worry about making sure I've got all the things with me that I want to have and this'll be my house and I'll be much more in control than I would feel if I was in hospital. That's the main thing, that I'll be much more comfortable here. If I'm relaxed it's bound to all go better and also I think it will be much easier for me as a first time mother – never having looked after a young baby before – to start doing that in my own home rather than under scrutiny in hospital with all the other pressures that there would be in hospital. And it will be much easier for my partner to be the father to the baby if he doesn't get sent off home just after it arrives.

My home's a place I feel relaxed and I feel that I would be able to follow my instincts there. It's a space I've got control over. I've sat in the sitting room thinking, oh, yeh, I'll have the fire on and that candle that we've got. Someone gave us a beautiful candle, and we can move the sofa back and it'll be quite comfy, and it's like, I can actually see it happening in this room.

There's the environment – being at home with people that I care about and who care about me is very positive. Labour is quite an emotional time, or a trying time. It's a time when you need supportive people and an environment that you know and like – and that makes such a difference. I think it certainly makes a difference to my labour because I have freedom from limitations for – well, for all three stages really. Sometimes they limit time in hospitals. Limitations on freedom of movement – I'd be very unhappy, you know.

I like the idea that they're here all the time as opposed to in hospital where you're on your own, and you've got to press the buzzer and nobody might come for ages if they're busy. So I like

*the idea of having your own captive, personal midwife that is
there. I find that quite reassuring.*

Interestingly, what I have not found in the thirty years of supporting
women planning home births, is a woman who was not concerned
about safety or refused to transfer to hospital under any circumstances. Disagreements over this are to do with the reasons for transfer and who makes the final decision. However, while women are
often incorrectly accused of being more attached to the experience of
birth than to their babies, professionals are not usually accused of
being attached to their professional ideology.

For women, home birth was about protection and reclaiming connections. Protecting the integrity of the woman and her relationship
with her baby within the family. Protecting her autonomy and self
esteem. Connecting her to her baby, her body, her spirituality and sexuality, and integrating the baby into the family. Home was a metaphor
for control and connection and hospital a metaphor for loss of control and separation. Many women felt that the ideology, organization,
policies, rules and spatial arrangements in hospital left little room for
birth to be a sacred, powerful or creative act.[20] These ideas about protection and connection make possible very different constructions of
safety, supportive relationships and ethics that I discuss in Chapters 4,
5 and 6.

In essence, this book is about how women attempted to move
through their pregnancies from their own unique ethical stances,
with some degree of integrity, dignity and control. It is about the
paradox of women feeling obliged to familiarize themselves with
obstetric knowledge, while at the same time searching out other
knowledges and sources of information and support, in the hope
of balancing the realities of our culture with their personal ethics.
They often felt obliged to find compromises which were not too
far removed from their aspirations, beliefs and knowledges and
close enough to their midwives' practices not to threaten these
relationships.

This book is also about the impact of the often uneasy compromises
resulting in varying degrees of distress which affected the woman's
sense of herself and her ability to be autonomous, and her
relationships with her baby and partner. It suggests that when women
and midwives are able to be autonomous, women can grow, and midwives can develop their knowledge and skills to make birth safer while
at the same time enhancing women's self-esteem. The experiences of
the two women who were attended by independent midwives and the

seven women who transferred to hospital to give birth contributed to these ideas in ways that could only be imagined or glimpsed at by other women.

So while the women I interviewed hoped that home births could fulfil their hopes and ideals, they had some awareness about the underlying obstetric beliefs that might impose constraints on these ideals. This book is a discussion about why this is the case, why we need to know about the thinking behind obstetrics and how we might be able to move towards beliefs and practices about birth that are more closely aligned with women's and their families' needs.

Notes

1 See, for example, Green et al. 1998b; Jacoby and Cartwright 1990; S. Kitzinger 1992; Ogden et al. 1997a, 1997c; Simkin 1991, 1992; Waldenstrom 2004; Waldenstrom et al. 2004.

2 See, for example, Alexander 1987; Andrews 2004a, 2004b; Bastian 1993a, 1993b; Bortin et al. 1994; Caplan and Madeley 1985; Damstra-Wijmenga 1984; North West Surrey Community Health Council 1992; O'Connor 1992; Ogden et al. 1997a; Oswin 1993; Spurrett 1988; Viisainen 2000a.

3 See, for example, Alment et al. 1967; Campbell and Macfarlane 1994; O'Brien 1978; Wright 1992.

4 Research in these areas has been done by Bastian 1993a, 1993b; Caplan and Madeley 1985; Damstra-Wijmenga 1984; McLain 1987; Madi and Crow 2003; Claudia Martin, personal communication, 1995. Claudia Martin was the co-director of Scottish Health Feedback.

5 Andrews 2004a; Leyshon 2004; Sandall et al. 2001b; van der Hulst et al. 2004.

6 See, for example, Lemay 1997; O'Connor 1992; Ogden et al. 1997a, 1997b, 1997c; Oswin 1993; Searles 1981; Viisainen 2000a, 2000b, 2001.

7 Halldorsdottir and Karlsdottir 1996; van Olphen Fehr 1999.

8 Davis-Floyd 1992: 293.

9 Viisainen 2000a: 72–73.

10 Griffiths 1995.

11 Cronk 2000.

12 Robinson 1998.

13 Edwards 1996, 2001.

14 Madi and Crow 2003.

15 Fraser 1992a; Meyer 2000.

16 Banks 2000: 200.

17 Kirkham 2003; Saunders et al. 2000.

18 McCourt and Page 1997.

19 MacVicar et al. 1993.

20 Adams 1994; Rabuzzi 1994.

1 Home birth?
What's the problem?

What did the women say?

One of the issues I want to address in this book is that while home birth is apparently supported by government and local policies in the United Kingdom, it remains an ambiguous and contested site. This profoundly affects birthing women, many of whom are disturbed by the medicalized approach to birth and lack of alternative approaches but find it difficult to make their voices heard. Carrying out multiple, in-depth interviews with women planning home births seemed a good way of raising some of these voices. While I want to discuss why women planned home births, what they thought about safety, and how they experienced the home birth services in other chapters, in this chapter, I describe how individual women experience the cultural ambiguity and conflict about home birth and some of the contributing factors to this conflict.

All the women I interviewed for this book and all the women I talked to about their plans to have home births are deeply concerned about the safety of their babies and want to move through birth in ways that best protect their own and their babies' integrity. To think otherwise is insulting and hurtful to these women. Those involved in maternity services also want to protect women and babies and provide the best evidenced-based care they can. They also feel insulted and offended when challenged. And yet different responses to women's plans occur even when women live only a few miles from each other. For example, one woman was told by her local midwives that she could not have a home birth because she had left it too late and there were already two other women planning home births in the month her baby was due. When this did not put her off, she was told that she was making an inappropriate, irresponsible decision without knowing all the facts. When this still did not put her off she was told that her child might die and that she might bleed to death before help could arrive. Another woman talked to her midwife about who might attend the birth of her baby:

> *I was asking her how I'd know who was going to be coming. And she said, 'Well, I'm the only one who's got a four-wheel drive' (cos it's due in the middle of winter) 'so I'll probably pull the short straw'. And I just looked at her, and she said, 'Oh I shouldn't have said that should I?' And I was like, no way, you really shouldn't have said that. So, she's just obviously really nervous about it.*

Another woman explained:

> *I contacted the midwives and one of them came out to see me. That was my first **very** disappointing experience. I was **very** disappointed because prior to that I hadn't expected much. I hadn't expected much from my GP, but I thought, right, this is one of the community midwives. This is someone who could deliver my baby. These are the people that I need to speak to. This is my lifeline. And I knew from books that I was likely to be dissuaded as it was my first baby. And actually that's exactly what she did.*

Yet, nearby, a woman who assumed that her midwife would tell her that home birth is dangerous received a very different response. Her community midwife sensed the woman's unspoken ideals and actively contributed to the woman realizing these:

> *The home birth came, I think, through a combination of things. But it was suggested. I mean, I didn't demand it or anything.*
>
> *Nadine: Would you have thought about it?*
>
> *Oh I would have liked to have had it.*
>
> *Nadine: You would?*
>
> *Yeh, but the current thought was – and I mean I nearly fell into the trap, and in fact I did. I fell into the trap of thinking. First birth? At home? Far too dangerous. Far too risky, you know. The midwives where I lived previously wouldn't even let me have a domino [domiciliary in and out] so why would I ask for a*

home birth. And that's the reason I didn't. And that was a big mistake on my part.

Nadine: So what changed your mind about that? What made you think it wasn't so dangerous after all?

My midwife offered it to me, and as long as she was confident to do it – what I didn't want was to have a midwife who wasn't confident about me having it at home, who was grudging me having it at home. That would be also a very anxiety sort of building thing. So that also wasn't an alternative. I think I needed to have everything in place with everybody happy doing what they're doing.

Another woman was delighted with and describes the impact of the support she received from her community midwife for her two home births following a traumatic experience of an induced labour in hospital with her first baby:

I suppose we're just lucky here that our local midwife is so keen on home births and does put the option forward and say it's a good idea. I mean, if you met opposition from your midwife it would probably be very easy to just go with the flow and end up in hospital even though you did want a home birth. I mean, your first time choosing it, you're not a hundred per cent sure that it's the right thing to do. But, you know, getting such a positive attitude off the midwife is a big help in keeping you to your decision. We're just lucky here that she is so positive.

How can such different experiences be possible in a health-care system that espouses evidence-based care and apparently values individual rights and choices? Is it possible that our health-care system does not recognize the challenge of pursuing diverse aspirations that can be difficult to reconcile?

What do others say?

Marsden Wagner, paediatrician and former director of Women's and Children's Health, World Health Organization (WHO), remarked at the first International Home Birth Conference in October 1987 in London, that debates about home births often generate 'more heat than light'.

I had already become aware of this when I planned a home birth in the Scottish Borders in 1976. I knew babies could be born at home, but my general practitioner (GP) informed me that if I persisted in my wish to have my baby at home, he would strike me off his list. When I did persist, I was struck off, and he and his colleagues in the area met to discuss my plans. They decided not to accept me on to their lists or provide support. The chief area medical officer was more supportive and assigned a midwife to me. Although experienced, the midwife seemed nervous about supporting my plans when all the GPs in the area were opposed to these. She advised me to transfer to hospital during labour due to her own anxiety rather than any complications.

While I had a lot to learn about birth ideology, the structure of maternity services, the vested interests of those in control of services, the politics of birth, statistical research and women's rights, the conflict around home birth struck me as extraordinarily puzzling. Why was home birth supposedly an option with a community midwifery service in place to support it, when there was such opposition to women giving birth at home?

Since then I have had two home births, been a national point of contact for women considering or planning home births and have led antenatal and postnatal classes in Scotland since 1985. I have thus had the privilege of listening to the home birth stories of hundreds of women. These stories are frequently marked by conflict and confusion. Over many years I have heard stories of hurt, anger and desperation from women who felt committed to home births, but experienced lack of support, even hostility. I also hear stories of joy, power and appreciation towards midwives when somehow all worked out well at the end of the day.

I will explain the historical basis for this conflict in the next two chapters, but meanwhile a useful way of looking at this conflict is in terms of different ideologies.

Are there really different ideologies?

Anthropologists were among the first people to begin to write about the existence of different knowledges. Rather then define these as incoherent or deficient, their work accepted that knowledges have their own internal consistencies based on people's belief systems.[1] While studying birth in different cultures, anthropologist of midwifery, Brigitte Jordan (1993) found that there were different knowledges and belief systems about birth. At the same time, sociologists of scientific knowledge have shown that knowledge does not stand outside culture, but is shaped by the core beliefs and values of any given community or society.[2] But of course, what became more apparent was that while knowledges have their own internal consistencies, some take precedence and others are marginalized.[3] Brigitte Jordan coined the term 'authoritative knowledge' to describe a dominant knowledge system which undermines other legitimate knowledge systems. In terms of childbirth, while acknowledging that belief systems are not necessarily fixed, discrete entities,[4] Robbie Davis-Floyd (1992) makes a useful distinction between 'technocratic' and 'holistic' belief systems about birth. In the British context these are often referred to as the medical model, as opposed to midwifery, social or woman-centred approaches to birth. Charlene Spretnak's (1999) definition of an ideology could describe obstetric ideology in relation to other birth practices:

> An ideology is simply the elevation of a particular set of perceptions, assumptions, and analyses to a normative belief system. It provides a framework by which adherents respond to events and developments. An ideology also makes it difficult to see beyond the framework, however, so events reflecting other perspectives may seem nonsensical.[5]

This entrenches a cycle of dominance. For example, drawing on Ludwik Fleck's work Jo-Murphy-Lawless, suggests that so-called scientific knowledge 'appears to be systematic, proven applicable and evaluated to the knower because it has been generated within the framework', while other knowledges appear 'unproven, inapplicable, contradictory, even fanciful.[6] This means that authoritative knowledges, such as obstetrics, are relatively closed systems which, by definition, cannot easily appeal to other knowledges. Only major paradigm shifts tend to have any impact on them, though they might take on other knowledges, and adapt and incorporate them as their own.[7] On the whole, they develop their knowledge base according to their own assumptions and develop a ritualistic series of practices to reflect these.[8] They respond to unexpected occurrences, disasters or failures by intensifying these rituals.[9] Jo Murphy-Lawless (1998a) gives an example of the power of beliefs from Irish obstetric literature that describes the death of a woman following the use of forceps.[10] Rather than questioning the safety of forceps (which one might expect), the incident reinforced the obstetrician's belief that forceps are beneficial for women during birth.

Technocratic and social ideologies of birth

While knowledge systems are constantly renegotiated, there are a number of important distinctions between technocratic (i.e. mechanistic) and social models of birth including: their views about knowledge, safety, the birth process and relationships.[11]

Those who subscribe to and practise in a technocratic model tend to assume that they are experts and that their professional knowledge is superior to that of pregnant and birthing women. They thus assume the moral role of decision-making and expect women to acquiesce.[12] Birth is defined in industrial terms where the woman's body is likened to a machine, birth is likened to a mechanistic process and the baby becomes the product.[13] This technocratic perspective focuses on obtaining a live product by attempting to reduce the perceived riskiness and uncertainty of nature, women's bodies and birth. The Irish Model of Active Management exemplifies this approach in which safety means carrying out a series of routine interventions at specific times that have little to do with the needs of the individual woman and her baby.[14] The resulting narrow, short-term view of obstetrics obscures the social impact of birth, the transition to parenthood and the long-term well being of the family.[15]

Social, holistic midwifery approaches to birth tend to relate to the woman as a knowledgeable decision-maker in the context of her beliefs, lifestyle and concerns. Birth is seen as safe unless complications occur, so the midwife contributes to the woman's confidence but remains watchful of her and the baby's well-being. She draws on a range of midwifery knowledges and skills,[16] and turns to obstetric tools only if they are needed. Birth is seen as a complex interaction between mind, body and spirit and the body rhythms and processes are acknowledged and supported. These more holistic approaches rely on a trusting relationship between the woman and her midwife and take into account the long-term physical and emotional well-being of the woman and her baby as well as the well-being of the family as a whole.[17]

Whereas obstetric ideology sees birth as only normal in retrospect, and focuses on risk and fear, social models see birth as normal unless problems arise and focus on safety and confidence. Describing this difference, Canadian home birth midwife Celine Lemay (1997) suggested that while in obstetrics, 'la maison n'est pas un lieu securitaire pour un accouchement' (the home is not a safe place for birth), in social models, 'l'accouchement à la maison est un choix securitaire pour des femmes' (home birth is a safety choice for women).[18] Finnish sociologist Kirsi Viisainen (2000a) suggested that in medical ideology, risk resides in the pregnant and birthing body, but in alternative ideologies, it resides in medical ideology: 'According to the medical model, physicians seek to control the inherently risky pregnant body, while according to alternative models women seek to control the risks they are subjected to in the hospital environment'.[19]

Robbie Davis-Floyd (1992) suggests that these issues go beyond the immediate control of birth and that the purpose of a technological approach is to do with socialization and a simultaneous demonstration and inscribing of societal values that tell us how to live our lives and how to relate to others and our environment.[20] The oppressive influence of technology has been made visible by feminist explanations about patriarchal fears of nature and how women's bodies threaten to undermine patriarchal ideology unless they are carefully managed.[21] But feminists have also observed that natural philosophies of birth can be equally oppressive if they prevent women from valuing and accessing appropriate technologies, obscure women's experiences, or prevent women from exerting their own autonomy.[22]

I elaborate on these themes throughout the book, but the above goes some way to explaining why home birth might be a contested site and why it remains a marginalized activity. Women certainly experienced this and it is confirmed by the statistics on numbers of home births. Though this is changing in some geographical locations, in many parts of the Britain it remains between 1 and 2 per cent.

How many women have home births?

The annual number of births in Scotland has been slowly declining since 1971.[23] There are just over 50,000 births each year in a population of around 5 million. The home birth rate of less than 1 per cent in many areas has not changed significantly over recent years.[24] It appeared from the General Registrar Office Annual Reports from 1963 to 1997, that the decline of home birth was particularly sharp during the 1960s and 1970s, dropping from nearly 22 per cent in 1963, to just over 1 per cent in 1973 and stabilizing at around 0.5 per cent in 1980 where it remained until the 1990s. The only area that had a higher home birth rate was East Lothian, in south-east Scotland. A dedicated team of midwives provided a more accessible home birth and domino service and reported that 2.3 per cent of the women in its catchment area had home births. The rate has remained steady since then. Edinburgh and Fife also now have home birth rates of around 2 per cent. The Scottish inquiry, carried out in conjunction with the 1994 confidential inquiry into home births in England and Wales,[25] showed that in that year around 300 women had planned home births and a further 300 women had unplanned home births in

Scotland.[26] Unplanned home birth means that either the woman did not engage with maternity services, or that she planned to give birth in hospital but had her baby unexpectedly at home.

In fact, the number of planned home births has not always been recorded, or has been included with unplanned home births, as well as births that have happened on the way to hospital in cars or ambulances for example. These statistics are still not differentiated in Scotland. Because unplanned home births often include premature or precipitate births, they are associated with high mortality rates among babies. Amalgamating the statistics for planned and unplanned home births misled (or was used to mislead) people into thinking that all home births are dangerous.

A Scottish policy review of maternity services paid little attention to home birth.[27] It stated that there was little demand and anticipated a small rise to 1 per cent in the foreseeable future. The main discussion focused on domino births as the best option for healthy women and babies, though in many parts of Scotland these are not offered. Later reports do not address home birth, except to mention that women's choice on place of delivery should be respected if possible.[28]

In order to gain more of an overview of general attitudes and policies on home birth in Scotland, I carried out a postal survey in 1994 requesting information about any documentation regarding the provision of home birth.[29] Fourteen of the fifteen Health Boards responded. Less than half the responses were reasonably positive, others were non-committal or negative. Guidelines ranged from a 'commitment to ensuring women have a choice of where and in what manner they deliver their babies', and in some areas, midwives were expected to receive requests for home births in a 'professional and sympathetic manner'. A number of guidelines stated that women should be provided with information about place of birth, but only one region included a leaflet for women. At the opposite end of the spectrum, one health board claimed that home birth was considered to be 'foolhardy by medical and nursing [*sic*] staff' and another suggested that a woman might have to defend herself in court, if a child was injured during a home birth. While information has been updated and is generally more positive, there remains a cultural ambivalence towards home birth. Even in 2004, a negative and misleading leaflet about home birth was being given to women in an area of central Scotland. When I pointed this out to a senior midwife there, she immediately withdrew it and replaced it with a more positive one, containing accurate, research-based information.

In England, while the home birth rate is around 2 per cent, there are significant geographical variations.[30] In 1998, 47 per cent of services had home birth rates of over 2 per cent.[31] In Torbay 23 per cent of women expecting normal births had their babies at home.[32] Higher home birth rates depend on midwife managers and community midwives actively supporting the idea of healthy women having their babies at home. When this happens the numbers of women from all backgrounds having home births increases.[33] There is an intention to increase the home birth rate to 10 per cent in Wales by 2007.[34]

Even in the current hospital-based birth culture, where most woman have not experienced home birth, somewhere between 8 and 22 per cent of women in Britain would consider home births.[35]

On the surface, home birth is a legitimate option, yet the low home birth rates suggest that there is a deep ambivalence towards it in many parts of Britain. However, the fact that home births increase when they are supported challenges the assumption that only a small number of 'elite' women want home births.[36] This is simply not borne out by the evidence – it is only the case when home birth is a difficult option to choose.

Home birth is a marginalized activity

At the beginning of the twentieth century only 1 per cent of women in Britain gave birth in institutions. But by the 1980s only 1 per cent gave birth at home.[37] The change was rapid and decisive and the women I interviewed certainly experienced planning a home birth as a marginalized activity:

> *Your whole life is spent being told that you have babies in hospital and that just seems to be the thing that you just presume. So I suppose a lot of women don't even consider having a home birth, just because it seems the norm to have them in hospital. It's what always seems to have been recommended and what the experts think you should do, or so-called experts think you should do.*

If for any reason this has not been internalized, societal norms quickly become apparent:

> *I think I've been quite surprised that other people have been so surprised. Like people at work have been so surprised that I'm having a home birth. Really, as if they've never heard of anybody ever having a home birth before, which I didn't realize it was so unusual.*

Women were aware of the cultural, geographical and historical specificity of obstetric ideology and how this might influence home birth, and those who plan it. For example, in many parts of the world birth at home is the only option available for most women. In some cultures it may be an acceptable alternative to hospital birth:

> *I'm just trying to keep the emotional temperatures around as low as possible. I don't know, I guess I'm just young and rebellious still. If I were a bit older then maybe I wouldn't feel so much that I had to prove a point. In my own country, certainly I wouldn't feel that way, because I mean, my mother's now married to a man, and his daughter had her baby at home and it was a very relaxed affair and no one batted an eyelid apparently. But, you know, it's the usual thing there – and just a very sort of matter of fact approach to birth, whereas here, I do feel it's quite dramatic.*

In others parts of the world, home birth is even more marginalized than it is in Scotland. A non-European women commented:

> *I mean, in Europe in general I think there's more an acceptance of home birth, or it's not so alien to have one. I mean, in my country there would have been no question of not going into hospital really. I mean, if I'd moved back and I said I wanted a home birth, they would probably have looked at me as though I was crazy or it would have been so hard to organize, you know, because, there's also this problem of who takes responsibility and malpractice suits and who's responsible for what. I mean, it would have been really hard. Midwives aren't trained to the extent they are here, and the doctor takes centre stage. And probably a doctor is too busy to come out to your home, so that the whole routine, the whole concept of what happens when you have a baby, just makes home births almost impossible. So I'm glad I'm here.*

But the women I interviewed were left in no doubt that in planning to have babies at home they were transgressing usual cultural norms. There was a general consensus that information about home birth and its availability was not 'handed on a plate' and that they had to search it out for themselves. Nearly all the women commented that a significant improvement in maternity services would be to provide women with the option of a home birth. But women attending the Birth Resource Centre pregnancy classes in Edinburgh, for example, continue to comment that they are not given information about the availability of home birth.

Home birth is not the only site of struggle

The current struggle and ambivalence about birth practices is reflected in maternity services overall. While many areas continue to centralize services in large obstetric units, others have retained or are opening small midwifery units, community hospitals or birth centres. Uneasy compromises include midwifery-run units situated alongside obstetric labour wards where midwives have limited autonomy, and small units where access criteria are kept unnecessarily strict. These units struggle to gain cultural acceptance and are continually under threat of closure.[38] The configuration of services remains in a state of flux.

During the 1990s in Scotland, many services were centralized and some of the smaller obstetric units catering for two thousand births or fewer per year, along with some of the community units closed. Many of these closures met with fierce opposition,[39] and occasionally campaigns against small unit closures have been successful.[40] Recently, a small number of community units have been opened or transformed in rural areas to provide services for women who would otherwise have to travel up to a hundred miles to have their babies in large obstetric units. These are usually in areas where midwives and sometimes doctors are committed to providing a service, or where there was a history of a small unit and a strong enough community voice to argue for its retention.[41] A few of the Scottish islands have small units with one or two maternity beds, but obstetrics' focus on risk led to fewer births and a reduction in skills and confidence, resulting in women on the islands and parts of the Highlands flying to their nearest obstetric unit at the thirty-eighth week of their pregnancies to await their labours. There are currently eighteen obstetric and twenty-four community units, with plans to close more of the smaller obstetric units.

Home birth services

While services vary, the first point of contact for maternity services in Scotland is often the woman's GP, even though a woman is entitled to book directly with a midwife, who can provide all her maternity care. The midwife practises by a set of rules and standards;[42] while she may advise the woman to see an obstetrician in certain circumstances, the woman can accept or reject this advice.[43] Some women planning home births contact their community midwives, but are asked to see their GPs 'out of courtesy'. Women are often unaware that GPs receive payment for antenatal and postnatal care and are thus reluctant to relinquish their interests in birth. But women need not see a GP for pregnancy-related care and it can be counterproductive if the GP is negative about home births. However, there are a small number of GPs who genuinely support birth in the community, and are often members of the Association for Community-Based Maternity Care.

Each of the fifteen health board regions in Scotland has its own guidelines and arrangements for providing a home birth service, organized and supervised by the senior midwives in the region and run by teams of community midwives. These teams vary from two or three midwives to over thirty. National Health Service (NHS) case-load midwifery, and one-to-one schemes that run elsewhere,[44] are not generally available in Scotland. Until recently, midwifery services were not always available in rural areas and midwives in these areas were often employed as the area nurse and/or health visitor so that their workload was taken up with nursing duties.

Regions are further divided, each area with its own interpretations of regional guidelines. This could depend on local resources, the views of senior midwives and obstetricians, and the beliefs, skills and commitment of individual practitioners providing the service.

Most of the woman I interviewed booked with teams of between six and eight NHS community midwives, and a few women had small teams of up to three midwives. (These teams are now larger, with up to twenty midwives per team.) The idea was for women to see a different team midwife at each antenatal appointment, so that she could meet each of the midwives on at least one occasion before giving birth. Most women found that this was variable in practice. For example, one woman saw the same midwife for her first five antenatal appointments and had not met at least two of her team midwives in very late pregnancy.

Independent midwifery services

The term 'independent midwife' usually applies to the few midwives in Britain who are self-employed and offer themselves for service to individual women. These midwives usually provide a one-to-one service, subscribe to a holistic midwifery approach to birth and are members of the Independent Midwives Association. While their training, rules, code of conduct, supervision and disciplinary body are the same as that of any other midwife, they are not bound by the policies and practices of individual NHS hospitals. They are therefore more able to rely on their own clinical judgement. They practise single-handedly, or with one or two other midwives, and are usually only able to offer a home birth service. Some had honorary contracts with hospitals and offered a domino service, but these contracts are now rarely given. This means that if a woman booked with them requires medical services, independent midwives can accompany her to hospital only as friends – a situation that many women and independent midwives find unnacceptable. NHS midwives occasionally practise independently in addition to their NHS work and in these circumstances usually make individual arrangements with women and their local supervisors of midwives. In some countries midwives combine independent work with part-time hospital work for financial reasons. This is the case for nearly all the home birth midwives in southern Norway, whom I met in Oslo in 2000, and some German midwives.[45]

While there are currently over seventy independent midwives in Britain, there have been few in Scotland over the last decades. One midwife practised independently from 1960 to 1999 in northern Scotland and two practised in Lothian in the early 1990s but stopped when insurance problems arose. The Scottish Independent Midwives (SIMS) group was formed in 1994 and has continued to campaign for small autonomous groups of midwives to provide services within the NHS.

Since the mid-1990s a small number of midwives has continued to practise independently in parts of southern and central Scotland. The experiences of the two women in the study of their independent midwives' ideologies and practices brought the issue of conflicting ideologies and its impact on women and midwives into sharp relief. However, the similarities and differences between NHS community and independent midwifery blurred any discrete boundary and it was the individual contacts between women and practitioners that were instrumental in shaping women's experiences of planning and having home births.

First points of contact or conflict?

With doctors

All the women I interviewed saw a GP and most were unaware that they could book directly with midwives. While some GPs simply referred women to community midwives with little comment, only one GP responded positively to the idea of home birth. Some women reported that they had wanted a home birth previously, but had been put off by a GP's negative response. Some women experienced negative attitudes but continued to plan home births:

> *I felt I needed support, so when my first child was expected I read and I went to my GP. But I wasn't involved with any other pregnant women and certainly no one that was contemplating a home birth. So when my GP said that they didn't do home births for first babies I really saw no other option. So I did raise it with the GP, the possibility was rejected and I didn't pursue it. In my second pregnancy I raised the possibility again. It was a different GP and he suggested that it wasn't possible. I just ignored him and called the community midwives and booked with them. By that time I was involved with people who as well as knowing were also supportive.*

> *I didn't know that you could go straight to the midwives and bypass the GP altogether. I thought that I would have to do it through my GP. And I was new to the practice anyway so home birth was just one of the things I asked about. And I got this five minute lecture about how irresponsible I was. I was really shocked by the GP's response. When I went to the practice I'd asked for a young woman who I could see in the mistaken belief that she'd be more sympathetic. I found it really upsetting at the time. I hate it when people rant and rave at me and also tell me that I'm being incredibly irresponsible. She was fairly heavy handed about it.*

In line with the evidence showing that obstetricians' approach may be harmful to healthy women and babies,[46] they tend to be less involved with women planning home births, unless complications occur. Many women are nevertheless encouraged to see one during pregnancy. While some were non-committal, from time to time, experienced obstetricians were more supportive of home birth than midwives. Occasionally women described negative, patronizing attitudes:

> *I went in to hospital and saw the same doctor that I saw when I was pregnant with my first child and he said exactly the same thing to me that he said the first time round. His classic statement when you say you wish to have a home birth is 'if you were my daughter or my wife I wouldn't let you do it'.*

> *I found him very insulting in his approach. He directly said I was being foolish. And when I went to hospital the second time, that*

was how he referred to me – three or four times in the conversation – 'I think you're being very foolish'. And he implied that I didn't care about the safety of my baby. 'I don't know where you get your research from but if I thought home births were safe then I'd be advocating them.' And he just gave me no credit for being an intelligent woman. He didn't give me credit for having read in the field or for the fact that it's me that's having the baby and of course the baby's safety is paramount to me.

As one woman explained, this kind of response is unhelpful. It fails to acknowledge that people make decisions from their own unique, ethical standpoints and that parents do not as a rule 'willingly risk the lives of their children'.

With midwives

Women often felt both anxious and hopeful before meeting their midwives for the first time. Given the marginalization of home birth, they felt that these first meetings would be a gauge for how supportive they could expect midwives to be and how likely it was that their plans for a home birth would materialize.

The women hoped for enthusiasm and support for their plans. But realistically, because of their own or other's experiences, they were unsurprised (but still disappointed) if this was not the case. Many women expected a 'fight', thus if the midwife was not actively against home birth, they were often pleasantly surprised. In other words, many women have low expectations of others when engaging in marginalized activities, so that any response which is not overtly hostile is a relief.

The women quickly realized that their community midwives were caught between different ideologies. While their regulating body tells them to support women,[47] their employers instruct them to work within local policies.[48] Local policies are usually obstetrically dominated and often prevent midwives from being enthusiastic about home birth. Instead, midwives are expected to begin the process of steering women through pregnancy and birth in accordance with these policies. They appeared to be required to tell women about the risks of home birth, (but not the advantages of home birth or the risks associated with hospital birth), and to ensure that women understand that they are responsible for their decisions to have home births:

She said she had to tell me about the dangers. Well, maybe that's not the exact expression she used. But, you know, what the problems may be should they arise. She said, 'I have to tell you this, just to let you know. It's in my job description and if I don't tell you, I'll be breaking my contract'

She was pointing out the dangerous side of it [home birth] and I was getting into a sort of argument with her. But then again, you see, I think she was just doing her job.

Having complied with their policies, midwives often then qualified what they had said, by reassuring women that they had not had problems in the past, and by being more positive about home birth. But women also made judgements about which midwives were supportive of home birth despite spelling out the risks and responsibilities and which midwives were less confident about home birth and were conveying their own fears through initial discussions about risk. While the policies and practices within which midwives work may be no more in accordance with their beliefs about birth than they are for the women, they may feel unable to question these.[49] Whatever they thought, most women experienced a combination of caution and support, which many described as positive, but which some experienced as 'lukewarm' or unsupportive.

The initial focus on risk criteria and women's responsibility reminded women that home birth is not an easy option and that because of the constraints they practice in, midwives may not be able to give them the support they needed. Some women began to feel distanced rather than engaged with midwives. As I discuss in Chapter 5, this is a problem, as women usually make decisions in the context of relationships rather than in isolation.

What does research tell us?

The lack of support for home birth does not reflect research findings on place of birth. Even within a medical research framework, the results of home births cited in medical and midwifery publications over many years shows that it is safe and holds a number of advantages for women and babies. Research initially focused on mortality rates of women and babies, but as maternal mortality rates declined, it looked at mortality and morbidity among babies, and morbidity in women. The consensus seems to be that home birth attended by skilled practitioners is safe for healthy women and babies in Britain and elsewhere.[50] Its advantages include women and babies receiving fewer interventions, including caesarean sections and women retaining more control over the birth process, and experiencing greater satisfaction.[51] Where problems have occurred it is usually when births at home are unplanned and without skilled attendants.[52]

Definitive findings within the scientific framework are difficult to achieve because it has been estimated that even if a randomized controlled trial (RCT) included 700,000 women at low risk of complications, only moderately reliable conclusions about perinatal mortality rates could be expected.[53] However, the Cochrane Review, which evaluates research considered to be of a high standard, concludes that home birth is safe.[54] Of course additional problems include that the RCT is often considered to be definitive by virtue of being an RCT rather than because it provides good research,[55] and that it is always the appropriate method for the topic under scrutiny. Helen Stapleton and Mavis Kirkham's (2004) qualitative research alongside an RCT raised searching questions about what can usefully be the subject of an RCT and what an RCT alone can tell us. The current practice of combining the results of RCTs (meta-analysis) has also been criticized.[56] Furthermore, RCTs cannot take individual circumstances into consideration, nor can they tell us how the individual will respond to a particular treatment or practice. Ann Oakley (2000) suggests caution rather than dogma and dialoguing rather than dichotomizing between quantitative and qualitative methods of research.

There is also some disagreement within feminism generally about how far the tools of patriarchy can disrupt and reconstruct oppression.[57] One of the difficulties when using the logic of a medicalized belief system to challenge it is that the economy is still one of flawed rationalism and any research is always created and measured against what is already dominant. Any challenge is therefore limited, and is likely to 'stretch' rather than change dominant beliefs. Women's concerns are still omitted and we can end up falling back on rather sterile arguments. For example, using statistics to argue the safety of home birth, does not address substantive issues of safety that women identified and that I discuss in Chapter 4. Clearly we cannot step outside our cultural heritages, yet feminism and postmodernism have contributed to seeing our culture differently with a view to changing ideological and societal norms and practices. The difficulty is that using the research tools of the dominant social group tends to contain and limit debate. It may protect deeply coercive beliefs and focus research on its concerns rather than those of others. In the case of birth, the dominant tools have questioned the belief that birth is safer in hospital, but have failed to develop understanding about women's concerns and experiences. For example, the onus is often on so-called subjugated groups and individuals to produce convincing evidence with which to challenge dominant views.[58] In terms of birth practices, Shelley Romalis (1985) points out: 'it is clear that there is an unequal burden of proof on any approach that diverges from conventional medicine'.[59] There is less onus on dominant ideology to justify or probe its own central tenets or ethics and if we are unable to shift the burden of proof, we risk focusing only on women.[60] In other words, focusing on the subjugated may leave dominant ideologies untouched.

Ironically while research supporting home birth has grown in both quantity and quality, home birth itself might currently be less of an option than it was, due to a recent reinterpretation of the legal status of community services and whether or not these are optional.[61]

Home birth under threat

The conversations I had with the women I interviewed were based on a shared assumption that home birth was protected in law through the provision of the community midwifery services.

When I embarked on this project, I assumed that the woman's right to have a home birth and be provided with care during pregnancy, labour and postnatally by a qualified NHS midwife was enshrined in law throughout Great Britain. This assumption was held by the women, those providing maternity services, and those providing information for parents about maternity services. Most information on women's rights and midwives' duties regarding home birth for parents reflects this belief.[62]

It has been generally believed that it is the duty of the most senior midwife in any geographical area to make adequate provision for women planning and having home births, so that there is always a midwife available to respond to calls from the community. If a midwife is called, whether or not the woman is officially booked for a home birth, it is her duty to attend the woman, whatever the woman's circumstances or health status.[63] Further, it was understood that the midwife would have support from both midwifery and medical services and that if she deemed it necessary, she could summon medical assistance. In practice, most midwives suggest that the woman transfer to hospital if medical help is needed.

These rights and duties were closely linked to the professionalization of midwifery during the early part of the twentieth century. Midwifery training was put in place and it became illegal for anyone other than an officially trained midwife (or medical practitioner) to attend births. Legislation outlawed the empirically trained 'handywomen' or 'bona fide' midwives, and made provision for all women to receive care at home from midwives with a recognized training. While there has never been any legal requirement for the woman to engage with maternity services, the oppressive regulation of birth is apparent in the publicized case of Brian Radley, a father who was fined £1000 for attending the birth of his own baby at home without assistance.[64] Indeed, Article 43(3) of a government (draft) order (2001) for the establishment of the new Nursing and Midwifery Council increased this sum to £5000. Due to the activities of the Association for Improvements in the Maternity Services (AIMS), however, it has now been established that this ruling should not be applied to family and friends who provide support to the woman during birth.[65]

The notion that there may not be a 'duty of care', or indeed any requirement to provide community services, was raised in an editorial in a widely read British midwifery journal.[66] This was taken up by the Midwifery Committee of the United Kingdom Central Council for Nursing, Midwifery and Health Visiting (UKCC) and legal opinions sought.[67] Apparently, since the National Health Service Act of 1977, when the term 'domiciliary' was omitted,[68] there has been a mistaken assumption that women have the right to the services of a midwife during labour outwith the hospital setting. This was communicated to voluntary childbirth organizations at a meeting convened by the UKCC in December 1999. Meanwhile, some NHS Trusts began to withdraw their domiciliary services. Both lay and midwifery organizations campaigned for home birth provision to be made mandatory again.[69] Although the Department of Health stated that it expected women's requests for home births to be supported,[70] it remained unclear how this could be enforced. Subsequent correspondence to AIMS demonstrated that opinion at government level is divided on this issue. Similar correspondence to a woman in England from the Department of Health highlighted a theme running through this book, that although choices are said to be available, there are few mechanisms to support them. This leaves the untenable anomaly that a woman has the right to have her baby at home but could be refused the services of a midwife. AIMS now receives calls most days from distressed women in late pregnancy who have been informed that resources are no longer available for their planned home births.[71] The NMC Midwifery Committee is currently seeking to remedy this situation.

As I explain in Chapter 6, although women are ambivalent about appealing to rights, the right to home birth supported by community midwifery services provides a degree of support and protection. It makes home birth more of a real possibility. Given the marginalization of home birth, the impact of placing more obstacles in its way can only be detrimental to women and midwives. On a number of occasions it was the midwives providing the service who facilitated home births by offering the service to women who had accepted that it was not possible, or supporting the growing confidence of those who initially booked for domino births. If community services are withdrawn this will no longer be possible.

Moving through pregnancy and birth is a challenging journey for women. For those committed to home birth, it could be all the more challenging. Women would be forced to weigh up complex moral responsibilities and obligations in a society that is unsupportive of home birth and all too ready to blame women who challenge its norms.

Home births without midwives

Some women will choose to have their babies at home despite the climate of opinion, and lack of legal or practical support. In Marie O'Connor's (1992) study, for example, one in nine women had their babies with the support of partners and friends, without the help of a midwife or doctor, in parts of Ireland where there was no provision for home birth. In North America, where midwives have all but disappeared, a small percentage of women continue to be attended by empirically rather than formally trained 'direct entry' or 'granny' midwives.[72] There is also a small but growing number of women who decide to give birth alone or with partners, often called unassisted birth.[73] This occasionally happens in Britain too.[74] Despite powerful attempts on the part of obstetrics in most western countries, it has proved impossible to erase home birth altogether. And even where medicine is powerful, politicians are reticent about enforcing hospitalization.[75]

Though some considered unassisted birth, none of the thirty women I interviewed chose to give birth without calling a midwife. The reasons they gave for considering this were to do with avoiding the particular services on offer (that they experienced as impersonal and over-medicalized) rather than wanting to give birth without the support of midwives.

So this book is about the importance of the availability of a home birth service that meets the needs of women planning home births. It explains why providing this service is difficult, because of the different beliefs about birth. It suggests that divergences between women and practitioners about what is best for them and their babies is about differences in ideology and who should have ultimate responsibility for decision-making. It explains that women's plans around birth are based on ethical concerns rather than choice and that focusing on choice without dismantling the powerful beliefs on which these rest is unlikely to be effective or helpful to women.[76]

Women and midwives are struggling to identify and voice their ethics in an increasingly complex postindustrial and sophisticated patriarchal society.[77] The short-term concerns of a market economy threaten to thwart any possibility of change, and obstetric (and increasingly, paediatric) authority continues to assert its priorities over women's moral and ethical considerations. Despite the rhetoric of choice and an apparent acceptance of the advantages of community-based care, the combined political and medical will is pushing towards standardization of services based on centralization and medicalization. The women in this study provide a profoundly thought-provoking challenge to the knowledge and rationality on which this trend is based.

Notes

1 Clifford and Marcus 1986.
2 Kuhn 1970; see also Davis-Floyd 1992.
3 Jordan 1997.
4 Davis-Floyd and Dumit 1997; Davis-Floyd and St John 1998.
5 Spretnak 1999: 12.
6 Murphy-Lawless 1998a: 256.
7 Kuhn 1970; Saks 1992: 198.
8 Davis-Floyd 1992; Murphy-Lawless 1998a.
9 Davis-Floyd 1992.
10 Murphy-Lawless 1998a: 151.
11 Davis-Floyd 1992; Schmid 2003.
12 Davis-Floyd 1992; Jordan 1997; Shildrick 1997.
13 Davis-Floyd 1992; Martin 1987, 1990.
14 O'Driscoll et al. 1993.
15 Kennedy and Murphy-Lawless 1998.
16 Davis-Floyd and Davis 1997; Roncalli 1997; Smythe 1998.
17 Lane 1993, 1995; Lemay 1997; Smythe 1998.
18 Lemay 1997: 81.
19 Viisainen 2000a: 51.
20 Davis-Floyd 1992; see also Spretnak 1999; Starhawk 1990.
21 Murphy-Lawless 1998a; Shildrick 1997.
22 Bourgeault et al. 2004; Cosslett 1994; Diprose 1994.
23 Expert Working Group on Acute Maternity Services 2003; Health Policy and Public Health Directorate 1993.

24 For recent figures for England, Wales and Scotland, see www.Birth ChoiceUK.com.
25 Chamberlain et al. 1997.
26 Tricia Murphy-Black, personal communication, 1995. Tricia Murphy-Black is Professor of Midwifery at the University of Stirling.
27 Health Policy and Public Health Directorate 1993.
28 Expert Working Group on Acute Maternity Services 2003.
29 Edwards 1994.
30 See www.BirthChoiceUK.com.
31 English National Board for Nursing, Midwifery and Health Visiting (ENB) 1999: 17.
32 National Childbirth Trust (NCT) 1999.
33 Leyshon 2004; National Childbirth Trust 1999; Sandall et al. 2001b.
34 Welsh Assembly 2002.
35 Department of Health (DoH) 1993; Scottish Health Feedback 1993.
36 Sbisa 1996: 366.
37 Campbell and Macfarlane 1994.
38 Kirkham 2003.
39 See, for example, McLaren 1990.
40 Jones 1991; Nicoll, 2004.
41 Leatherbarrow et al. 2004.
42 Nursing and Midwifery Council (NMC) 2004.
43 Beech 2003.
44 McCourt and Page 1997; Sandall et al. 2001b.
45 Sandall et al. 2001a: 127.
46 Enkin et al. 1989.
47 Nursing and Midwifery Council 2002.
48 Clarke 1995; Edwards 2004a, 2004b.
49 Kirkham 1999b, 2004; Stapleton et al. 1998.
50 For Britain, see, for example, Campbell and Macfarlane 1994; Chamberlain et al. 1997; Davies et al. 1996; Ford et al. 1991; Northern Regional Perinatal Mortality Survey Coordinating Group 1996; Shearer 1985; Tew 1985, 1998. For other countries, see Ackermann-Liebrich et al. 1996; Anderson and Murphy 1995; Crotty et al. 1990; Durrand 1992; Eskes and van Alten 1994; Gaskin 2003; Howe 1988; Mehl et al. 1976; Olsen 1997; Schlenzka 1999; Tew and Damstra-Wijmenga 1991; Treffers and Laan 1986; Tyson 1991; van Alten et al. 1989; Wayne et al. 1987; Wiegers et al. 1996; Woodcock et al. 1994.
51 Chamberlain et al. 1997; National Institute for Clinical Excellence (NICE) at www.nice.org.uk/pdf/CG013NICEguideline.pdf; Olsen and Jewell 2001; van der Hulst et al. 2004.
52 Burnett et al. 1980; Haloob and Thein 1992; Murphy et al. 1984.
53 Ford et al. 1991.
54 Olsen and Jewell 2001.
55 Gyte 1994; Johnson 1997; Shipman 1988.
56 Gyte 1994; Macfarlane 1997; Olsen 1997.
57 Friedman 2000; Lorde 1984.
58 Hooks 1990.
59 Romalis 1985: 198–199.
60 Alldred 1998; Spivak, in Diprose 1994: 23; Stanko 1994.

61 Rosser 1998.
62 Beech 1991: 43–45; Health Education Board for Scotland 1998: 48; Thomas 1998: 4–5; Wesson 1990: 52.
63 Rosser 1998.
64 Donnison 1988: 195–196; Robinson 1982.
65 Beech 2003: 41.
66 Rosser 1998.
67 United Kingdom Central Council for Nursing, Midwifery and Health Visiting (UKCC) 2001: 3.
68 Rosser 1998.
69 See, for example, Beech 2001.
70 Cooper 2000.
71 For information on how to respond to this see Beech 2003: 35, or www.aims.org.uk.
72 For interesting explanations and accounts of these midwives, see Benoit et al. 2001; Bourgeault et al. 2004; Chester 1997; Gaskin 1990; Rooks 1997.
73 Shanley 1994.
74 Sumpter 2001.
75 Wagner 1994: 327.
76 Edwards 2004c.
77 Thompson 2004.

2 What do we know?
What does she know?
Can anyone know anything?

> To a stunning extent, the interests of one half of the human race have
> not been thought about through history: men have not thought about
> them and women have been kept in ignorance . . . If we adopt uncrit-
> ically the framework, the tools, the scholarship created overwhelm-
> ingly by and for men, we have already excluded ourselves . . . We are
> being forced to try to discover new intellectual constructs because
> many of those we have don't fit our experience and were never
> intended to.
>
> Elizabeth Minnich[1]

How can we talk about women's experiences?

Beginning the journey

Readers who are interested only in home births may wonder why they
need to know anything about feminism and postmodernism. Some
researchers also question why we need to get embroiled in high-falutin'
theoretical discussions and criticize those who fly off into realms of
apparently incomprehensible philosophical jargon.[2] Why not get on
with the women's stories? Do they not speak for themselves? Are they
not self-explanatory? Well, yes and no. We can read any number of
home birth stories. Some of them tell us about oppression, some about
empowerment and some about triumphs over adversity, but few
explain the marginalization of home birth and what these struggles and
triumphs are all about. It is only by creating a close dialogue between
women's experiences and what theorists have discovered that we can
tell more confident stories about stories that help us understand what
these are all about and why they matter so much. I have introduced
some of the main themes of the women's stories and now I introduce
some of the main themes of the philosophical ideas I used.

My priorities were threefold: to develop a theoretical framework that would enable women to recount their experiences in their own words (in so far as words are our own), to enable me to understand both the similarities and differences between their experiences, and to retain a politically liberatory stance. This chapter explains how I did this.

This book is about women's journeys through the transformation of childbearing. It is also about my journey through the transformation of feminism and postmodernism.[3] These parallel journeys create different meanings of birth by posing searching questions about the assumptions we often make about knowledge. But if I and the women wanted to question an entire body of knowledge, we needed to know why we were doing this. If we wanted to create knowledge based on other assumptions we needed to know what these were and how different knowledges come about. The reader also needs to be able to follow our journeys in order to place herself or himself within these dialogues.[4]

Scratching the surface

Having done the usual literature searches using systematic reviews and electronic databases such as Medline, BIDS (Bath Information and Data Service) and local library systems,[5] I searched the Index Medicus and MIDIRS (Midwives Information and Resource Service). I followed up references from the material I gathered. I even carried out a broader search, amassing anything and everything to do with home birth – past and present, here and elsewhere. I studied parliamentary and Health Department documents for England and Wales, and Scotland from 1904 to 1994, which had anything to say about place of birth.[6] Overall these promoted medicalization, hospitalization and finally centralization of birth, progressively phasing out domiciliary care until the apparent sea change in 1992 in the Winterton Report.[7] This focused on demedicalization, decentralization, greater use of midwifery, and support for women's choices, including that of home birth.

I considered the apparently anomalous situation in the Netherlands, where the home birth rate has been consistently higher than in other westernized countries, remaining at 25–30 per cent from the early 1990s until the present time,[8] and attempted to gain some understanding about this. I concluded that although birth is perceived as normal, and that midwifery is indeed a strong profession in the Netherlands, home birth has been retained largely because of supportive state legislation rather than because birth ideology is significantly different there. Strict medical risk criteria and identifying abnormality are as central to birth ideology in the Netherlands as they are in the United Kingdom.[9] This view was confirmed by the talks given by Dutch midwives in the Netherlands at the Fourth International Home Birth Conference in Amsterdam, in March 2000. There was a sense that home birth is hanging in the balance in the Netherlands. Debates about the medicalization of birth and cost implications are increasingly similar to those in the United Kingdom, technological interventions are increasing and there was a shortage of midwives that is currently being addressed. Differences around pain perception which have contributed to home birth remaining an option are slowly changing, as a Dutch newspaper article, entitled 'Pain or prick', demonstrated.[10] A recent sociological study of birth in the Netherlands suggests that home birth is perhaps more secure than it was and that the Dutch approach to political decision–making through involving the community makes it unlikely that midwifery or home birth could be quickly or easily undermined (De Vries 2004).

I acquainted myself with the contrasting situation in North America, where midwives all but disappeared and home births are relatively rare.[11] This suggested that the change in place of birth was closely linked to the change in attendants and their ideology at birth. I searched the literature for historical accounts and commentaries about the development of obstetrics, and the simultaneous suppression of midwifery practice. Beneath the surface, a host of gender issues vied for attention. Feminism beckoned.

I considered not only home/midwife birth and hospital/medical birth, but also the possibilities of home-like births in hospital,[12] and hospital-like births at home.[13] I examined literature about freestanding birth centres in England and elsewhere in Europe,[14] and in North America.[15] This challenged sharp distinctions between home and hospital birth and questioned the natural/technological dichotomy.[16] This time, scratching the surface brought to light the issues of uncertainty and diversity central to postmodernism. I could not ignore its call.

Moving towards feminism

I was well aware of criticisms of the hospitalization and medicalization of birth. I was after all one of its critics. I could see that maternity services were less based on women's needs than on those of obstetrics. But this was based on experiential knowledge and a basic understanding that patriarchy was implicated in the development of obstetrics – particularly clear in Jean Donnison's (1988) meticulous documentation of the demise of female midwifery and the rise of male obstetrics. Journeying through the different facets of feminism provided the insight that ideological, structural and material arrangements in all areas of life, including birth, are consistently and thoroughly saturated by patriarchy in its many different guises.[17]

I was deeply impressed by some of the phenomenological studies I read.[18] Phenomenology pays a great deal of attention to the detail of people's lives as they live them in their bodies, through time and place and in relation to others.[19] I was particularly impressed by the understanding, sensitivity and respect shown to women and their experiences of birth and motherhood by Vangie Bergum (1989) in her critical study on the transformation from woman to mother and by Juliana van Olphen Fehr (1999) in her study on the caring relationship between women and midwives.

Given the embodied nature of pregnancy and birth, I was also drawn to one of the central tenets of existential phenomenology, that of 'locating consciousness and subjectivity in the body itself'.[20] In other words we need to acknowledge that our bodies are sensitive and integral to our experiences of being who we are, rather than separate, unfeeling attachments. Iris Marion Young's (1990a, 1990b) inclusion of women's bodies in her accounts alerted me to the disappearance of or ambivalence about women's bodies in the accounts of many postmodern feminists. We cannot hope to talk about women's experiences of childbearing without focusing on the embodied realities of those experiences. Any ambivalence about women's bodies constitutes a disservice to women. The trouble was that while I could see that phenomenology and other critical approaches could be useful,[21] I realized that they were not quite sensitive enough to women's experiences and bodies and had a tendency to refer to 'human' when in fact the human involved was decidedly male.[22] Because obstetrics is a manifestation of patriarchal values, it is in a position of control over women and their bodies.[23] I therefore needed a framework that could focus on women's experiences and their bodies, and locate them in the largely invisible, often oppressive, complex matrix of social relations.

Given the priorities I mentioned at the beginning of the chapter, feminism seemed ideal. It is in the business of examining women's experiences with a view to transforming society. As midwife researcher Valerie Fleming (1994) suggested, 'the overt goal of feminist research is to make visible women's experiences and, by so doing, reveal and correct the distortions which have maintained women's unequal social position'.[24] Feminist research challenges negative stereotypical images of women that exclude and oppress them, providing interpretations of their lives that are both supportive of and plausible to them.[25]

Bringing women back into the picture

There are different definitions of feminism and approaches to feminist research, many of which still hold currency. It is difficult to say where it began, because while women over the centuries have understood the consequences of patriarchal structures on their sex, they have struggled to make their voices heard.[26] Feminisms are about making these voices heard and letting the so-called silence tell its own story.[27] Silence is perhaps too absolute a term because it ignores women's resistance. But it was a useful tool because it highlighted the fact that amid the cacophony of competing voices about birth, women's views about their priorities and needs were left largely undocumented. Thus a feminist approach has meant seeking out the voices of the women who took part in my research. But different strands of feminist research have sought out women's voices in different ways. The widely held view in the 1960s that advocated research on women, by women, for women,[28] often assumed that they had been omitted as an oversight and took an 'add women and stir' approach.[29] The approach that developed from this was called feminist empiricism. It believed that sexism could be eliminated from the research process through rigorous attention to objectivity and attributed 'bad science' or 'bad sociology' to individual researchers who had allowed sexism to enter the process.[30] This seemed inadequate for a number of reasons. First, the so-called 'oversight' was clearly not coincidental,[31] second, it adds women onto 'malestream' research without challenging the thinking behind this,[32] when challenging this is what this book is all about, and third, the researcher remains removed from the process,[33] rather than part of the dialogue.[34]

A different response to raising the profile of women was the feminist use of standpoint theories.[35] These theories rest on the belief that subordinated groups of people are epistemically privileged (i.e. that they have knowledge that those in power are unlikely to have). They 'are likely to have insights . . . about their own experience',[36] as well as 'insights into the dominant mind-sets'.[37] In other words, who and where we are in the world affects what we can know,[38] but those in powerful positions often have a more restricted understanding of the world than others because:

> The dominant culture is known to us all. We are continually bombarded with its worldview, the symbols of its values, and those outside it learn its beliefs and nuances in order to survive. But

when we are inside the dominant culture we do not have to learn about the cultures, the values, the realities of others.[39]

Standpoint theories seemed initially promising. Unlike the empiricism that I have just described, standpoint accepts that knowledge production is situated and political, and it is therefore as interested in the views of the researcher as those of the research subjects,[40] It has been successfully used by feminists to prioritize and authenticate women's experiences. Yet there are a number of problems. For example, the assumption that oppressed peoples can somehow stand outside dominant cultural norms, does not fit with women's experiences of obstetric ideology as pervasive and difficult to see beyond. More troubling for my work is that women of colour, non-heterosexual women and women in less prosperous circumstances accused standpoint theories of failing to respond to their very different experiences.[41] Any inability to acknowledge diversity seemed problematic given women's desires not to be stereotyped. This reminded me that the researcher must be aware of her own assumptions,[42] and that her assumptions can prevent her from understanding other women's views. As Ann Opie (1992) pointed out, 'ideology can obscure as well as enlighten'.[43] Indeed, none of us can underestimate the power of our assumptions, as we 'can never know the level to which we have internalized and identified ourselves with the available images of Woman'.[44]

Whatever one concludes about the potentials and limits of feminist empiricism and standpoint theories, it is clear that the main concern of these feminist approaches is unquestionably liberating women. While more complex notions of what feminisms are and do continue to develop, this remains the cornerstone of all feminist research.

Looking towards postmodernism

The 'posties' have been influential since the 1960s, but defy being attached to any historical moment or political stance.[45] Postmodernism also defies being confined by any one definition. Its main impact has been to challenge the modernist myth that there are objective truths that hold constant wherever we are, whoever we are and whenever we happen to inhabit our planet. It claims instead that everything we know and do arises from the particularities of our lives. This challenge has added to the complexity of feminist research and has caused a great deal of angst among some feminists.[46] As they have grappled with how to represent women without stereotyping them, how to talk about their oppression without ignoring their abilities to resist it, and how to work with other axes of oppression, such as race and poverty for example, the potential of postmodern theories have become evident. I decided I might position myself somewhere between standpoint and postmodernism, to take advantage of postmodernism's acceptance of different knowledges, and diversity, without questioning the very notion of knowledge, or the existence of the category 'woman'. I thought that this would enable me to acknowledge a collective resistance to obstetric ideology without stereotyping women. I saw the possibility of reconstructing the story of obstetrics (often told as one of unmitigated success) and the story of midwifery (often told as one of unmitigated failure), by unearthing the messiness and partiality of these stories and finding less told stories. For example, while the suppression of midwife-attended births at home in most of western Europe and North America over the nineteenth and twentieth centuries looked superficially uniform, this masked the dissenting voices and places of resistance that I discuss in Chapter 3.

But because the philosophical foundations for our work is crucial to the interpretations we make, I felt that without a deep understanding about the debates between feminisms and postmodernism, I was unable to judge whether or not a position between standpoint and postmodernism was a misleading or useful compromise. On the basis of this deeper understanding, it became clear that 'hybrid' theories,[47] which accept that knowledge production is situated, but argue for retaining some modernist concept of reality and value,[48] are illogical. Linda Nicholson (1999) describes this kind of thinking as part of the legacy of modernity whereby 'we have inherited both the idea that culture changes and the idea that constructs that rise above such changes are possible'.[49] This being the case, I moved closer to a feminist reading of postmodernism but wanted to consider the specific charges brought against it.

Rolling out the charges

Criticisms of postmodernism centre on the apparent disintegration of any notion of meaningful historical analysis, the disintegration of any commonalities (and thus the means to identify woman or oppression as meaningful categories), the disintegration of feminism and critical voices, the subsequent lack of political direction, and finally the complete disintegration of absolutely everything into text and chaos. In other words, the death of history, women, politics, knowledge and everything else. These are serious charges.

Does postmodernism mean the death of history? It has indeed posed questions about the authenticity of historical analysis. In particular, it has challenged the notion of historical unity, linearity and progression,[50] or that history can be interpreted through the eyes of the present. Postmodernism claims that history is disjointed and that interventions can have unexpected, even unwanted consequences because of the many coexisting influences at any moment in time. For example, the introduction of the British NHS in 1948 did not plan to phase out home births and independent midwives, but making doctors and hospitals more accessible, combined with the influences of science and medicine, and poverty, contributed to this happening.[51] The question is whether or not abandoning history as a chronological series of events means abandoning history altogether. Radical feminist historian Joan Hoff (1996) fears that the logical conclusion of post-structuralist theory is the annihilation of history, and along with it herstory: a herstory that feminists have so painstakingly reconstructed,[52] and rely on as a tool for liberation and a place for cultural insights.[53]

Does postmodernism signify the death of the category 'woman' and political analysis? This book rests on the belief that the category 'woman' exists and that women are an identifiable, subordinated group but may have unique experiences of this subordination.[54] But some feminists are worried that postmodern feminism is a contradiction in terms,[55] because postmodernism fragments categories. This would mean that feminists could not provide a critical analysis of women's oppression, indeed, could not exist at all[56]. If, 'to undertake feminist research is to place as central to the inquiry the social construction of gender',[57] and the suggestion is that gender can no longer identify itself, we have a problem.

Does postmodernism entail the death of everything, especially knowledge? And if it does not, why is this so? On the one hand, Katja Mikhailovich (1996) asks 'whether deconstruction inevitably leads to relativism or nihilism (basically the end point of which is, nothing exists, nothing really matters, and anything goes), and if not, then when, and where do we stop deconstructing?'[58] On the other hand, drawing on Kate Soper's work, Alison Assiter (1996) points out that postmodernists cannot appeal 'to the very values they are rejecting',[59] by claiming a single truth – that there are no truths.[60]

Postmodernism still seemed to me to offer a number of possibilities for women engaged in marginalized activities who are often stereotyped. Its focus on exploring the gap between stereotypical woman or the 'fantasy' of woman, and the complexities of actual women, meant that I could engage more closely with women's individual experiences[61]. Its focus on power, and questioning of knowledge,[62] offered more potential for examining the power structures and the truth claims of so-called rational scientific knowledge on which obstetrics and its practices are based. It could be exposed as a belief system among others and "reason" itself examined. While Rene Descartes' statement 'I think therefore I am' put reason beyond question, postmodernism brings it back again and thereby questions dichotomous thinking (male/female, reason/emotion etc.) on which patriarchy sustains itself. If dichotomous thinking can be displaced,[63] our thinking could more easily integrate life's messiness and create spaces for women to construct their own meanings of childbirth (based on emotional and embodied knowledge as well as the intellect), that are profoundly different from the narrow, obstetric definitions provided for them. It seemed worth answering the questions: Are all these deaths I discussed unavoidable? Can postmodernism be read in any other way? Can it be infused with feminist morality and materiality?

Answering the charges, uncertainly

I remained convinced of the potential of postmodernism and unconvinced that 'it is a capitulation in the face of our problems'.[64] The unease engendered by postmodern uncertainty seemed to be a response to modernity's need for certainty. In any case, not knowing the level of partiality in one's work does not make it any less partial and as Margrit Shildrick (1997) pointed out, deconstruction is not synonymous with destruction, and openness need 'not be interpreted as weakness, nor as indecision, but rather as the courage to refuse the comforting refuge of broad categories and unidirectional vision'.[65] Indeed, as Jane Flax (1990) suggested, 'if we do our work well, reality will appear even more unstable, complex and disorderly than it does now'.[66] In short, I rejected the relativist and nihilist view of postmodernism (that it is only destructive), and thus rejected the idea that it leads to the death of history, women, politics and knowledge. I interpreted postmodernism, not as a free for all, but as a collection of disparate, deconstructive discourses which on their own are incomplete but provide a set of theoretical tools. My task was therefore to produce an ethically sustainable reading of postmodernism based on individual women's morality and materiality and maintain a 'with women' political stance.

In fact, whether or not I located this book in a modernist framework and appealed to objectivity, truth, reality, or any other so-called legitimizing authority, the effects of postmodernity have destabilized the foundations of modernity to a point of no return. This book is a dialogue between me, the women and theory. The reader too is part of this dialogue.[67] I can only strive not to misrepresent those I listened to, trust that the end result is acceptable and coherent to the women involved and hope that I have described my journey well enough for the reader to place herself or himself somewhere in this dialogue.

As I moved towards postmodernism, the world looked less like a map to be discovered and more like transient maps under perpetual construction. While transient maps may be more difficult to follow than a single stable map, I knew they could lead to a deeper understanding of how women's accounts contribute to a tapestry of knowledge. But I needed to come back to four aspects of the debates above: knowledge, experience, power and bodies. First, I needed to know more about how situated knowledges come about and how to authenticate them within the limitations postmodernism has thrown up. Second, having accepted that knowledge is more than the sum total of intellectual thinking, I needed to understand how our experiences contribute to that knowledge and on what grounds we can rely on these because there is no reason to believe that our experiences are more or less stable than our intellects, or that the words we speak are somehow free of cultural constraints. Third, if I wished to claim that women are both oppressed and resistant to oppression in a myriad ways, I needed to understand more about the workings of power. Finally, in asserting that childbirth is a thoroughly embodied experience, I wanted to find ways of focusing on women's bodies that acknowledge both the similarities and differences between them.

Knowledge

Can women know?

Epistemology refers to the assumptions behind where and how we look for knowledge and what then counts as knowledge.[68] What we believe about epistemology profoundly affects how we view women and their experiences. Those who believe that pure male reason, free of all emotion and any other so-called distractions is the only sound basis for producing knowledge, will also believe that women's knowledge is unreliable and lacking. This kind of thinking dismisses women's knowledge about themselves and their experiences, and undermines the knowledge they have.[69] For example, several of the women I talked to knew when they had conceived, but were disbelieved. On one occasion, I accompanied a woman to a gynaeco-logical appointment. As we sat alone in a waiting area, a nurse appeared and called for Mrs Brown. She returned some minutes later and repeated her call for Mrs Brown. Finally, she approached us, and asked if my friend was sure she was not Mrs Brown. Brigitte Jordan (1997) describes a scenario in which health professionals assumed that they knew better than the woman, whether or not her baby was about to be born. Privileging rationality over emotion and the mind over the body vastly reduces what counts as knowledge, because it prevents women's experiences, for example, from being part of that knowledge.[70]

As I have already put forward, I believe that women have a great deal to say about their experiences and that male-based epistemology makes it difficult for them to develop and express their knowledge. I thus turned to feminist epistemology that understands this dilemma, knows that women are knowledgeable, and knows that knowledge comes from their intellects, emotions, bodily sensations, imaginations, past experiences and other attributes that create who we are and what we know.[71] In other words, pure reason is a modernist fantasy because it cannot be separated from the individual or culture. Indeed, aspiring to it limits our access to knowledge. So, feminist epistemol-ogy rejects the idea of the neutral researcher, claiming instead that both researcher and subjects are shaped by any number of social forces.[72] We are always embedded in a context, so knowledge is always contextual.[73] This is why the debates in this chapter are so important because they tell us about this context and how to work with it as best we can. They tell us how we can talk more confidently about women's experiences while acknowledging the limitations of what we do. They tell us that we can only ever contribute to a chang-ing tapestry of knowledge rather than build on a solid mass of truth.

Does knowledge come from relationships and dialogue?

Those that believe that knowledge comes from applying pure male reason, also tend to believe that knowledge is produced by isolated individuals. Again feminist work shows that this is not the case. Instead it suggests that knowledge production is a communal, ongo-ing process that arises through dialogues that we all contribute to.[74] While feminist debates in this area can be complicated, they alert us to the fact that we need to be aware of the similarities and differences between people and groups of people. Feminist debates lend weight to the particularities that postmodernism speaks about and the importance of bringing together all of our voices in the dialogue of knowledge.[75] This is particularly relevant when considering women who plan home births who are both marginalized and homogenized.

Some feminist theorists have looked at how marginalized dialogues can be included more easily, and suggest that not only is knowledge produced though dialogue, but that the environment in which that dialogue occurs impacts on knowledge. Brigitte Jordan (1977) showed that women were more or less likely to know whether or not they were pregnant depending on the expectations of their ability to know by those around them. Her findings suggest that women's knowledge can be muted or fostered depending on how, where and by whom it is sought.[76] This kind of knowing that is embedded in place and relationships (relational knowing) has huge implications for both researchers and health practitioners who work with childbearing women.

Detailed work in the area of women's decision-making,[77] and in knowledge acquisition,[78] showed how women take account of others' thoughts and feelings and often share and acquire knowledge best through conversations, life events and their involvement with community activities. They need to feel supported and at ease. Perhaps missing in this original work was the critical thinking about why most women develop relational and caring ways of thinking and being, whether or not this is their only mode of thought and being, and whether or not this is a good thing.[79] So while Mary Belenky and her colleagues (1986) and Carol Gilligan's (1985) earlier work plotted women on a knowledge or decision-making line, more recent work with girls and young women by Elizabeth Debold and colleagues (1996) suggests that women hold multiple knowledge positions because of the conflict between authoritative knowledge and their own experiences that contradict this. This internal conflict may make women seem and feel less knowledgeable than they actually are. Debold suggests a different interpretation of the knowledge positions identified by Belenky and colleagues:

> Girls' conflicts between their own experience and their increasing knowledge of cultural expectations at early adolescence may lead them to give up on developing methods for knowing (that is, procedural knowing), and in so doing, either accept what authorities say as true (received knowing) or to attempt to hold onto a personal truth (subjectivist knowing).[80]

This explanation tells us that women's development of knowledge and morality is a complex response to unavoidable dominant forces that can cause divisions and tensions within the individual.[81] So while Belenky and colleagues (1986) suggested that women's ways of thinking and being are innately caring, flexible, and able to sustain ambiguity and complexity, Debold and her colleagues (1996) suggest that women have no choice, if they are to retain any sense of their own integrity. One of the ironies of enforced relationality is that if relationships need to be maintained, disagreements that threaten these may be difficult.[82] Thus while relationality enables women in some ways it can disable them in others:

> Even when women held strongly to their own ways of doing things, they remained concerned about not hurting the feelings of their opponents by openly expressing dissent. They reported that they were apt to hide their opinions and then suffer quietly the frustration of not standing up to others. Some women described feeling either petulant, private resentment of others or self-admonishment for being so unassertive'.[83]

The work on relational knowing had a number of implications for my work. First, it suggests that how I approached interviewing women mattered and would impact on the quality of the material I gathered.[84] Second, it suggests that I needed to listen carefully to the tensions within and between women's accounts, and third, that I needed to focus as much on external structures that oppress women as on their internal psychological development, and consider how these interact.[85]

Experience

Does experience speak for itself?

I have talked about women's experience as a necessary and legitimate ingredient of knowledge. Because this is a contested area, I need to say more about what this means and how we can use it to challenge accepted knowledge and generate new knowledges.[86] This book is very much about the centrality of women's experiences, as described by feminists such as Liz Stanley and Sue Wise (1993):

> The essence of feminism for us is its ideas about the personal, its insistence on the validity of women's experiences and its arguments that an understanding of women's oppression can be gained only through understanding and analyzing everyday life, where oppression as well as everything else is grounded.[87]

But postmodernism suggests that we need to view experience with the same situatedness and partiality that I have attributed to other aspects of knowledge production. There is no such thing as 'raw' experience,[88] because, just as we create our culture, it also creates us.[89] Experience and culture are woven together, thus experience cannot speak for itself.[90] In other words, as I said at the beginning of this chapter, we do indeed need to engage with philosophical debates because women's stories do not just speak for themselves.[91] Without all the other stories, these provide only a limited account. In fact we already have accounts of birth,[92] which demonstrate the complex ways in which culture impacts on women's experiences of birth. Tess Cosslett (1991, 1994), for example, identified how women internalize both 'medical' and 'natural' views on birth and how these can obscure their own experiences (though, in my view this did not fully acknowledge the dominance of medical birth discourses). Tina Miller (1998) made similar observations about how women internalize cultural norms and suppress their own experiences in her research on childbirth and motherhood. As Sandra Burt and Lorraine Code (1995) point out, we tread a fine line between 'the old tyranny of authoritarian expertise that discounts women's experience . . . and a new tyranny of "experientialism" that claims for the first-person experiential utterances an immunity from challenge, interpretation or debate'.[93]

Can we trust our voices?

Of course experiences are mainly recounted through our voices and the same sorts of tensions that postmodern feminists have debated in relation to experience apply to voice:

> Subjects are not attributed authenticity outside (dominant) culture. Instead, we can present them as finding 'their voices' within and through the network of meanings made available to them, including where they resist the dominant meanings ascribed them.[94]

Postmodern feminists therefore suggest that we should represent women not only 'in a different voice',[95] but also in many different voices.[96] And because, as I explained above, women may embody different or conflicting experiences and knowledges, the individual voice is also many voices.[97] Those who believe that we must have only one rational voice and that other voices are irrational distractions may believe that accepting multiple voices negates any meaningful notion of the knowing person. But this is not the case.[98] It merely accepts that identity is complex and that we are always in a process of becoming who we are, rather than pre-formed and that our voices reflect this. This is why the idea of process during child-bearing is so crucial. If institutionalized obstetric care prevents women from questioning, revisiting and revising decisions during their pregnancies, it prepares women to rely on experts and their ideologies enabling them to autonomous thought and action that being a mother demands.[99] Acknowledging a certain level of fluidity within the person does not mean abandoning any notion of integrated identity. For example, Susan Greenwood (1996) identified a search for wholeness and identity among the women she worked with, which was in 'stark contrast to the postmodern fragmentation of the self'.[100]

These ideas about voices enabled me to listen to the voices of all the women in my study and hear rather than mute the coherencies, contradictions and ironies that form the rich weave of knowledge. They enabled me to hear disparate as well as collective voices.[101] Like Susan Greenwood, I too heard the search for some kind of wholeness among women planning home births and their dislike of the discontinuities and fragmentation they associated with obstetric hospital birth: a wholeness that can contain but not stifle the unique experience of the disintegration and reintegration that marks a rite of passage such as birth. Finally Marjorie DeVault's (1994) comments about 'speaking up carefully' suggest how we can use our voices authoritatively and ethically, to prioritize women's experiences within a postmodern feminist framework:

> A voice that will be thoughtful and self-reflective – not imposingly authoritative, but clear and personal – the voice of an author who invites others to listen and respond, aiming more toward dialogue than debate. I want to write about others *care*-fully, in both senses of the word, with rigor and empathetic concern.[102]

What do words tell us?

We express our voices through language and just as knowledge and experiences are rooted in culture, so too are the words we use. Language is not a transparent naming of 'things'.[103] As Paula Treichler (1990) pointed out:

The word *childbirth* is not merely a label provided us by language, for a clear-cut event that already exists in the world; rather than describe it, it *inscribes* and makes the event intelligible to us. We cannot look *through* discourse to determine what childbirth really is, for discourse itself is the site where such determination is inscribed.[104]

As I have explained, our culture has been created more by men than by women. This means that language is far from neutral and that 'a particular vision of social reality is inscribed in language – a particular vision of reality that does not serve all of its speakers equally'.[105] This underlying linguistic bias alienates women from and shapes their experiences by imposing male concepts and terms through which they must think of their worlds.[106] 'Man-made' language makes it difficult for women to think about, talk about and write about their experiences.[107] This is certainly the case in relation to childbearing because the authority of the medicalized, technical language of obstetrics has a profound influence on women's experiences and how they relate to their bodies.[108]

But as postmodern feminists and others have shown us, language 'both gives us our world and yet keeps us from being imprisoned in it'.[109] Fortunately for us, there is some degree of linguistic manoeuvrability, because although 'language creates us', it is 'also created by us' and 'descriptions of experience are always revisable'.[110] So while 'languages predispose speakers to view the world in particular ways . . . such a world view is not all-determining'.[111] Other stories *can* be told,[112] but to tell them we need to look very carefully at the context in which women describe, decide and act in relation to pregnancy, birth and motherhood.[113] We must also accept that words and meaning are contentious.

These feminist insights about language lend further weight to the idea that our work is thoroughly political and never neutral.[114] They also demand that we examine how language reproduces dominant ideologies, and look for 'new terms to express women's perceptions and experiences'.[115] The discussions in feminist theory made me all the more aware of listening to how the women and I used medicalized language, and where we created new meanings. This led to my redefining of obstetric meanings of 'safety' in Chapter 4, 'continuity' in Chapter 5 and 'choice and control' in Chapter 6.

Power

Can women empower themselves?

The discussions in this chapter, so far, are implicitly about power – the interplay between domination and resistance. Postmodern feminists and others have found it difficult to understand how power circulates. They have thus found it difficult to find ways of representing both how women (and others) are profoundly disempowered by a culture that marginalizes them, and yet manage to breach these constraints and empower themselves.[116] We therefore must treat terms such as 'woman-centred' with caution:

> In 'woman-centred' research, women are acknowledged as active, conscious, intentional authors of their own lives. As an ideal this notion of 'woman-centred' research is appealing. As a description of reality, however, the term 'woman-centred' is not entirely satisfactory because it seems to suggest that women can occupy a powerful authoritative and controlling position in their lives: lives often hemmed in by social arrangements and structured inequalities not of their own making.[117]

We must keep in mind the tension between 'downplaying' the impact of patriarchy and women's abilities to resist it, and resist the tendency to do one or the other: '*either* we limn the structural constraints of gender so well that we deny women any agency *or* we portray women's agency so glowingly that the power of subordination evaporates'.[118] These insights confirm that the more we understand about the basis of our oppression and how we internalize this,[119] the more we can resist it: 'Patriarchy has created us in its image. Once we see that image, however, it no longer possesses us unaware. We can reshape, create something new'.[120] This tension, between over or underestimating women's victimization,[121] is crucial to work with as best we can, because our knowledge of it contributes to how well we listen to and interpret women's experiences.

Recalling Drucilla Cornell's (1995) words on page 47, while we cannot know how far we have internalized the norms of our times, we can gain insight into how these might influence our thoughts and actions. This idea that cultural norms are part of who we are and how we live our lives implies that power circulates in complex ways. It seems to be both everywhere and nowhere and exerted by 'everyone and yet no one in particular'.[122] This makes sense of women's descriptions of practitioners' apparent lack of awareness of either the power that policies exert over them or the consequent power that they exert over women. For example, one of the women I interviewed reported that a midwife's usual procedure of holding the baby's head as it birthed caused her a great deal of pain. When the woman shouted at her to stop, the midwife continued. The woman commented that it was 'understandable' because the midwife 'didn't know any better'.

Another strand of feminist discussions about power suggests that while feminism talks about dominance and marginality, it has not always been sensitive to the particularities of power. This is because of a concern on the part of some feminists that accepting the existence of uneven, shifting networks of power may undermine our abilities to resist domination collectively. This is not the case.[123] We can accept that 'some women share some common interests and face some common enemies' but that these may change and 'are interlaced with differences, even with conflicts'.[124] In terms of my work, understanding that there are general and specific patterns of oppression that may change over time is important. It means that we can work towards creating feminist theories based on multiplicity and difference rather than dissecting people along fixed lines. It means that we can acknowledge the usefulness of forming loose groupings,[125] around issues like home birth that can act on the shared goal of making home birth more available, but accept that individual women might not share other commonalities, and might engage with obstetric ideology in different ways. For example, the women I interviewed considered the advantages and disadvantages of both alternative and authoritative birth ideologies and took varying positions on these.

Of course, these discussions imply that power affects our bodies as well as our intellects. Indeed feminists have pointed out that power impacts most concretely on the body.[126] Seemingly simple acts such as showing a practitioner a rash, or a practitioner placing a stethoscope on a person's chest, are 'the stuff of power'.[127] This meant taking note of the women's descriptions of obstetric practices – being 'strapped up', 'hooked up', 'tied on' and 'held down' for example. While these may seem relatively innocuous, obstetric and gynaecological practices tell women that they should be selfless and compliant.[128] But in the same way that language does not uniformly oppress our ability to speak about ourselves, power need not always oppress our bodies.[129] They can equally well 'become sites of struggle and resistance'.[130] Taking into account that women's bodies are a 'platform upon which social politics are choreographed, resisted and negotiated',[131] enabled me to hear what women had to say about the violation of their bodies through obstetric practices. It also enabled me to hear women talk about their powerful, knowing, sensual, and spiritual pregnant and birthing bodies. I discuss this in Chapter 6.

While women are usually described as passive recipients of male desire,[132] this is largely because 'the expression of female voice, body and sexuality are essentially inaudible when the dominant language and ways of viewing are male'.[133] French feminists such as Luce Irigaray and Helene Cixous have talked about female desire and the female body as a site for pleasure, and the sexuality and sensuality of the pregnant and birthing body is discussed in some of the more recent birth literature.[134] This literature stands in contrast to the disembodying, desexualizing discourse of obstetrics. This is not to say that it denies the pain of birth or suggests that childbearing and mothering are or should be pleasurable for all women, but that the potential for this has been muted through the muting of women's bodies and their bodily desires and powers.

At the end of the day, there is no obvious agreement on power issues. But the women's stories confirmed Diana Meyer's (2000) view that the 'stark opposition between dominant and subordinate positions' does not exist in practice because few people have wholly privileged or subordinated identities.[135] So I align myself with those who believe that our culture is not 'wholly and seamlessly phallocentric',[136] but who know that it remains remarkably resistant to our attempts to change it, as can be seen throughout this book.

Bodies

Can we bring back women's missing bodies with some integrity?

It would be anathema to research women's experiences of birth without thinking more carefully about the 'matter' of bodies. While Mavis Kirkham (1999a) has written about embodied midwife knowledge, the idea that knowledge may be contained within our bodies has not been widely theorized. Until recently, sociology has neglected bodies. Much of western thought could be said to be distinctly disembodied.[137] This has had implications for health-care practices because the male body can remain relatively absent if it is healthy. Its presence is then thought to signify illness.[138] Women's 'leaky' menstruating, birthing, breastfeeding and menopausal bodies make themselves very present,[139] and this presence has contributed to their bodily processes becoming increasingly medicalized. The disembodied rhetoric of health care talks at cross-purposes to women's bodily experiences. If health-care practices could accept the presence rather than the absence of the body, women's unique reproductive cycles and changing bodies could become part of a health(y) discourse rather than one of pathology.[140]

While sociology of the body is now more popular, feminists are still very wary about including women's bodies in their work. Acknowledging that women's bodies could play a part in their discussions about knowledge and oppression worries feminists.[141] Those who have considered how women's bodies inform their knowledge and subordination have often been accused of biologism, essentialism, ahistoricism and naturalism (i.e. fixed gender differences), that prevent any way out of women's subordination. The trouble is that muting the body mutes both oppressive bodily practices and the power of women's birthing bodies. It stops us finding the words to express the oppression and knowledge of our bodies,[142] and understanding more about the how our bodies interact with knowledge and oppressive practices.[143] Meanwhile, muting knowledge about oppressive bodily practices does not stop these practices impacting negatively on women's lives.[144] In other words, just as refusing to acknowledge the politics of research does not make it less political, failing to acknowledge the materiality of the body does not make it less material. Instead, it leaves women's bodies vulnerable to modernist beliefs about the body. These include that it is 'corporeal raw material',[145] little more than inanimate mass or fixed, 'brute matter'.[146] This goes some way to explaining the emphasis on technical proficiency within our health-care system, and the ease with which invasive practices are carried out on pregnant and birthing bodies. Health care appears to have little knowledge that when carrying out its business on bodies, 'the integrity of the patient as a person may be at stake'.[147]

For women, practices on their bodies affect not only the fleshy substance of those bodies, but also how they feel about themselves. As Rosalyn Diprose (1994) suggests, 'significant bodily changes' effect changes in the self.[148] This may explain why abuse of the body is so keenly felt as violating personhood and why self-esteem is implicated.[149] Just how the body and mind interact is difficult to understand.[150] But the women I talked to tended to describe being in relation to their bodies rather than possessing them. Like other women, they talked about their hopes to integrate mind and body through birth,[151] but often experienced a distancing from their bodies. This has echoes with other circumstances in which women distance themselves from their bodies. For example, women describe sexual harassment as though they were bystanders, outside their bodies.[152] Indeed invasive birth practices are often described in similar ways to violating sexual experiences,[153] and the splitting of mind and body that occurs could be interpreted as a self-protective mechanism. I thus took care to listen to women's accounts of bodily practices that they experienced as harmful and invasive and those that seemed acceptable or helpful, as well as the context in which these were experienced. So ignoring women's bodies (or ignoring that they are different to men's bodies) was clearly not an option but at the same time moving beyond essentialism seemed essential! The former mutes women's bodily experiences while the latter mutes differences between those experiences. Both positions are trapped in the same dualistic, falsely generalizing paradigm.[154]

Once again postmodern feminists offered some hope. While postmodern theories on their own do not necessarily address the substance of bodies, feminist readings of postmodernism accept the '"real" bodies of women' because being a woman's body impacts on our experiences. This acceptance need not suppress embodied differences between women.[155] Just as I claimed that Gilligan's (1985) voice should be many voices, so the female body is many bodies and any similarities between them 'may be interlaced with difference': our bodies shape our experiences, but so do other variables.[156] Nor need we accept that women's bodies are unchanging. Indeed, postmodern theories show that physiology and anatomy are socially constructed and that we 'see' the body through socially and historically specific lenses.[157] This means that while birth activists, midwives and others have challenged obstetric assumptions and introduced midwifery practices based on alternative interpretations of physiology, these alternatives are no more stable and applicable at all times to all women and babies than obstetric interpretations. The body changes through its interactions with culture and culture is changed by bodies.[158]

To conclude this chapter, feminist thinkers in debate with postmodernism have successfully developed critical feminist theories in which we can examine patterns of oppression and resistance. These thinkers remind us to acknowledge the tensions, complexities and contradictions that ultimately enrich our understanding of our worlds. They remind us to be vigilant and humble, knowing that our work is rooted in specific times and places.[159] They enable us to make authoritative claims that remain open to change: our 'fictions' or 'stories' may be coherent but not forever true.[160] They help us understand how women's bodies are part of the dialogue about knowledges and practices. Thus while postmodernism does not lead automatically to the inclusion of all women, a feminist reading of it leaves space for the exploration of difference and avoids closure. Feminist thinkers have also unearthed the deeper structural layers of society to reveal that separation rather than connections is the main organizing concept through which life, birth and motherhood are constructed.[161] These crucial concepts form the warp against which the interpretations of this book are woven.

Notes

1 Elizabeth Minnich, quoted in Reinharz 1992: 11.
2 Stanley and Wise 2000.
3 In fact, I did not confine myself to any one discipline or methodology, as it is often at the intersections of these that new knowledge is created. I became 'bricoleur' (Shildrick 1997: 5) and 'nomad' (Braidotti 1997: 60), moving across midwifery, medicine, sociology, philosophy, anthropology, psychology, politics, postmodernism, feminism, ethnography and phenomenology, in order to stay close to the concerns of the women and the contexts in which these were shaped. While this entails some 'awkwardness', 'border dwellers occupy an epistemically favourable vantage point, for the virtues and the defects of each community are easier to spot from the borders' (Meyer 2000: 155). This borderland created space in which to consider the diversity of women's experiences. This in turn moved birth discourses beyond the natural/technological polarities.
4 For a useful and readable introduction to debates about knowledge, see Wickham 2004.
5 The systematic reviews included Chalmers and Haynes 1994; Clarke and Stewart 1994; Dickersin et al. 1994; Knipschild 1994; Murphy-Black 1994a, 1994b.
6 Scottish, English and Welsh policy documents included CRAG/SCOTMEG 1993, 1994a, 1994b 1994c, 1994d; Department of Health 1993; Health Policy and Public Health Directorate 1993; House of Commons (Health Committee) 1992; House of Commons (Social Services Committee) 1980; Maternity Service Advisory Committee 1982, 1984, 1985; Ministry of Health 1930, 1932, 1954, 1956, 1959, 1961, 1970, 1979; Scottish Home and Health Department 1965, 1973a, 1973b, 1980, 1988.
7 House of Commons 1992.
8 Eskes and van Alten 1994; van der Hulst et al. 2004.
9 Declerq et al. 2001. For general research and commentaries, see Declercq et al. 2001; De Vries 2004; Eskes and van Alten 1994; Kloosterman 1984; Smulders and Limburg 1988; van Lieburg and Marland 1989; van Teijlingen 1992; van Teijlingen and van der Hulst 1995. Some of these specifically discuss how the Netherlands has maintained a strong midwifery presence, for example, Declercq et al. 2001; Eskes and van Alten 1994; Treffers et al. 1990; van Teijlingen 1992. The issue of state legislation is addressed by Torres and Reich 1989; van Teijlingen 1990, 1992; van Teijlingen and van der Hulst 1995. De Vries 2004 discusses how these are interwoven in Dutch society.

10 Pasveer and Akrick 2001; Rothman 2001; van Teijlingen and van der Hulst 1995 provide different perspectives on the changing use of technology and its impact on birth and women's bodies. Oakley and Houd 1990; Rothman 1993; van Teijlingen 1994 discuss how pain has been viewed in the Netherlands and compare this to responses to pain in other cultures. De Vries 2004 provides a detailed sociological view of how home birth is embedded in Dutch society in a variety of ways.

11 Rooks 1997.

12 Macvicar et al. 1993.

13 Hall 1999.

14 Kirkham 2003; Saunders et al. 2000.

15 Chester 1997; Rook 1997.

16 See, for example, Annandale and Clark 1996, 1997; Campbell and Porter 1997.

17 Spretnak 1999.

18 Anderson 1991; Bergum 1989; Field et al. 1994; van Manen 1990; van Olphen Fehr 1999.

19 Van Manen 1990.

20 Young 1990a: 161.

21 Denzin and Lincoln 1994.

22 Martin 1990; Soper 1990; Stacey 1991.

23 Murphy-Lawless 1998a; Roberts 1981: 19.

24 Fleming 1994: 64.

25 Griffiths 1995 and Okely 1994 discuss exclusion and a number of feminist collections and articles provide a range of research findings that challenge dominant ideology. See, for example, Burt and Code 1995; Charles and Hughes-Freeland 1996; Evans 1985; Fine 1992; L. Hunt et al. 1989; S. Hunt and Symonds 1995. The double strategy is addressed by Rosi Braidotti (1997: 61), who describes the essence of feminist theory as 'a two-layered project involving the critique of existing definitions, representations as well as the elaboration of alternative theories about women'.

26 O'Neill 1998; Reinharz 1992: 12.

27 Clair 1997; Morgan and Coombes 2001. Elizabeth Minnich describes feminism as a response to the realization that 'to a stunning extent, the interests of one half of the human race have not been thought about through history' (quoted in Reinharz 1992: 11). Thus uncovering silence, practising 'vigilance for traces of the untold story' and 'learning to see what is not there and hear what is not being said' (Burt and Code 1995: 32, 23) are very much the work of feminists. Michelle Fine and Susan Merle Gordon (1992: 23) suggest that, because women maintain these silences, 'Feminist research must get behind "evidence" that suggests all is well'. Mary Maynard and June Purvis (1994: 24) suggest that one way of doing this 'is to use our theoretical knowledge to address some of the silences in our empirical work'. I would add, *and vice versa.*

28 Stacey 1991: 111.

29 Oleson 1994: 159.

30 Harding 1987: 183.

31 Braidotti 1997: 64.

32 Eichler 1988.

33 Harding 1987: 183.

34 Although feminist empiricism still holds currency nowadays, it is clearly located in modernist, patriarchal thought based on definitions of reason and liberal views of equality that I suggest later in this chapter, cannot be supported. Ironically, its failure to recognize or challenge the oppression of so-called scientific methods was the very reason for its relative success (Harding 1993: 53). Yet at the same time, it raised questions about the anonymity of the researcher, how research is constructed and whether or not traditional empiricism can indeed see beyond a male view of the world (Harding 1987: 184). It thus laid the groundwork for the more recent feminist debates.

35 Standpoint theory is usually attributed to Hegel's realization that master and slave must have different perspectives on the world because of their different places within it (Bar On 1993: 83). Standpoint theory highlighted general differences between groups of people depending on their place in the world and the inequalities between them.

36 Charles and Hughes-Freeland 1996: 27.

37 McLennan 1995: 396.

38 Harding 1993: 54–55.

39 Starhawk 1990: 319.

40 Harding 1993: 70.

41 Code 1993; hooks 1990; Oleson 1994.

42 DeVault 1994.

43 Opie 1992: 66.

44 Cornell 1995: 97.

45 Jencks 1995.

46 Many feminists are reluctant to abandon modernism (Assiter 1996; Bell and Klein 1996; Brodribb 1992). Alison Assiter (1996), for example, argues against postmodernism because of its perceived instability and apolitical (and therefore oppressive) stance. Because of this, feminism and postmodernism have often 'kept an uneasy distance from one another' (Fraser and Nicholson 1990: 19). Bringing them together has been seen as both 'promising and dangerous' (Nash 1994: 65). Some feminists lean towards Lorraine Code's (1993: 41) 'mitigated relativism' in order to examine but not lose gender constructions and relations. In a similar vein, Michele Barrett (1992: 216) comments that 'feminism straddles the modernist and postmodernist divide, refusing to abandon values on which the modernist project of liberation is founded but also recognizing the validity of different women's experiences and the different ways of knowing and being that these encompass'. These debates are not confined to feminism, but take place across a range of disciplines: see, for example, Doran 1989; Knorr-Cetina and Mulkay 1983.

47 Nicholson 1999: 6.

48 Code 1993: 21; McNay 1992.

49 Nicholson 1999: 9.

50 Foucault 1972.

51 See also Robinson 1995.

52 Radical feminists take a mistakenly narrow view of postmodernism as destructive and 'paralysing' because they believe that 'a male-defined definition of gender that erased women as a category of analysis emerged as a major component of American post-structuralism' (Hoff 1996: 393).

Typically, the view is that postmodernism denies history any reality because all that exists is the moment, 'therefore historical agency – real people having an impact on real events – is both impossible and irrelevant' and research is powerless to reveal anything of substance from the chaos or non existence of history (Hoff 1996: 395–396).

53 Starhawk 1990.

54 Meyer 2000.

55 Benhabib 1995.

56 This is discussed by Butler 1995; Fraser 1995; Hartsock 1990; Holmwood 1995; McLennan 1995; Nash 1994; Phillips 1992, among others. The arguments by those who adhere to a narrow view of postmodernism have become ever more critical. Kate Soper (1990: 13) asks whether the apparent dissolution of feminism and its political critique complete a patriarchal circle, leaving women once again, silenced and vulnerable. In other words, postmodernism is seen as the 'cultural capital of late patriarchy' (Brodribb 1992: 21), 'drift[ing] inexorably to the male point of view' (Ronni Sandroff, in Hoff 1996: 406). Katja Mikhailovich (1996: 343) asks us if we can afford 'the erasure of words like oppression, exploitation and domination'. And if, as Joan Hoff (1996: 408) suggests, politics is replaced by linguistics and reality by texts, Christine Delphy (1996) doubts that textual analysis can relate to the materiality of women's lives. Standpoint theorist Dorothy Smith (quoted in Mann and Kelley 1997: 404) deplores what she sees as the acceptance of relativism because:

> Judgemental (or epistemological) relativism is anathema to any scientific project and feminist ones are no exception. It is not as equally true as its denial that women's uteruses wander around in their bodies when they take maths courses, that only Man the Hunter made important contributions to human history . . . that sexual molestation and other physical abuses children report are only their fantasies – as various sexist and androcentric scientific theories have claimed.

Other committed feminist theorists (for example, Benhabib et al. 1995; Nicholson 1990, 1999; Shildrick 1997) are, however, carefully integrating a postmodern feminist approach to research.

57 Fleming 1994: 64.

58 Mikhailovich 1996: 342.

59 Soper, in Assiter 1996: 5.

60 Standpoint theorists make similar assertions, that 'without some degree of epistemic grounding, without some coherent notion of the knowing, acting subject, distinctive political projects and articulations of *any kind* cannot be sustained' (McLennan 1995: 393). Feminists are also concerned that without attention to power differentials, the kind of consensus or 'conversations' (Rorty 1991) that some postmodernists appeal to are open to dominant ideologies and groups enforcing their own consensus or conversations (Code 1993: 24).

61 Cornell 1995.

62 Foucault 1980.

63 Shildrick 1997: 111.
64 Holmwood 1995: 415.
65 Shildrick 1997: 3.
66 Flax 1990: 57.
67 Rosenblatt 1978.
68 Maynard and Purvis 1994: 18.
69 Belenky et al. 1986; Brown et al. 1994; Jordan 1977; Murphy-Lawless 1998a: 211, 220–223 show how women's knowledge is subjugated. Code 1993 and Dalmiya and Alcoff 1993 discuss the so-called 'view from nowhere' or 'neutrality' of knowledge production.
70 McNay 1992: 13.
71 Griffiths 1995; Mackenzie 2000.
72 Code 1993; Harding 1993; Stanley and Wise 1990.
73 Haraway 1988; Nicholson 1999.
74 Code 1993; DeVault 1994; Nelson 1993; Potter 1993; Stanley and Wise 1990.
75 Mauthner and Doucet 1998.
76 Belenky et al. 1986.
77 Gilligan 1985.
78 Belenky et al. 1986.
79 Nicholson 1999.
80 Debold et al. 1996: 95.
81 Debold et al. 1996: 87.
82 Belenky et al. 1986: 70.
83 Belenky et al. 1986: 84. This kind of theory (often called ethics of care) that suggests that women are essentially different from men because they are by nature caring and nurturing risks falling into 'essentializing' or over-categorizing women (Flax 1990: 52; Nicholson 1999; Shildrick 1997: 122) and forgetting that so-called 'feminine' difference is often a response to oppression (Di Stefano 1990: 71).
84 Finch 1984; Kirby and McKenna 1989.
85 Fine and Gordon 1992. In fact, as Diana Meyer (1992) eloquently argues, much feminist psychology must be viewed with caution because in trying to define women's psychology, it has unwittingly taken on board male-based theories of development.
86 Maynard and Purvis 1994.
87 Stanley and Wise 1993: 136.
88 Maynard and Purvis 1994: 24.
89 Roseneil 1996: 88.
90 Scott 1992: 37.
91 Miriam Glucksmann's (1994) research on the experiences of women assembly workers is a good example of how theory and experience can combine to provide a more useful explanation of women's subordination.
92 Davis-Floyd and Sargent 1997; DeVries et al. 2001.
93 Burt and Code 1995: 36.
94 Alldred 1998: 161.
95 Gilligan 1985.
96 Nicholson 1999: 28.
97 Mair 1977; Ribbens 1998.
98 Butler 1995: 42; Meyer 2000.

99 Cronk 2000.
100 Greenwood 1996: 109.
101 Shildrick 1997: 133.
102 DeVault 1994: 3.
103 Scott 1992.
104 Treichler 1990: 13.
105 Ehrlich 1995: 45.
106 Eichler 1988; Smith 1987: 86.
107 Spender 1980; see also DeVault 1990; Stanley and Wise 1993.
108 Martin 1987; Murphy-Lawless 1998a: 54.
109 Cornell 1995: 76.
110 Griffiths 1995: 55.
111 Ehrlich 1995: 47.
112 Murphy-Lawless 1998a: 247–250.
113 Alldred 1998: 154.
114 Nicholson 1999: 75.
115 Ehrlich 1995: 47–51.
116 Meyer 2000; Stoljar 2000.
117 Brown et al. 1994.
118 Fraser 1992a: 16–17; see also Cowan 1996: 65–67.
119 Bartky 1997.
120 Starhawk 1990: 67.
121 Fraser 1992b: 191.
122 Bartky 1997: 142–143.
123 Cowan 1996: 82; Eisenstein 1989: 16; Shildrick 1997: 94.
124 Fraser and Nicholson 1990: 35.
125 Fraser 1992b; Young 1997a.
126 McNay 1992: 16.
127 Armstrong 1987: 70.
128 Scully 1994.
129 McNay 1992.
130 Grosz 1993: 199.
131 Fine and Gordon 1992: 27.
132 Fine and Gordon 1992; Starhawk 1990.
133 Fine and Gordon 1992: 38.
134 See, for example, Adams 1994; Gaskin 1990; Gregg 1995; Hall and
     Taylor 2004; Irigaray 1985; Kahn 1996; Kitzinger 2000; Lorde 1997;
     Jeanine Parvati-Baker, in Chester 1997; Rabuzzi 1994; Starhawk 1990;
     van Ophen Fehr 1999.
135 Meyer 2000: 160.
136 Fraser 1992a: 17.
137 Longino 1993: 104; Shildrick 1997. When bodies have been considered
     (in the 'lived experience' of phenomenology, for example) they are usu-
     ally male bodies, or supposedly neutral bodies that turn out to be male:
     see Gatens 1996: 23–24; Grosz 1993; McNay 1992; Marshall 1996:
     255; Soper 1990: 13.
138 Leder 1990.
139 Shildrick 1997.
140 Shildrick 1997.
141 Grosz 1993: 195.

142 Gatens 1996: 26.
143 Grosz 1993: 187.
144 Shildrick 1997.
145 Shildrick 1997: 13.
146 Gatens 1996: 61; Marshall 1996: 255.
147 Shildrick 1997: 18.
148 Diprose 1994: 116.
149 Griffiths 1995.
150 Marshall 1996: 261; Shildrick 1997.
151 Noble 2001; Rabuzzi 1994.
152 Brodkey and Fine 1992: 82.
153 Kitzinger S. 1992.
154 Different aspects of these debates are covered by Barkley 1998; Flax 1990: 53; Gatens 1996: 68; Marshall 1996; Nicholson 1999: 68–69; Shildrick 1997; Soper 1990: 13; Rabuzzi 1994.
155 Shildrick 1997: 102, 179.
156 Nicholson 1999: 57–58.
157 Armstrong 1987; DeVries et al. 2001; Jordon 1993; Murphy-Lawless 1998a; Davis-Floyd and Sargent 1997.
158 Featherstone et al. 1991: 13–15; Pasveer and Akrich 2001.
159 For example, while there is evidence of a widening gap between rich and poor in Britain (Hogg 1999: 114; Townsend et al. 1992), this work is set in a predominantly white, affluent, industrialized country. It cannot begin to speak for those women who lack basic sanitation, food, housing, education, employment, and access to appropriate health services, those who suffer the devastating effects of poverty and ill health, whose traditional birth practices have been dismantled. It does, however, challenge the mistaken belief that maternal and child mortality and morbidity can be improved only by the introduction of industrialized birth technologies and practices (Murphy-Lawless 1998b).
160 Foucault 1972; Code 1998.
161 Adams 1994; Rabuzzi 1994; Spretnak 1999; Starhawk 1990.

3   How have we got here?
Historical and current perspectives

> One consultant is said to have congratulated a 1926 conference for having 'travelled today very far from the old view that a confinement is an interesting domestic occurrence which should be celebrated in the family like Christmas or a birthday party'.[1]

Using some of the debates in the previous chapter, I now consider the context in which obstetrics replaced midwifery as the authoritative ideology on childbirth in Britain. I look at how it developed its knowledge and practices, how it was challenged, how it impacted on women's views on birth and how it influenced the development of midwifery. I also examine how it continues to shape birth knowledge and practices.

Critical histories of midwifery and obstetrics are well documented.[2] My focus is on making visible and reflecting on the many competing, contradictory and complementary storylines that run through this history. In essence, I want to consider the transition from the long-standing female-based traditions of birth to the recent medicalization and hospitalization of birth in Britain, and how the two continue to interact. First, I look at some of the influences which paved the way for the development of obstetrics.

How patriarchal thinking paved the way for obstetrics

The subordination and control of women

Although the term 'patriarchy' has perhaps been overused, blamed for all women's ills, and in some quarters thought to be a thing of the past, Carol Pateman (1989) and Sandra Bartky (1997) suggest that patriarchal values and practices are so integral to society and the subordination of women, they are almost invisible and therefore still very powerful. Feminists have traced how early mechanisms for women's subordination originated through creation myths, and became embedded in culture.[3] Thus patriarchy continues to be a major determinant nowadays.[4] The subordination of women in modern patriarchal society both strengthened and was strengthened by dichotomous thinking which established hierarchical distinctions between for example 'reason and emotion' and 'public and private'. This kind of thinking laid the groundwork for industrialization, capitalism and professionalization to flourish and benefit men rather than women.[5] Jean Donnison (1988), Iris Marion Young (1990b, 1997a) and Anne Witz (1992), among others, provide nuanced debates about these processes, and how democracy works to favour the already powerful, denying women and other marginalized groups access to policy-making. Until the successful suffragette movement, women literally had access to policy-making only through powerful men.[6] The long struggle to secure the right to vote resulted in women over 30 years of age being able to vote in the 1918 election. It was only in 1928 that women over 21 were able to vote. But feminist political theory demonstrates that having a vote does not ensure that women's concerns will even reach the political agenda, let alone be heard and responded to.

As feminist interpretations of creation myths suggest, control of midwifery and birth took place on the back of a long history of men controlling women. Women's sexuality and morality were particularly regulated from at least the twelfth century by the Church. While midwifery practices and women's bodies were not controlled in the way they are at the present time (because the outcome of birth was believed to be in the hands of fate or God), birth, death and midwives were tightly controlled. For example, appropriate rituals had to be closely followed at births and deaths, and midwives themselves were expected to conform to the beliefs and morals of the day.[7] As modernity took hold in the seventeenth century, its beliefs enabled obstetric thinking to arise. This redefined childbirth and its management.[8]

The dichotomous roots of obstetric thinking

It has sometimes been thought that technological developments gave rise to science and industrialization, and that the invention of obstetric forceps promoted the ascendancy of medical men over female midwives.[9] But it is usually beliefs that give rise to technology and how it is used.[10] Without the scientific belief system underpinning modern medicine, the damage perpetrated by forceps that I referred to on page

23 could not so easily have been construed as teething problems in need of refinement.[11]

Broadly speaking, modernity meant assuming that applying a certain definition of rationality (which I challenged in Chapter 2) to our world provides a more accurate understanding of reality and thus provides the means to manipulate and control it more effectively – to our ultimate benefit.[12] It is this multiflawed philosophy that promulgated a set of beliefs that made the suppression of midwifery more probable and the rise of medicine more possible.

This way of thinking assumed that the world could be dichotomized (reason/emotion, culture/nature, mind/body for example) and that these dichotomies could be aligned with male/female distinctions, where all that is privileged is attributed to the male category. This in itself was not a completely new idea. Feminist anthropologists have argued that in all cultures women are subjugated by a culture/nature dichotomy, where they symbolize nature.[13] But modernity's overall categorization of hierarchical values systematically defined and disadvantaged women and benefited a small group of men. Modernity's assumptions provided the basis for the development of medicine as we know it. The modern mind's belief in rationalism and faith in science[14] apparently 'freed birth from the constraints of nature and opened it to improvement'.[15] This belief provided the conceptual framework that legitimized obstetric knowledge and practices and initiated the technology to create its tools of the trade.

The dislocation of mind and body is an important storyline in the development of obstetrics. Again this was not entirely new. Sociologists of the body and feminists tell us that women's bodies and bodily functions have been considered to be threatening to social order for much of history and that the womb has been the focus of attention all over the world.[16] Ordering the body orders society.[17] Hierarchical dichotomous thinking cemented the mind/body split, however, and as I described in Chapter 2, attributed reason to the mind, left the body as inanimate, brute mass, and thus paved the way for its mechanistic construction central to the ideology and practice of obstetrics. The body was the material site on which to defy the constraints of and improve on nature.

Capitalism and poverty

Sociologist Anne Witz (1992) suggests that the transition from what she calls pre-modern to modern practices of medicine took place in a 'structural matrix of patriarchal capitalism'.[18] In pre-modern times women practised healing in domestic settings and both healing and medicine were based on informal, experiential knowledge. At the end of the eighteenth century, an expanding middle class with disposable income made the expansion of formalized medical services in the public sphere possible. The subsequent restructuring of medical markets promoted medical men and demoted women healers because patriarchal order demands male control of market economy in order to control the generation of and access to wealth. This meant appealing to a gendered discourse on the appropriate division of labour, whereby caring was left to women and medicine to men. It meant establishing a knowledge base for medicine, controlling its education, creating a powerful medical profession (which was done partly by uniting different branches of medicine in the Medical Registration Act of 1858), moving medicine into the public arena, maintaining control over that arena and excluding women. Once all this was accomplished, attending births became a route for men into the more lucrative practice of general medicine.[19]

Other capitalist stories circulated. While the state had had little interest in childbirth except to regulate midwifery, it was suddenly catapulted onto its agenda when ruling men were alarmed into thinking that the British race was in a state of deterioration following the humiliating defeats of the Boer Wars in 1899–1902 and reports that significant numbers of young men were ineligible for recruitment into the army because of poor physical health. This was later apparently refuted, but concerns about the nation's health persisted.[20] Statistics showed that despite a decrease in overall death rates and a drop in birth rates, infant mortality showed no improvements between 1838 and 1900.[21] The government's interest in infant mortality arose from concern about the availability of fit young men to sustain British interests abroad and provide labour for industry at home following the Industrial Revolution. It suited medical and governmental agendas to assume that health problems could be solved by medicine. This avoided addressing the more difficult cause of ill health – poverty. Just as 'dealing with the social conditions which might contribute to maternal ill-health was never going to be the bailiwick of obstetrics',[22] it was not going to be that of the state's either. Medicalization, hospitalization and centralization made much more sense in a modernist patriarchal society where 'rationality' was the main driving force. Sharing similar values,[23] it was highly likely that medical men and men in government would concur, as they did, on these issues.

Is the rationality of obstetric thinking irrational?

To establish itself as the new authority on childbirth, medicine gradually created a division between normal and abnormal birth and claimed that it should manage all abnormal births.[24] It then blurred this division and took control of both normality and abnormality.[25] In other words, birth was redefined from being a 'natural state to being always potentially pathological',[26] giving obstetrics sole claim to authoritative knowledge over all births.

Eckart Schwarz (1990) identified how the normal/abnormal boundary was collapsed by definitions of abnormality in British obstetric textbooks from 1960 to 1980. The definition of abnormality changed from a relatively narrow definition (usually based on 'mechanical failures' during birth dealt with through operative and surgical techniques), to an expanded one. This expanded definition incorporated a discourse of prevention, where abnormality was defined 'as a gradational deviation from the physiological norm'. Obstetrics moved from providing last-minute rescues to being in charge of the smooth running of 'all systems'.[27] This perpetuates the powerful belief that birth contains within it the constant potential for abnormality and that normality exists only 'after a last possibility for a pathological symptom has been eliminated'.[28]

The term 'normality' (used from the 1820s) is perhaps a misnomer as it has little to do with individual women and their unique patterns of labour and birth.[29] Under the influence of science, maths and statistics, it describes a theoretical 'norm' (Friedman's curve or a textbook labour). This norm comes from recording and plotting cervical dilation and fetal descent against a timeframe in a group of women. It is still used to assess the progress of women's labours nowadays. In the rush to rationalize, measure and quantify, medical men in the nineteenth century decided 'that the absolute length of labour beyond which it becomes dangerous, can be determined by a set rule and that it is in the power of the practitioner to judge how to achieve delivery to meet that set rule'.[30] If labour 'deviates' from this timeframe, oxytocin is used to speed it up.[31] And if birth does not occur within a designated length of time, forceps are used to expel the baby. A stark example of this timeframe comes from Ireland where 'a formal decision was taken on 1st January 1972 to restrict the duration of labour to 12 hours. After this date, no provision was made on the official record for labour to last a longer time'.[32]

Defining the body as an unfeeling, inflexible, mechanical mass that I described in Chapter 2 was crucial in the development of birth practices based on technology and tools rather than on skilled midwives' hands and able women's bodies. The pelvis and surrounding tissues were assumed to be rigid rather than flexible and women's bodies were assumed to be defective, unreliable, weak machines in need of help.[33] Thus episiotomy replaced perineal massage, syntocinon replaced the use of gravity in labour and active management replaced physiological approaches to the birth of the placenta:

> The irresistible conclusion is that the body works differently according to the ideological frame of reference within which it is thought to be captured and that the problem is one of cognition, which is itself bound up both with the way the production of knowledge is an exercise in power and with the way autonomy and agency are established.[34]

Part of the obstetric project was persuading society to accept its knowledge and practices. It then had to move birth into hospital where it could practise on women's birthing bodies more easily. It initially took control of poor law hospitals where it could further its development.[35] It gradually built on this move to hospital, promoting risk and fear and creating its own 'ideologie securitaire' based on surveillance, medicalization and hospitalization.[36] It incorrectly defined home birth as particularly risky and hospital as the only safe place for babies to be born. The decrease in perinatal mortality rates coincided with the increase in hospital births and embedded the mistaken belief that hospital birth is safer than home birth in the fabric of society.

The obstetric construction of risk applies only to the risk of death. Social concerns are not its concern. It concentrates on its technical proficiency rather than on women's needs. 'Les besoin emotifs ne present pas tres lourds face aux risques' (emotional needs carry little weight in the face of risks), or in the words of a North American doctor, 'we don't believe in taking an added risk in order to satisfy an emotional need'.[37] The:

> search to defeat death with obstetric techniques, aided by a preset bundle of risks, has become the equivalent of the philosopher's stone for obstetrics, to the extent that the whole of the current system of childbirth management is determined by this frame of reference.[38]

Obstetric thinking successfully convinced society about the unpredictability and uncertainty of birth which it alone could manage:

The outcome of every first labour is rather uncertain since there is no reliable method of knowing beforehand which will be easy and which will be difficult, although it is now possible to give statistical probabilities in groups of cases with certain characteristics.[39]

The use of the word 'risk' in medical journals in Europe and the United States has reached 'epidemic proportions'.[40] The concept of risk is now linked into the politics of managing changing populations and resources. The convergence of different strands of risk, in medicine and the new public health discourses,[41] has on the one hand forced obstetrics to dialogue with community care and consider moving services into the community. On the other hand this convergence has increased the emphasis on risk and developed self-management practices through which individuals monitor themselves.[42] The emphasis on risk has transferred obstetric practices and technologies into the community, extending the institutional 'umbilical cord' through ultrasonography and telemonitoring.[43] Not surprisingly, medical ideology attempts to control decisions about what can and cannot be 'managed' in the community. Thus risk is focused on birth while antenatal and postnatal care can be supervised in the community.

What do critics say?

Are normality and abnormality definable?

Sociologists and critics of all sorts have a lot to say about the shaky foundations of obstetric abnormality, time and risk on which obstetrics developed and maintains itself. They claim that obstetric thinking is thoroughly socially constructed from the moment of observation to the theorized concept, law or premise – and thoroughly flawed.[44] They claim that its distinction between normality and abnormality is illogical:

> Logically, the abnormal cannot be identified without a clear scientific definition of the variations of normal. Obstetrics lacks this because the risk concept implies that all pregnancy and birth is risky and therefore no pregnancy or birth can be considered normal until it is over. In other words one cannot claim both the ability to separate normal from abnormal during pregnancy and the inability to determine normality until after birth. The wide variation which occurs in the healthy experience of childbirth is too large for a single, uniform definition of 'normality', which can be used to define 'abnormality'.[45]

Does clock time make sense in relation to bodily processes?

Critics claim that clock time has taken precedence over nature's time and is used to control people in medical and other settings.[46] Feminist 'Sandra Bartky points out that in the disciplinary regimes of modern society, "the body's time . . . is as rigidly controlled as its space"'.[47] Control of time renders bodies 'docile'.[48] It is central to the 'pathway from the person to the patient'. It reinforces professional power and decreases patient autonomy.[49] It causes interventions in the birth process 'where the only pathology is that the duration of the process is considered to be excessive'.[50] But institutional time also manages uncertainty (the spectre of modernity) and the anxiety this causes. As a resident in training commented in Diane Scully's (1994) study, 'If I section her, I don't have to worry about it'.[51] Institutional time transforms women's time into a series of averages, measurements, sizes and weights,[52] bringing order to women's 'disorderly' leaky bodies and bodily processes: processes that are deemed out of time and place.[53] As I mentioned in Chapter 2 disorderliness and leakiness are disconcerting to male integrity.

Speed and efficiency are very much part of modernist practices. But speeding up labour and birth often fulfils the needs of busy institutions and the training needs of professionals rather than improving birth for women and babies. For example, Patricia Kennedy (1998) points out that speeding up labour through Irish Active Management conveniently managed the 'bottleneck' identified by Irish obstetricians.[54] In her study in England, Sheila Hunt (1995) observed an emphasis on moving women from the pre-labour to postnatal wards as efficiently as possible.[55] In North America, Diane Scully (1994) noticed that the single foremost skill required of residents in training was speed.[56] She also noticed that they were under pressure to perform a minimum number of procedures in prearranged blocks of time in order to move through their training successfully. As understaffing in maternity hospitals becomes chronic, in a curious twist of values, speed takes precedence over quality of care, and quality assessment becomes a misnomer for measuring efficiency. Student midwives are thus currently assessed on their ability to perform tasks quickly. The short-term view of time masks longer-term harmful consequences of obstetric practices. A contrasting view of time exists in the Native American community, where the group considers the consequences of its decisions on the community in seven generations' time.[57] In our own culture, the long-term consequences of birth practices remain largely unresearched and undocumented and when they have been considered, the findings are often unpopular. For example, Bertil Jacobson and colleagues' research on the harmful effects of drugs in labour on babies in later life has been largely ignored.[58]

Not surprisingly, the focus on controlling time, managing uncertainty, and increasing speed and efficiency merge as birth becomes imminent. Sheila Hunt and Andrea Symonds (1995) and Franca Pizzini (1992) commented on the speeding up or intensity of action at the time of birth: a 'speeding up of gesture and movement, an increase in the number of staff present and a kind of frenzy of activity' that can lead to the following experience,[59] where a woman believes that something must be wrong with her healthy baby:

> As soon as I started pushing, there was hysteria in the room, everyone was frantic and screaming at me to PUSH! I thought to myself, 'Something must be wrong! They've seen lots of births – they wouldn't be acting this way if everything was okay.' When my baby was coming out, someone asked, 'Do you want to touch him?' I said 'No' because I thought he was dead. I assumed he was dying or dead for them to be in such a panic about my pushing faster. When he was born and put on my belly, I was afraid to look, or to touch.[60]

In fact as Barbara Adam (1992) suggests, intervening with finely tuned bodily processes that 'are not only orchestrated into a coherent whole, but are also synchronized with the rhythms of the environment' may predispose us to physical and mental ill health.[61] And adhering to linear clock time locks us into a worldview based on urgency, time-management, deadlines, a sense of time 'running on and out' and ultimately fear. She calls for 'temporal time, the symbol of life' to be much more prominent in our society.[62] Distinctions between physiological, psychological, social and perhaps other time specific to pregnancy and birth may also be useful.[63]

Can costs be counted in different ways?

Financial implications of policy are high on the political agenda and it is frequently assumed that medicalization and technocratization is more cost-effective than social approaches. Yet, research suggests that low-tech midwifery services have good outcomes and are at least as cost-effective as obstetric services.[64] Dutch research suggests that cost and ideology are intimately connected and that cost is calculated in different ways depending on beliefs.[65] Research into the wider, long-term costs of maternity services has not been carried out. For example, during the course of my work with AIMS, I, and other colleagues have witnessed negative experiences of childbirth having long-term health effects on women, men and children necessitating repeated visits to GPs, specialists, psychiatrists or counselling services over many years. In 1996, a panel on cost-effectiveness in health and medicine set up by the US Public Health Service recommended that cost-effectiveness analysis:

> Needs to take a more comprehensive view by framing the analysis from a social perspective, assessing effectiveness and costs to society at large, and highlighting all the impacts of an intervention and not just those which pertain to a narrow perspective.[66]

Going back to the research

As I suggested on page 34 research tells us that home birth is as safe as hospital birth for healthy women and babies. However, this research often de-emphasizes women and babies' well-being by focusing only on mortality. When morbidity is included, home birth studies actually show that women and babies are subjected to significantly reduced levels of intervention and morbidity and that women have more control and are more satisfied. Marjorie Tew (1998) even concluded that home birth is statistically safer for most women and babies, even when they have complications. The attempts to prevent her completing and publishing her work suggest that this is too threatening a concept,[67] yet her findings are supported by other findings. A large study and literature review in California on the outcomes of births at home, in midwife-run birth centres and in obstetric units concluded that midwives' perinatal outcomes are consistently as good as those of obstetricians and that women having midwife care have fewer interventions.[68] The study confirmed that natural birth approaches resulted in slightly better outcomes at all levels of risk. The researcher suggested that:

> We need to keep in mind that the natural approach, while operating today in the United States under suboptimal conditions, still is able to produce these results. We would expect the natural approach, when being part of a shared maternity care system and supported by society's beliefs to produce even better results.[69]

What is risky?

There are criticisms of risk as a concept, as well as criticisms about how obstetrics defines risks and what it omits to mention. For example, as a concept, whether risk is located in environmental issues, technological developments, bodies, medicalization, or elsewhere, a number of commentators suggest that its main function is to ensure compliance with dominant forces. In Britain, for example, the initial focus on individual health was a response to imperialism. In the twenty-first century, as resources become finite and the population grows older, maintaining a healthy workforce has become an important capitalist commodity. The boundary between healthy and unhealthy has collapsed (in much the same way that obstetrics collapsed the boundary between normal and abnormal). Everyone is seen to be 'at risk' and exhorted to avoid those things that are assumed to contribute to ill health and to do the things that we currently believe contribute to good health. The ever more complicated, statistical calculations of risk are increasingly less comprehensible to the lay person, but nevertheless infiltrate more and more of the lifeworld,[70] and result in high levels of self-management and self-control in order to avoid illness and death. Frank Furedi (1997) criticizes this pitting of risk against potential, claiming that it leads to passivity and cultural docility. While I disagree with his view that violence towards women, children and minority groups is being exaggerated, his ideas about risk decreasing potential echoes with other views about positive aspects of risk.[71] These suggest that while in other situations, taking risks is valued and seen as heroic, the medicalization of birth excludes women giving birth from heroism.[72] Indeed, the notion of powerful birthing women is anathema to patriarchal domination and control.

In terms of actual risk, there is no agreement about where risk originates, what constitutes a risk, how to measure it, or how to respond to it.[73] The definition of risk might change over time,[74] and what is seen as a risk in one belief system might contribute to safety in another. Yet notions of risk are powerful determinants of behaviour:

> According to Carter, the authority of risk assessors lies in their power to make the distinction between safety and danger – this separation constitutes a boundary which defines a space in which the dangers are more controllable. Finnish obstetricians and policy-makers clearly had drawn the safety boundary line between home and hospital. In hospital the medically acknowledged uncertainties and risks of childbirth are under the control of the profes-

sionals. Parents who give birth at home deliberately cross this socially and culturally constructed boundary. In the medical discourse they are defined as a 'risk group' because of their non-compliant behavior. The language referring to home birth as risky can be seen as a social coercion technique to keep everyone in compliance with the system.[75]

Some sociologists identified technology itself as a risk.[76] Others suggest that professions and their technologies pose risks.[77] For example there are iatrogenic risks associated with technology and pharmacology.[78] Despite this, medicine has remained relatively free of criticism.[79] The criticism that exists usually questions medicine within its own terms of reference,[80] as the Cochrane database demonstrates. This has been useful, for example, those who criticized continuous electronic fetal monitoring can now refer to accepted guidelines to support their criticisms,[81] and some midwives are developing their own midwifery practices in institutional settings.[82] But more nuanced understandings about the interface between institutions and individuals is needed.[83]

The focus on risk is clear in the new antenatal screening technologies, though it is not always clear that these are often used to steer women towards aborting babies with apparent abnormalities.[84] These technologies provide women with individual risk scores that are often difficult to interpret for the individual woman. Women are then divided between discredited high and low risk categories throughout their pregnancies. Decisions about care are based on these risk assessments.[85] Murray Enkin and colleagues (1989) warn that 'the introduction of risk scoring into clinical practice carries the dangers of replacing a potential risk of adverse outcome with the certain risk of dubious treatments and interventions'.[86] Indeed, the relentless pursuing of risk during pregnancy has been cited as a potential risk itself because it can induce stress.[87]

Concluding an extensive review of the research on place of birth, and research on outcomes of births in California during 1989–1990, sociologist Peter Schlenzka (1999) suggested that 'the already apparent disadvantages of the obstetric approach have such large order of magnitude, that in any clinical trial it would be considered unethical to continue with the obstetric "treatment"'.[88] It is clear that obstetric interventions result in extensive morbidity following birth,[89] but this remains muted. Research and commentaries indicate the multifaceted consequences of birth practices.[90] These are difficult to understand and research to date has tended to focus on women's psychological vulnerabilities. However, it is crucial to understand the complex impact of birth when women are telling us that they have experienced long-lasting, life-changing consequences – especially when these include lowered or enhanced self-esteem.

From a global perspective some critics suggest that risk scoring is unpredictable of events and insensitive to the demographic, social and cultural circumstances of individual women.[91] They suggest that professionalization and institutionalization pose the greatest risk to women in isolated, poor communities. They urge us to focus on poverty and the circumstances of women's lives, to support existing and new low interventionist birth technologies, and to assist in the appropriate training of individuals so that there are the right skills in the right place at the right time.[92] A recent publication on maternal deaths in Britain clearly indicates that poverty and social exclusion put women at risk of dying wherever they are and that the policies above could be usefully applied to industrialized as well as other countries.[93]

Managing risk through obstetric time and technologies (Active Management) remains largely discredited when used routinely.[94] The 'majority of infant deaths occur outside the grasp of obstetrical knowledge' and are mainly to be found in material and social poverty.[95] Health is likely to be improved by addressing poverty and social exclusion, rather than focusing on sophisticated technological solutions and impossible expectations of self-care.

There are examples of alternative definitions of risk and safety among Aboriginal and Inuit peoples in Australia and Northern Canada where the women no longer leave their communities to give birth. This different weighing up of risk and benefit is documented in Betty-Anne Daviss' (1997) account of birth practices among some of the Inuit peoples. A collective decision was made by the tribal council to return birth to the community. It considered that the well-being and survival of the community was as important as the survival of individual babies. The argument was that the occasional death of a baby was acceptable in order for the community as a whole to survive. 'We are willing to include that [the possibility of death] because sending birth out of our villages is killing our society. We need to birth with our people in order to survive as a culture and we will take responsibility for any losses'.[96] Interestingly, there is no evidence to suggest that fewer babies are likely to die if women are removed from their communities or that more are likely to die if they remain there. Accounts of the !Kung women in Africa suggests that the heart and strength of communities may be profoundly affected by its cultural approach to birth.[97] The skills and autonomy continually passed on to women and those involved in birth practices sustain the community in ways that may be difficult to understand, but may nonetheless be crucial to its survival. For example, Jo Murphy-Lawless reported at the European Midwifery Congress for Out-of-Hospital Births in Aachen, Germany (September 2000) that a community in Bolivia rejected the opportunity to trade their skills, knowledge and autonomy about birth and death, for what they saw as disempowering and thus inappropriate medicalization.

The medical view cannot easily acknowledge other social constructions of birth. By not seeing birth as part of community life, it limits itself to seeing only what happens inside its hospital walls. Even premature and precipitous births, which are more likely to happen in the community fall outside its remit – and thus limits the provision of safety. Research in Finland also noted an increased mortality rate following the centralization of services in remote areas.[98]

What does the state say?

The state generally accepts medical ideology and practices. However, it also criticizes these from time to time. For example, it did not escape the attention of Janet Campbell, Senior Medical Officer of the Ministry of Health set up in 1919, that women who had interventions during labour were more likely to develop puerperal fever;[99] the home continued to be seen as a safe place for birth in normal circumstances.[100] However, despite the nutrition campaigns of the 1930s, the government increasingly looked to medical rather than social solutions, reluctant to 'uncover a mass of sickness and impairment attributable to childbirth, which would create a demand for organized treatment by the state'.[101] Linkages between poverty and ill health are unwelcome by governments.[102] Thus improved training for attendants was recommended,[103] along with more obstetric beds for those who needed or would accept institutional confinement.[104] The status of midwives was ostensibly supported but in reality undermined by recommendations that doctors should be in overall charge.[105] Similarly small, local maternity homes, attentive to women's social and emotional needs were apparently supported,[106] but then phased out as obstetric safety took precedence.[107] Overall the medicalization and mechanization of birth has been irresistible and the state response has been to attempt to humanize an inhumane system by 'educating' women and 'refining' obstetrics,[108] rather than to question its hegemonic ideology.

An interesting fracture occurred in the early 1990s, when a Conservative government sought to reduce the power of doctors through linking the practice of medicine more directly into market economy and promoting a politics of individual choice. Though the initial report recognized poverty as a cause of ill health and inequity during childbearing,[109] the final report omitted poverty and focused on the less contentious issue of choice.[110] However, one of the premises on which the report justified choice was its claim that safety is not an absolute concept. There was a tentative suggestion that there may be qualitative meanings of safety and that birth has the potential to be an 'enriching' experience.[111] Exemplifying both resistance to and acceptance of societal values, and a pragmatism appropriate to a Conservative government, the report stopped short of deconstructing risk and safety, and instead promoted choice through the provision of midwifery models of care. But without fully developing a social model of birth, midwifery models of care can be discounted because they are attached to women's choice rather than safety. For example, as I discuss a number of times, while continuity of carer is linked to choice rather than understood as integral to safety and well-being, lip service will continue to be paid to the importance of relationships between women and midwives. The report's attempt to transform the medical model of birth into a social/midwifery approach has been largely unsuccessful because choice carries no weight in the face of obstetric risk. In addition, medicalized views of risk assessment and management are embedded in the fabric of capitalist societies, where risk and insurance have formed a powerful alliance.[112] So while points are awarded to hospitals that demonstrate compliance with medical protocols, independent midwives are unable to obtain insurance because a social/midwifery definition of safety carries no currency.

What did midwives have to say?

Despite the systematic deskilling and undermining of midwives, some midwives have refused to be silenced or deskilled. It has typically been assumed that midwives were easily subsumed into the obstetric project because they had no recognized body of knowledge, were often illiterate, and had no group identity.[113] They have been accused of lacking political awareness and failing to professionalize in the face of competition.[114]

Feminist historians, sociologists and midwives tell more complex stories of resistance, acceptance and pragmatic or enforced compromise.[115] The portrayal of midwives as ignorant, naive and apolitical is both simplistic and oppressive.

While unsuccessful, campaigns to form midwifery societies in

Britain began as early as 1616 and 1635.[116] Visionary midwives were politically active in maintaining and developing midwifery. For example, in the seventeenth century, Elizabeth Cellier argued for midwifery training through colleges, emphasizing the benefits of female experiential midwifery.[117] In the same century, Mme Angelique Marguerite Le Bousier du Coudray travelled through France teaching midwifery for three decades.[118] Diaries, archives and commentaries,[119] for example, show that midwives had an understanding about birth physiology, skills to reduce mortality and morbidity, and concerns about relying on invasive tools such as forceps.[120] While the mechanistic view of the birthing body took hold, midwives continued to promote working with the woman and her body to assist birth – helping her to change position to enlarge the space in her pelvis for example, using birthing chairs, massage, nutrition and their hands to aid long or slowing labours.[121] These conceptually different ways of working relied on an understanding of the woman's body as both able and flexible, rather than passive and rigid. It is obstetrics' need to cut across the birth process,[122] rather than work with it that roots the obstetric and midwifery approaches in different traditions.[123] This focus on cutting across women and birth endangers women's and babies' physical and emotional well-being.[124]

The depiction of the midwife as an ignorant, dirty, dangerous, poverty-stricken old woman, (personified in Charles Dickens' character, Sairey Gamp) 'owe more to medical disdain than historical accuracy.[125] Midwives came from different walks of life,[126] many were literate and from the middle classes.[127] They were often well trained through apprenticeship schemes, involved in many areas of women's health (especially sexual health) and respected members of their communities.[128]

The Midwives' Act of 1902 in England and Wales and that of 1915 in Scotland were landmarks in the gradual subordination of midwifery (and therefore birthing women). While the Act ostensibly set out a mechanism for public protection, it actually established the control of midwifery by medical men.[129] This control has been both accepted and resisted throughout the twentieth century. As late as the 1930s community midwifery-based models of care flourished.[130] These operated until at least 1948 in what has been described as the 'heyday' of the domiciliary midwife.[131] Of course, this was set against a steadily increasing number of hospital births from 15 per cent in 1927 to 54 per cent in 1946. Following a government white paper in 1944, both the College of Midwives and the Central Midwives' Board expressed concerns that obstetric discourse was proving to be so influential, that the midwife's role was being eroded to that of 'handmaiden'. They suggested that the normality of birth and the midwife's ability to provide a service for women were being lost sight of.[132] But at the same time, a textbook for midwives asserted that independent midwives had been 'superseded . . . It would now be considered a retrograde step for a midwife to take sole charge of an expectant mother, thereby depriving her of the scientific expert care only the obstetric team can provide.'[133] Yet midwives have continued to maintain and develop their skills.[134] They provide consistently good outcomes, even when they attend some of the poorest women.[135] Midwifery research has also increased over the last few decades. Some of the first, formal midwifery research on routine procedures such as episiotomy showed these to have detrimental effects on women.[136] While midwifery mainly engages with obstetric knowledge by providing 'better' scientific research (similar to feminist empiricism), it is beginning to develop its own research agenda based on developing its own knowledge.[137] Midwifery research on the third stage of labour in the home setting has even questioned the unexamined assumption that the hospital setting has no impact on research findings.[138] The results were different from those where the research had been carried out in hospital. This is not to say that all midwifery care is good and all obstetric care harmful, but that the potential of midwifery remains underdeveloped.[139]

The costs of obstetric thinking

Restricting women's autonomy

Modernist values, concerns about the nation's health, even philanthropic concerns rather than women's voices contributed to changes in childbearing practices. Overall, 'the goal of women-centred health care has been defeated because of a tendency within medicine to trivialize and psychologize women's own accounts and analyses of what their needs are'.[140] In addition, 'professionals and policy-makers have always tended to abstract childbirth from the fabric of women's lives'.[141] So while women's concerns are to do with the 'ongoing experience of being a mother to a child',[142] and include personal values as well as physical outcomes,[143] 'obstetrics remains in a position to practise an immortality strategy quite separate to the needs and desires of pregnant women'.[144] Obstetric thinking and practices have subjugated women's concerns, power and strengths immeasurably but paradoxically, because they have reshaped many of these concerns and expectations, they might also be experienced as a gain by some women.

The consequences of obstetric thinking and practices are not necessarily obvious to women or to the commentators who have tried to understand their concerns. For example, women did not necessarily see the connections between modernity and their own poverty and ill health.[145] So the portrayal of 'early twentieth-century women's groups [being] content to exchange their power to determine the meaning of childbirth as a domestic event in return for increased safety and pain-relief',[146] as a neutral trading of conveniences, or the view that hospital birth was led by women themselves is too simplistic a notion. It fails to understand how women made decisions about birth in the context of their knowledge and lives. Women's acceptance of hospital birth, with its postnatal stay and meals could be interpreted as a response to the grinding poverty of their day-to-day lives, rather than or as well as their acceptance of obstetrics' definition of safety. Not surprisingly, campaigns by women's organization such as the Women's Cooperative Guild, the Women's Labour League and the Fabian Women's Group focused on the relief of poverty and better health care for women where 'better' often meant more medicalized:

> Each successive proposal paid more attention to the need to provide poor women with the best skilled medical assistance available. In 1914 the demand was for trained midwives; in 1917, for a trained midwife and easy access to a doctor, with specialist care and hospital accommodation where necessary; and by 1918, for a doctor to supervise every case and enough hospital beds to accommodate those in poor home conditions.[147]

The childbirth organizations that arose from the 1950s onwards (the Natural Childbirth Trust in 1956 (now the NCT), the Society for the Prevention of Cruelty to Pregnant Women in 1960 (now AIMS) and a host of other groups based on specific issues such as miscarriage or home birth for example) began to question the assumptions of obstetrics.[148] For example, while pain relief remains a controversial issue, there was some understanding that the view of women as weak and fragile was implicated with it.[149] Home birth also remains a controversial issue, but there was a recognition that women had little control over birth in hospital.[150] Just as there was then, there is still much debate about how women's concerns can best be brought onto the maternity care agenda.[151]

While some organizations were more critical of interventionist birth practices than others, feminists have remained ambivalent about the issues embedded in industrialized childbirth, because of the reluctance to engage with the body and reproduction that I mentioned in Chapter 2. Yet the obstetric interpretation of women's bodies as out of time and place mutes their individual bodily rhythms, their knowledge and their social and psychological diversities. Institutionalized time produced by professionals and machines inevitably leads to interventions. While women may feel unable to reject this powerful interpretation of birth, they 'may also recognize the violence being done and the doubtful utility of its application to each single case'.[152]

This underlying violence is a consistent theme in both patriarchy and obstetrics. Subordination and control inevitably involve a certain level of violence.[153] There are numerous examples, but the witch hunts between the fourteenth and seventeenth centuries that killed thousands of women, particularly healers and midwives, are a shocking enactment of this.[154] There are few recent discussions about obstetric violence, but where women have been able to talk about it, they describe experiences not unlike those of women who have been sexually abused.[155] As Jo Murphy-Lawless (1998a) observes, the 'deep violence to us carefully handled as science' makes it almost invisible because it is benignly interpreted as rescuing women and babies from risk and death.[156]

Whatever women's views, dominant ideologies are influential.[157] As I suggested in Chapters 1 and 2, bodies themselves can be socialized to follow the trajectories designed for them.[158] Examining maternity care, researchers have found that women are indeed coerced and manipulated to accommodate obstetric views and practices and are often persuaded that this was in their best interests.[159] The deal is: 'You can have your baby any way you like as long as you understand that I must step in when the safety of you and the baby is involved'.[160] If the woman remains unconvinced, fear is often used to persuade her 'into handing over her pregnant body to the authority of the hospital'.[161] Women may also be subjected to reprisals if they resist obstetric 'advice'.[162]

Does choice lead to autonomy?

The rhetoric of choice in maternity services has been grafted on to the restrictions in autonomy that I have just described. Thus it could be said that choice is 'a social construction that makes people feel free even in the context of oppression and supports the status quo: capitalism and patriarchy'.[163] Choice during childbearing is curtailed not only by poverty and social exclusion, but also by a restricted obstetric menu. Women have not contributed to this menu, do not necessarily know the values on which it is based, and cannot easily change it.[164] Women are coerced, steered or manipulated to choose what others want and expect them to.[165] Even when women are well informed and know their rights, most will not make choices that might antagonize their carers:[166]

> No choice is a free choice when others have feelings, beliefs and values about the choice that is made. The choice becomes much more than 'will I do this or that'. It is about 'will doing this bring other consequences with it, will it harm a relationship, will it offend, will it create barriers to on-going help?'[167]

From the discussion in Chapter 2, it is clear that the assumption in medicine that choices are made in isolation, using male-defined rationality, completely ignores that when women make decisions they usually take others' views and feelings into account.[168] The notion of choice also mutes very real power differentials between doctors and women. As Margrit Shildrick (1997) pointed out, 'the dominant material, physical, psychological power of men over women is simply unacknowledged in the fiction that the transaction is between two equal moral agents'.[169] More importantly, the patriarchal assumption that women are irrational excludes them from being moral agents in the first place. They are presented with predetermined 'choices' that prevent them being able to make moral decision on their own terms.[170] This kind of choice coupled with impersonal services focuses on communicating information adequately. Information is assumed to be correct, so communication is thought to be a neutral bridge between information giving and autonomy rather than the powerful tool of coercion it often is. Differences in opinion between professionals and women are thought to be a result of poor communication, or the woman's inability to understand the information she is being given.[171] For example, Rosaline Barbour (1990) describes how one father told her: 'We've come to see the consultant about Helen being induced . . . and, frankly, it'll be over my dead body.'[172] Both this man and another attending for the same reason later revealed that the inductions were to take place, as the doctor had satisfied them with the medical explanation he had provided. Impersonal (faceless) services reduce communication, as I discuss in Chapter 5. Birth plans have become the main strategy for women to attempt to put forward their views. Childbirth organisations transformed the Association of Radical Midwives' 'letter to the midwife' into birth plans and were designed to help women resist interventions that they did not want.[173] But hospitals quickly produced their own birth plans, to make sure that women's choices remained within local practices and policies.

Choice is seen as important because it is supposed to lead to control and 'feeling in control is central' to birth experiences.[174] However, it is clear that women have relatively little control and are usually swept along by dominant ideology. While they need external control i.e. control over their environments and what is done to them, ironically, they are expected to exert internal control over themselves.[175] This is what psychoprophylaxis was all about.[176] Interestingly lack of external control is thought to be a problem only in hospitals. 'It is this external sense of control which is most likely to be experienced as lost immediately a woman enters the hospital institution. Hence, for some women maintaining control may mean having their babies at home'.[177] 'The social relationships between the childbearing woman and her carers are different when the birth occurs in the woman's home, where she is in control and her carers are guests';[178] when they give birth at home, 'they own the whole shop and can be in charge of the whole enterprise'.[179] The women I talked to suggested a more complex relationship between control and place of birth, and that control at home was relative rather than absolute. As Maggie Banks (2000) observes, women may indeed only be 'truly autonomous' at home, but when they talk about 'I had to . . .' or 'they made me . . .' this is clearly not the case.[180] While polarized debates often place hospital and home birth at the centre of the divide between obstetric and social meanings of birth, the powerful rhetoric of choice, communication and control may result in the hospital being brought into the home, as the women I talked to described.

The gap between the rhetoric and reality of autonomy is perhaps most starkly obvious when we look at enforced caesarean sections. In 1987, Angela Carder was dying of cancer while carrying a 25-week-old baby. Against her wishes and those of her family, and knowing that the operation would probably kill her, she was subjected to an enforced caesarean section in order to save her baby. She and her baby died soon after the operation.[181] This and a number of other enforced caesarean sections seemed generally to be going a step too far for both lay and medical communities.[182] Carrying out enforced caesarean sections transgresses deeply held beliefs about the rights of the individual that underpin liberal democracies. These beliefs, however, do not prevent the day-to-day coercion of women and the increasingly punitive attitudes towards those women who challenge obstetric and societal morality.[183] The debate about autonomy is set in a complex milieu of competing ethics, the drive to improve and extend technology and the costs to society of preserving life.

How is morality defined?

Where obstetric thinking dominates, a woman cannot help but view birth through its lens, no matter what she believes.[184] And if she considers defining her own meaning of birth, she is obliged to examine her motives, morality and responsibility in the context of obstetric risk that tells her she is selfish, immoral and irresponsible.[185] Risk and morality are so defined by obstetric thinking that if women reject the belief that compliance with obstetric regimes reduces risk, they are blamed for any untoward event; this same message to comply with surveillance and treatment can be seen in feminist discussions about hormone replacement therapy and cervical screening.[186] Thus when death or damage occur in hospital, moral questions remain unasked, but when they occur at home, the woman and/or the midwife are deemed immoral because of their risk-taking behaviour.[187] In a curious inversion of usual assumptions, women who hand themselves over to practitioners are deemed to be more moral than those who expect to take some level of responsibility for themselves and their babies.[188] So it is difficult for women to reject obstetric morality and develop their own birth ethics.[189] In order to avoid retribution, many adopt uneasy compromises or take a 'pragmatic' approach somewhere between their own beliefs and those of obstetrics.[190]

So while modernity's morality prevents women from making ethical decisions based on their own ethical concerns,[191] obstetric morality limits their abilities to make and act on decisions that they believe are best for themselves and their babies.[192] In other words, it prevents them from being who they are and making decisions about birth and death,[193] as I discuss in Chapter 6. Indeed obstetrics' narrow thinking and its claim to morality has led it to the erroneous conclusion that it alone is in a position to safeguard the interests of babies (yet at the same time it often has no hesitation about coercing women into aborting babies with apparent abnormalities). This increasingly exclusive focus on babies reduces the woman from 'a complete physical and emotional being' to an 'active uterus'.[194] This means that crucial decisions about babies' lives and deaths are increasingly in the hands of medicine and technology, without reference to the ethical or quality of life considerations that parents might have.[195]

Meanwhile obstetrics remains silent about the physical, emotional and spiritual abuse it perpetrates. It says nothing about how it appropriates women's bodies and their babies, how it coerces women and undermines their confidence in their abilities to be pregnant and give birth, and how it reduces their autonomy. Instead the focus is on the individual woman's responsibility to submit to surveillance and take care of herself in ways that obstetric thinking deems appropriate.[196] There is no guarantee that self-care practices are beneficial or that they are harmless, and many of these practices are accessible only to those who are economically privileged.[197] Focusing on individual responsibilities in this way also tends to de-emphasize the impact of dominant ideologies on women's autonomy.[198] In other words, dominant ideology is more likely to prevent home births than how individual women look after themselves.

In the search for autonomy, one of our challenges is to avoid muting women's experiences by imposing medical or naturalistic interpretations of birth. In other words, we need to consider how to engage with technology without erasing women's autonomy or polarizing obstetric and social birth practices.[199] Another challenge is to encourage the authoritative circulation of women's knowledge, often dismissed as 'old wives' tales'.[200] Related to this, we need to challenge the tendency for obstetric thinking to interpret positive experiences of birth through a currency of luck, rather than accept the knowledge and skills of women and midwives. Birth literature, poetry, and accounts of births in birth centres and at home are usually freer of the obstetric gaze and can provide alternative readings of birth that portray women's autonomy and ability.[201]

Relationships between women and midwives

How do midwives engage with women?

In privileging obstetric over social birth practices, midwives' knowledge and skills and how they relate to women became muted. Obstetric thinking attempts to restrict midwifery to the detection of abnormality through set practices of surveillance (midwifery by numbers) and a nebulous form of emotional 'support'.[202] There is thus a false sense that the midwife, her skills, and how she is has little impact on how the birth process unfolds. Women and midwives challenge this view and urge midwifery to define what it is and does and make itself more visible.[203] Researchers in midwifery have suggested that midwives can provide therapeutic relationships,[204] caring relationships,[205] and professional friendships;[206] they bring a range of qualities to these relationships.[207] These complex interactions are often referred to as support and this support is considered to be beneficial.[208] Indeed, support from midwives can improve outcomes,[209] and social support has also been shown to decrease the length of labour and the need for interventions.[210]

But we need to know more about support, how and why definitions of support vary and whether or not they coincide with women's views about what they need. For example, Active Management promotes continuous support for women during labour and birth. But this is to ensure compliance with its methods, retain control of the woman and assist her to remain in control of herself. As the painful scene described by Elizabeth Baines articulates, the costs of compliance with obstetric management includes alienating the woman from her own body and knowledge.[211] In attempts to counteract the impacts of stress and poverty, social support has been provided by midwives for women who have had premature or low-birth weight babies, and those living in poverty.[212] Few midwives have considered Nicky Leap's (2000) approach of encouraging women to draw on their own social networks before and during birth, so that ongoing practical and emotional support is in place after birth. So how support is provided depends a great deal on the beliefs and skills of those providing that support, and how far they are able to engage with women's individual circumstances. The way in which midwives have become professionals has a bearing on these issues.

Does professionalization distance midwives from women?

Historical accounts of midwifery suggest that midwives were initially regulated in much the same way as other trades through training and certification.[213] As science and technology gained currency, so too did professionalization. Midwifery was forced to compete by organizing itself. As I alluded to earlier, it was disadvantaged by having to do this in a gendered political climate, depending on 'proxy male power'.[214] It was dominated by medicine that deemed it inferior and outmoded – but a necessary inconvenience because it served poor women.[215]

Professionalization was part of a process of demoting existing beliefs and practices and establishing the 'modern' beliefs and practices of science based on reason.[216] As midwifery struggled to survive by moving towards professionalization during the nineteenth century,[217] it was obliged to define itself through modernity's 'scientific' knowledge, and align itself with the dominant values of the day rather than with the women it had always served.[218] Ironically, while it professionalized in order to gain its own Act and thereby increase its status, oppressive morality and humility became the order of the day. Those midwives who questioned the restrictions imposed on them by professionalization and medical control, or who continued to align themselves with women were persecuted.[219] This conflict of allegiances has intensified over the last few decades, resulting in midwifery aligning itself ever more closely with the 'powers that be'.[220] Midwives are currently in the untenable 'piggy-in-the-middle' position between employment legislation, evidence-based care, local policies and practices, and women.[221]

The combination of professionalization, medicalization and hospitalization introduced deep divisions between women and midwives. Historian Susan Pitt (1999) noted that the seemingly innocuous change in terminology from midwives being 'on the district', to being 'in the community' in the years between 1948 and 1970 indicated a profound change in the relationships between midwives and birthing women. 'On the district', the midwife was a more autonomous figure in the same geographical and social network as birthing women and their families. 'In the community', she became an outreach worker for a hospital service. She was no longer part of the community and surveillance became part of her job.

Rising birth rates within the more 'streamlined', factory-like hospital services of the 1960s and 1970s further fragmented relationships between women and midwives. Midwives increasingly worked in specialized areas and the sharp rise in the use of interventions in the 1960s and 1970s meant that although midwives attended most births, they were unable to use their clinical judgement.[222] A more distant relationship developed, with midwives carrying out doctors' orders and processing women through birth rather than supporting the process of birth by relating to individual women.[223]

As midwifery has adopted the values of modernity and its definition of what it means to be a professional, it has limited the way in which midwives engage with women. Many midwives have been encouraged to see knowledge in restricted ways and to see themselves as experts who must impose their expert knowledge on women.[224] Thus advising, monitoring and providing technical competence are seen as appropriate activities for the professional midwife. These reduce the likelihood of caring relationships based on mutuality and partnership developing.[225] In other words the contribution of personal 'biographies' (histories, qualities, skills and experiences) to knowledge, that I described in Chapter 2, is muted.[226] The restricted view of professionalism reduces the level of engagement between women and midwives and limits their abilities to develop their own authoritative knowledge and this knowledge is often dismissed as mysterious and untrustworthy – anathema to science. It deprives midwives of the support women can give them when relationships develop, as the campaigns to support apparently dissident midwives in Europe and North America attest to. Unless we rethink the

values on which professionalism is based and collapse distinctions between science/experience, rational/emotional, competency/care, doing/being, and so on, current concepts of professionalization cannot easily help women and midwives engage in meaningful relationships that acknowledge women's concerns and differences.[227]

The current concept of professionalization cannot easily understand the richness of relationships and how trusting relationships contribute to safe birth. The more sterile continuity of care is thought to be adequate and appropriate.[228] Yet, when women experience care from known and trusted midwives, they appreciate the many benefits.[229] The harm perpetrated by the kind of professionalism that encourages distance between women and midwives was brought home to me in an article by a woman who planned for her mother (a midwife) to attend her birth. These women were put under pressure to abandon their plans by senior midwives who believed that relationships between close relatives are not distant (professional) enough and that it is thus inappropriate for a close relative to attend a birth.[230] In another example recounted to me, a woman was rebuked for attempting to engage with her pregnant midwife over their shared experiences of pregnancy. She was told that the midwife was there to discuss the woman's pregnancy only.

While we know that relationships are central to knowledge and empowerment,[231] detached professionalism has muted important work on engagement and caring in midwifery and nursing.[232] The neglect of relationships reflects the values of patriarchal thinking and how it has impacted on how we organize our lifeworlds. As feminists point out, the focus on detachment rather than engagement means that we have:

> Learned a great deal about the development of autonomy and independence, abstract critical thought and the unfolding of a morality of rights and justice in both men and women. We have learned less about the development of interdependency, intimacy, nurturance and contextual thought.[233]

In an effort to organize itself, in order to secure its future, midwifery largely absorbed the knowledge and values of obstetrics and abandoned its own. It continues to stay within the boundaries sanctioned by obstetrics. Thus the professionalism it aspires to cannot easily provide a space in which women and midwives could expand their knowledges about childbearing, develop midwifery practices, or reconstruct their own subjectivities.

Do relationships have anything to do with safety?

I have suggested that obstetric thinking reduces women's autonomy. I have also suggested in this chapter and the previous one that trusting relationships based on respect, reciprocity and mutuality increase autonomy. That safety might also depend as much on relationships as on technical expertise remains even more muted by current models of maternity care. Considering this possibility leads to a view of safety that is rather different to obstetrics' view of safety. In this view safety is less of a stable entity and more of a process. This process is influenced by the ongoing dialogue (or lack of dialogue) between the woman and her midwife.[234] The woman is safe and feels safe when the midwife engages with her beliefs and concerns. Trusting relationships, autonomy and safety seem utterly inseparable in this way of thinking. Julianna van Olphen Fehr (1999) has focused on how the relationship continuum between woman and midwife through pregnancy, enables the woman to move physically, emotionally and spiritually safely through childbearing. The advantages of the engaged professional friend and the risks to women and babies posed by the emotional poverty of medicalized professionalism became self-evident to me when I witnessed my sister's struggle to carry and birth her twins with practitioners who were unable to engage with her concerns and saw her as an obstacle to the safe removal of her babies. The two skilled independent midwives who finally attended her, trusted her decisions and used their midwifery skills to work with her and her body to maintain both the safety and the integrity of her and her babies. Successful outcomes based on the forging of engaged relationship and skill are frequently dismissed as anecdotal. But these 'anecdotes' carry within them an understanding of the social meaning of birth. They show how midwifery skills work with the woman and her emotional and bodily processes that avoid inflicting the muted violence of obstetrics so rarely spoken about.[235]

Of course we must be wary of romanticizing relationship and muting other aspects of it, such as the potential for 'burnout' among midwives,[236] or the power differentials that leave the 'practitioner woman relationship open to the tentative hopes of the women being overridden by the practitioner'.[237] Some practitioners may be judgemental, abuse their power and blame the woman,[238] especially when she is struggling with poverty and marginalization. However, without acknowledging the potential of relationships, we perpetuate a reliance on faceless others, choice, communication, birth plans and control. All of these fail to address women and midwives' autonomy

and their abilities to determine their own ethics and practices around birth.[239]

Where does all this lead us?

From a feminist view, the underlying problems in obstetrics stem largely from the disconnections, distances, disassociationsm and dualisms of modernity, how it views decision-making and how it defines what it means to be a person. From a modernist lens, obstetric ideology and practices are entirely logical. They arise from the disassociations of mind, body and spirit.[240] From the woman's point of view, they mute her concerns and prevent her from shaping maternity services in line with these. Women and midwives have been hampered in their attempts to forge a coherent and authoritative alternative to obstetric thinking for a number of reasons. We have 'the difficulty of contesting the scientific approach, for it is a deeply privileged one, deeply embedded in our culture'.[241] Similarly, Kirsi Viisainen (2000a) points out, that while feminist research has attempted to bring issues of concern to women to light and create different views of childbirth, it simultaneously shows 'how deeply influential medical thinking has been on the western understanding of childbirth'.[242] In fact we lack feminist constructions of birth,[243] and there have been tensions between traditionalism and feminism.[244] However, debates challenging obstetric birth are occurring among women and midwives and feminist principles are being used to reframe birth ideology.[245] So the frequently used term 'woman-centred' may well provide a way out of obstetric thinking and become a reality, but without further theorizing about what it could mean, it remains a largely empty concept.

The next three chapters contribute to this theorizing based on women's views about what safety and risk mean for them, how they define supportive relationships with midwives, why they find obstetric ethics to be unethical and how birth impacts on them as women. In the next chapter on safety, the women question the knowledge on which obstetric risk and safety are based and describe how their concerns are part of a different definition of risk and safety.

Notes

1 Lewis 1990: 22.
2 Arney 1982; Donnison 1988; Murphy-Lawless 1998a; Towler and Bramall 1986.

3 Pateman 1989: 38; Rabuzzi 1994; Spretnak 1999; Starhawk 1990.
4 Pateman 1989.
5 Pateman 1989: 45; Witz 1992.
6 Witz 1992.
7 Donnison 1988: 14; Marland 1993b.
8 Murphy-Lawless 1998a.
9 DeVries 1989.
10 Arney 1982; DeVries 1989; Oakley 1984.
11 Murphy-Lawless 1998a: 151.
12 Oakley 2000.
13 Ortner and Whitehead 1981.
14 DeVries 1989.
15 Arney 1982: 25.
16 Braidotti 1997; Douglas 1966; Featherstone et al. 1991; Martin 1987, 1990; Shildrick 1997; Turner 1987.
17 Douglas 1966.
18 Witz 1992: 66.
19 Donnison 1988.
20 Inter-Departmental Committee 1904.
21 Oakley 1984.
22 Murphy-Lawless 1998a: 76.
23 Wagner 1994.
24 Arney 1982; Oakley 1984; Witz 1992.
25 Arney 1982: 25.
26 Oakley 1984.
27 Schwarz 1990: 52–55.
28 Murphy-Lawless 1998a: 168.
29 Murphy-Lawless 1998a: 162–171.
30 Murphy-Lawless 1998a: 88.
31 Schwarz 1990: 54.
32 O'Driscoll, in Kennedy 1998; 13.
33 Murphy-Lawless 1998a; Turner 1987, 1991.
34 Murphy-Lawless 1998a: 258.
35 Donnison 1988; Robinson 1990: 70.
36 Lemay 1997: 83–84.
37 Lemay 1997: 88.
38 Murphy-Lawless 1998a: 174.
39 Baird, in Schwarz 1990: 51.
40 Nettleton 1997: 215.
41 Cartwright and Thomas 2001.
42 Murphy-Lawless 1998a; Peterson 1997.
43 Davis-Floyd 1992.
44 Murphy-Lawless 1998a: 158–162.
45 Wagner 1994: 99.
46 Adam 1992, 2000; Armstrong 1987; Frankenberg 1992; Murphy-Lawless 2000; Pizzini 1992; Thomas 1992.
47 Bartky, quoted in Murphy-Lawless 1998a: 208–209.
48 Foucault 1977.
49 Frankenberg 1992.
50 Pizzini 1992: 72.

51 Scully 1994: 193.
52 Pizzini 1992; Thomas 1992.
53 Douglas 1966; Thomas 1992: 64.
54 Kennedy 1998: 13.
55 Hunt and Symonds 1995.
56 Scully 1994: 162.
57 Starhawk 1990.
58 Jacobson 1988; Jacobson and Bygdeman 1998; Jacobson et al. 1990.
59 Pizzini 1992: 73.
60 England and Horowitz 1998: 138.
61 Adam 1992: 161.
62 Adam 1992: 163.
63 Pizzini 1992: 68.
64 Jewell et al. 1992; Kirkham 2003; Lincoln 2004; McCourt and Page 1997; Sandall et al. 2001b; Saunders et al. 2000; Schlenzka 1999.
65 Butter and Lapré 1986.
66 Schlenzka 1999: 58.
67 Tew 1995: 31.
68 Schlenzka 1999.
69 Schlenzka 1999: 174.
70 Peterson 1997.
71 Lemay 1997; Murphy-Lawless 1998a.
72 Lemay 1997: 90.
73 Lane 1995: 66; Peterson 1997: 201.
74 Peterson 1997: 202; Smythe 1998: 39.
75 Viisainen 2000b: 810.
76 Nelkin 1982.
77 Giddens 1991.
78 Downe et al. 2001; Illich 1976; Wagner 1994; Which? Way to Health 1990.
79 Lane 1995: 54; Scambler 1987.
80 Enkin et al. 1989; Strong 2000.
81 Royal College of Obstetricians and Gynaecologists (RCOG) 2001.
82 Central Sheffield University Hospitals 1998.
83 Lupton 1997: 103; Peterson 1997: 203.
84 Gregg 1995; Rothman 1986.
85 Enkin 1994; Strong 2000.
86 Enkin et al. 1989: 30.
87 Strong 2000; Teixeira et al. 1999.
88 Schlenzka 1999: 175.
89 MacArthur et al. 1991.
90 Banks 2000; Green et al. 1998b; S Kitzinger 1992; Lyons 1998; Ogden et al. 1997c, 1998; Rothman 2001; Simkin 1991, 1992.
91 Maine 1991; Murphy-Lawless 1998a, 1998b; Wagner 1994.
92 Maine 1991; Murphy-Lawless 2003.
93 Confidential Enquiry into Maternal and Child Health 2004.
94 Schwarz 1990: 56–57; Thornton and Lilford 1994.
95 Murphy-Lawless 1998a: 233; Murphy-Lawless 2003; Oakley 1992.
96 *Compleat Mother* 2001, 61: 22.
97 Biesele 1997.

98 Viisainen et al. 1999.
99 Janet Campbell, quoted in Tew 1998: 196–197; see also Lewis 1990; Ministry of Health 1930, 1932.
100 Ministry of Health 1930: 38.
101 Lewis 1990: 23–24.
102 Hogg 1999: 114.
103 Ministry of Health 1954: 124.
104 Ministry of Health 1956: 212; see also House of Commons 1980; Maternity Services Advisory Committee 1982, 1984, 1985; Ministry of Health 1959; Scottish Home and Health Department (SHHD) 1965, 1988.
105 Ministry of Health 1959.
106 Cumberlege 1948: 77.
107 Ministry of Health 1970.
108 Ministry of Health 1970.
109 House of Commons 1992.
110 Department of Health 1993.
111 Department of Health 1993: 10, 23.
112 Cartwright and Thomas 2001.
113 Dalmiya and Alcoff 1993.
114 Declercq 1994; Turner 1987.
115 Bourgeault et al. 2004; Green et al. 1998b: 64.
116 Donnison 1988; Witz 1992.
117 King 1993.
118 Gelbart 1993.
119 Marland 1993b; Murphy-Lawless 1998a; Schrader 1987; Wilson 1995.
120 Murphy-Lawless 1998a: 97.
121 Filippini 1993; Murphy-Lawless 1998a; Schrader 1987; Wilson 1995.
122 Murphy-Lawless 1998a: 171–173.
123 McAdam-O'Connell 1998: 25.
124 Murphy-Lawless 2003.
125 Dickens 1844/1998; Harley 1993: 31.
126 Ortiz 1993.
127 Evenden 1993; Harley 1993; Hess 1993.
128 Evenden 1993; Filippini 1993; Harley 1993; Hess 1993; Lindemann 1993; Marland 1993a; Weisner 1993.
129 Donnison 1988; Robinson 1990: 65.
130 Peretz 1990.
131 Peretz 1990; Robinson 1990: 71.
132 Robinson 1990: 73.
133 Margaret Myles in Schwarz 1990: 58.
134 Cronk 1992, 1998a, 1998b; Sutton 2001.
135 Allison 1996; Donnison 1988.
136 Sleep et al. 1984.
137 Downe 2004; Kirkham 2000.
138 Pritchard et al. 1995.
139 Schlenzka 1999.
140 Kennedy and Murphy-Lawless 1998: 8.
141 Lewis 1990: 15.
142 Murphy-Lawless 1998a: 47.

143 Lewis 1990: 15.
144 Murphy-Lawless 1998a: 48.
145 Davis 1978.
146 Lewis 1990: 26.
147 Lewis 1990: 19.
148 Beech 1990; Durward and Evans 1990; Kitzinger 1990; Reiger 2000.
149 For a discussion about pain and its relief, see Anderson and Leap 2004; Leap 1996.
150 Durward and Evans 1990.
151 Kitzinger 1990: 101.
152 Pizzini 1992: 70.
153 Foucault 1980.
154 Ehrenreich and English 1973: 24.
155 Kitzinger 1992.
156 Murphy-Lawless 1998a: 103.
157 Lukes 1974; Mackenzie 2000; Meyer 1992.
158 Pasveer and Akrich 2001: 232.
159 Green et al. 1998b; Holloway and Bluff 1994; Jordan 1997; Kirkham 2004; Lane 1995; Levy 1998; Machin and Scamell 1997; Shapiro et al. 1983; Trevathan 1997.
160 Romalis 1985: 190.
161 Smythe 1998: 58.
162 Green et al. 1998b; Hewson 1994; Jones et al. 1998; Robinson 2004a, 2004b; Scully 1994.
163 Gregg 1995: 27.
164 Browner and Press 1997; Cartwright and Thomas 2001; Kirkham 2004; Kitzinger 1990; Lazarus 1997; McAdam-O'Connell 1998; Mander 1993, 1997; Mason 1998; Wagner 1994.
165 Davis-Floyd and Sargent 1997; DeVries et al. 2001; Green et al. 1998b; Kirkham 2004; Levy 1999a; Machin and Scamell 1997.
166 Romalis 1985; Smythe 1998.
167 Smythe 1998: 232.
168 Belenky et al. 1986; Gilligan 1985.
169 Shildrick 1997: 86.
170 Edwards 2004c.
171 Kitzinger 1990: 109.
172 Barbour 1990: 203.
173 This 'letter to the midwife' was initially developed by members of the Association of Radical Midwives and then further developed into a birth plan by childbirth activists.
174 Green et al. 1998b: 160.
175 Green et al. 1998b; Kitzinger 1990: 107–108.
176 Wright 1964.
177 Green et al. 1998b: 19.
178 Campbell 1997: 4.
179 Martin 1987: 143.
180 Banks 2000: 214–215.
181 Hewson 2004.
182 Dolan and Parker 1997; Goldbeck-Wood 1997.
183 Hewson 2004.

184 Davis-Floyd 1992; Martin 1987; Murphy-Lawless 1998a: 229; O'Connor 1992; Viisainen 2000b.
185 Lemay 1997; O'Connor 1992, 1998; Viisainen 2000a, 2000b, 2001.
186 Harding 1997; Howson 1995.
187 See, for example, Anderson 2004; Bourgeault et al. 2001: 54; Wagner 1995.
188 Green et al. 1998b: 24.
189 Davis-Floyd 1992; Martin 1987.
190 Viisainen 2000a: 81; 2001: 812.
191 Belenky et al. 1986; Gilligan 1985.
192 Murphy-Lawless 1998a: 253.
193 Murphy-Lawless 1998a: 240–241.
194 Kennedy 1998: 10; see also Arney 1982; Duden 1993; Beard, in Oakley 1984.
195 Murphy-Lawless 1998b: 226.
196 Viisainen 2000b: 802.
197 Harding 1997; Lane 1995; Peterson 1997.
198 Benson 2000; McLeod and Sherwin 2000.
199 Murphy-Lawless 1998a, 1998b.
200 Cosslett 1994; Dalmiya and Alcoff 1993.
201 Adams 1994; Cosslett 1994; Kirkham 2003; Kirkham and Stapleton 2004; Noble 2001; Rabuzzi 1994; Thomas 1997.
202 Green et al. 1998b; Robinson 1990.
203 Edwards 2004a, 2004b, 2004c; Thompson 2004.
204 Siddiqui 1999.
205 Halldorsdottir 1996; Halldorsdottir and Karlsdottir 1996; Mander 2001; van Olphen Fehr 1999.
206 Pairman 2000.
207 Halldorsdottir 1996; Halldorsdottir and Karlsdottir 1996; McCrea et al. 1998.
208 Waldenstrom 2004; Waldenstrom et al. 2004.
209 Rooks 1997.
210 Hodnett et al. 2004; Mander 2001.
211 Elizabeth Baines, quoted in Adams 1994: 53.
212 Davies 2000; Evans 1987; Oakley 1992; Oakley et al. 1996.
213 Donnison 1988; Marland 1993b; Witz 1992.
214 Witz 1992.
215 Donnison 1988; Witz 1992.
216 Oakley 2000.
217 Heagarty 1997.
218 Heagarty 1997; Kirkham 1996; Pitt 1999.
219 Heagarty 1997: 74–79.
220 Kirkham 1996.
221 Clarke 1995; Edwards 2004a, 2004b; Murphy-Lawless 1991; Schwarz 1990.
222 Robinson 1990: 76–79.
223 Hunt and Symonds 1995.
224 Davies 2004.
225 Wilkins 2000.
226 Thompson 2004; Weiner et al. 1997.

227 Fielder et al. 2004; Pairman 2000; Thompson 2004.
228 Green et al. 1998a; Hundley 2000; Lee 1997; Murphy-Black 1993.
229 Edwards 1998; Fleissig and Kroll 1997; Fleming 1996, 1998; Flint 1991; Kirkham 2000; McCourt 1998; McCourt and Page 1997; Page 1992; Pairman 2000; Perkins and Unell 1997; Price and Williams 1998; Sandall 1995; Sandall et al. 2001b; Smythe 1998; van Olphen Fehr 1999; van Teijlingen et al. 2003.
230 Ann and Heidi 2001.
231 Belenky et al. 1986; Gilligan 1985; Ruddick 1989.
232 Halldorsdottir 1996; Halldorsdottir and Karlsdottir 1996; van Olphen Fehr 1999.
233 Belenky et al. 1986: 6–7.
234 Smythe 1998.
235 Murphy-Lawless 1998a; Rothman 2001; van der Hulst and van Teijlingen 2001.
236 Sandall 1997.
237 Smythe 1998: 174; see also Fleming 1994, 1998; Guilliland and Pairman 1995.
238 Robinson 2004a, 2004b.
239 Thompson 2004.
240 Davis-Floyd 2002; Spretnak 1999.
241 Murphy-Lawless 1998a: 45.
242 Viisainen 2000a: 53.
243 Savage 1990: 340.
244 Davies 1996; Daviss 1999.
245 Downe 2004; Guilliland and Pairman 1995; Stewart 2004a; Thompson 2004.

4 What's safe and what's risky?

Safety is not an absolute concept. It is part of a greater picture encompassing all aspects of health and wellbeing.[1]

In this chapter, I look at how women engaged with obstetric definitions of risk and safety. I explain how women's broader concerns of giving birth to and integrating a new family member challenged the narrower concerns of obstetric ideology. As the women weighed up the costs and benefits of home and hospital birth and identified the positive attributes of home birth, they developed a more complex concept of safety. This included the notion of safety as an ongoing process, an engaged dialogue between skilled midwives and the woman's own knowledge, and the protection of the woman–baby relationship. Women's explanations shed light on how to promote safe birth in a western context, by developing an authoritative social approach to birth, based on women's and midwives' collective knowledges.

This discussion about risk and safety is located in a relatively affluent country with accessible medical services. In Scotland, relatively few babies die and even fewer women die.[2] Death is rare enough that although the women were aware of its possibility, they expected to survive. The impact of this on women's views and experiences is profound and I can only attempt to imagine what it might be like to face the debilitating poverty and ill health that many women do all over the world, and the constant reminder that death occurs all too often during childbirth. So while uncertainty is ever present, the women in this study were able to focus on confidence rather than fear, as they did not generally fear for their lives or those of their babies. Yet, paradoxically, the decrease in danger has been met with a greater emphasis on risk and the pervasive message that obstetric units are safe and homes are risky places in which to give birth. Obstetrics generates 'free-floating' fear,[3] making it difficult to engage with risk and potential in more meaningful ways. This free-floating fear is connected to the growth of a 'risk society' where we are saturated with the pervasiveness of risk and the uncertainty about it.[4] Because of this, we are obliged to negotiate between the knowledge that science has produced open-ended long-term effects and the understanding that we cannot measure these effects or prevent or repair their damage. The juxtaposition of birth being less risky in terms of mortality and the greater cultural focus on risk means that those women who are most sceptical about obstetric ideology are most likely to be accused of placing themselves and their babies at risk, despite evidence to the contrary. It is this pervasive free-floating fear that exacts a 'coercive contract',[5] in which compliance with obstetric advice is seen as responsible and questioning that advice is defined as immoral.

Obstetric ideology frequently uses women's desires to do their best for their babies and families to persuade them to override their carefully considered ethical judgements. For example, one woman described a conversation with a doctor during a previous pregnancy, when she told him about her carefully considered decision to give birth to her breech baby vaginally. He immediately focused on the unlikely worst case scenario and accused her of selfishness in order to persuade her to change her mind. He asked her:

> *It's like, have I considered that this baby could be brain damaged, you know. I should be considering this, and don't I think I'm being a little bit selfish in not considering how my mother and my brothers and sisters and my other two children will feel about this.*

Of course, questioning authoritative meanings of birth is challenging for both the researcher and women, as we are all profoundly touched by our culture. But staying focused on the women's accounts, and listening to how they talked about their experiences and feelings showed me just how far women are able to create their own meanings.[6] Letting women lead me into hitherto unimagined realms opened up concepts of risk and safety that are invisible within dominant obstetric ideology, but that are nonetheless compelling and crucial if we are to find ways of developing safe alternatives to obstetric birth. This muting of knowledge by obstetric ideology is exactly the kind of muting that I discussed in Chapter 2.

Whatever their views about birth, it goes without saying that the women were passionately concerned about their own and their babies' safety and that there was no question about abandoning safety as a central concern. It became increasingly clear, however, that obstetrics does indeed distil complex issues of safety in narrow ways that mute other aspects of it. As the women discussed the advantages of home birth and the disadvantages of hospital birth, they included aspects of birth that are unacknowledged in modern obstetrics. While most research on place of birth looks at mortality and morbidity, birth outcomes for these women included their own and their families' physical, emotional and spiritual health and well-being. Their definitions of safety dissolved the arbitrary divide between short-term physical health and long-term well-being because birth takes place in the context of their life journeys. In other words, the narrow focus of obstetrics was in sharp contrast to the women's broader aspirations to create a more integrated safety, where physical health is not disconnected from well-being.

Challenging the authority of authoritative knowledge

The construction of obstetric risk is cast in the interacting patriarchal discourses I discussed in Chapter 3 and is therefore deeply implicated with belief systems and morality.[7] It forms part of our cultural authoritative knowledge.[8] It would be difficult to explain the extraordinary suppression of research showing the potential range of benefits for women and babies of a social approach to childbearing and the potential harms of obstetric procedures, other than in terms of power relations. As I suggested earlier, knowledge pathways are anchored through dominant belief systems and knowledge is generally sought to confirm those beliefs rather than necessitate their reconstruction in ways that might alter the societal balance of power.[9]

However, despite the development and control of elitist knowledge based on supposedly verifiable scientific truths, the suppression of competing ideologies, and the incorporation of obstetric ideology into the fabric of society, women continue to voice their concerns and challenge authoritative knowledge: they question its logic, assumptions and ethics. Thus in planning home births, they raised questions that challenged the construction, certainty and safety of obstetric policies and practices. Many women's views were located against a wealth of experience about the shortcomings of medical certainty and the de-emphasizing of women's health in modern medicine:

> *I was rushed in for an appendectomy and it turned out not to be appendicitis and I just had a horrendous six months after that*

with antibiotics and tests and trying to find out what it was. And I just thought, they just don't know loads of things really and in terms of women's gynaecology, aren't that interested. And so I think around maternity it's kind of similar really.

I would like to challenge some of the things people say. Like for example that the monitoring machine is completely safe. Nobody knows. You can't say that. They use it and any doctor will say it's safe to use. And they have no right to say that. What they should say is that there's inconclusive evidence, but as far as they know it's okay.

Even when apparent statistical certainty exists, this cannot simply be applied to the individual woman and baby, and may be interpreted in different ways depending on the perspectives, circumstances and concerns of the individual:

I mean, what he [obstetrician] said to me was that there's a definite 5 per cent chance that your uterus will rupture. And I said, that's fine isn't it, cos there's a 95 per cent chance that it won't, you know. So where's your argument then? And it's like, if I was coming to have an operation that might better my life or not, you'd be going – but it's 95 per cent effective wouldn't you? And so what's the difference? So I can't see why they can't be positive about my birth.

Indeed, one of the initial ways in which women challenged authoritative knowledge was through its own internal logic. Although decision-making processes are complex and women planned home births in diverse personal/social milieux, all the women engaged with obstetric risk and referred to research findings to support their views.

Engaging with statistical research

Of course women's concerns were broader than statistics and included how qualitative issues may impact on birth as the following quotation demonstrates:

At first I thought, no. There's no need to have anything different. I'll just go through the normal medical procedure. But as things went on, I think it was a combination of gaining confidence in the fact that childbirth is something fine, is something natural and something beautiful. So I started to feel less that it was a medical procedure and more something that could be a really wonderful experience. And I think then the second part was actually going to hospital antenatal classes which I found very difficult. I always came away feeling really quite depressed from them. I found I couldn't relate to the atmosphere there, which was very much fear orientated, and talking about how many drugs we can fill ourselves with, and how we can blot out the whole experience. And I think in the end, I just felt there's no point in me going through that. It seems so foreign to me, and the home birth seemed just a far more sensible thing to do, as long as it was medically viable. And when I talked to my GP and so on, there seemed to be no medical reasons why I shouldn't.

But dominant ideology dictates that statistics is the currency through which debates about home birth take place and women found it reassuring to find that research supported their decisions. Some women sought out more research than others, but all talked about the necessity of meeting the selective empiricism and beliefs about home birth embedded in obstetric ideology with statistics, for themselves as well as for others:

I think the things that I found useful were studies that I read that were very clear about it's no safer in hospital than it is at home. I think that I'm a great believer in well conducted studies and good statistics and things. So I think that sort of statistical information helps.

They quickly identified one of the paradoxes in obstetric ideology: that even using obstetrics' own tools, logic and figures, the statistical research on place of birth appeared to demonstrate to them that home birth is safe for healthy women and babies. Thus, if questioned about risk and safety, all the women responded through the accepted discourse of statistics, and pointed out that medical ideology rests on beliefs that its own research does not support:

I mean we often talk about it with friends etc., because they'll comment: 'You gave birth at home, oh, it wasn't very safe'. And I'll say – well you won't find a statistic that will tell you that it's safer to give birth in hospital. 'Oh, I don't know . . .'. No, no, listen to me. You won't find a statistic. You cannot prove it is safer to give birth in hospital. 'Oh', they'll say. 'Right'.

For those women who had approached birth sharing the dominant cultural assumptions about the greater safety of hospital, planning home births involved rethinking these assumptions, and engaging with research and alternative views:

> *I started reading books and finding out a bit more about it, and actually a lot of the books were saying that you're actually safer off having your child at home than you are in hospital – the risks are a lot less. I didn't actually have the facts the first time round, if you know what I mean. I didn't actually know about what the facts were. You're just always told that it's safer to have your baby in hospital and the risks are less and all this. But actually, reading the book, the actual research doesn't seem to prove that. It seems to point towards, that even if you're a high risk mum you have a much better chance of having a baby that's okay [at home]. So I think the medical profession likes to hide behind figures and say – oh you're much better off in hospital, because they can have more control over things.*

Clearly, good statistical analyses can give us invaluable information about generalities and trends in populations. As Mary Maynard (1994) points out, quantitative research on violence against women increased knowledge about the extent of the problem.[10] But it was the additional qualitative research that informed us about the nature of this violence. Thus, while statistical research was seen to be useful, it needed to be contextualized and combined with other knowledges and interpreted through women's concerns as well as those of obstetrics. Otherwise research-based evidence remains empty and oppressive.[11] So while women spent time reading and considering statistical research, like women in other studies,[12] they saw the need to differentiate between general research findings and individual, embodied women, like themselves:

> *I'm not just anybody, you know. I am above average health and fitness probably. My diet is a lot better than most people's. My confidence is probably a lot higher, and my knowledge of birth. And to bunch me in with everybody else without looking at me as an individual, I thought was a very unfair thing. To say that 33 per cent of women need intervention without looking at everything individually, I thought they were being very unfair. But then that's what systems do. You aren't an individual at that level.*

In short, they did not think that statistics could be applied to individual women in any direct or meaningful way. They appreciated the research findings because they lent support to their plans and helped gain the support of partners and other family members. However, many of the women's decisions appeared to be based on a sense of moral rightness and forms of knowledge that went beyond research findings.

It is difficult for an ideology to accept challenging findings. Accepting these threatens to undermine the already shaky foundations on which it rests. So obstetrics tends to ignore some of its own internal inconsistencies by continuing to promote hospital birth and defining women who plan home births as irresponsible. The obstetric focus on risk and physical outcomes alone has led some practitioners to consider themselves to be more responsible for babies than women themselves. Women's concerns are then cast as selfish desires for 'nice experiences'. This redefinition of women's concerns as frivolous and irresponsible in comparison to the serious and responsible concerns of obstetrics allows the coercive contract in obstetrics to retain currency:

> The obstetrician must respect the wishes of the mother and father, but only as far as it can be done without risking the health of the mother or the baby. Finally the obstetrician must be the expert who dares to set limits on 'experience hunting' and take full responsibility for the birth.[13]

Yet from the women's perspective, obstetrics' prioritizing of some perceived risks (usually those it has defined itself) and muting others (usually those defined by women), showed a very different side to its apparently ethical stance. As women pointed out, parents do not wantonly place their children in danger:

> *I wouldn't do anything to risk damaging my unborn baby obviously. But I'm doing what I think is right. And sometimes that's not what everyone else thinks is right.*

And they firmly rejected the view that they were deliberately taking risks. Indeed, neither they nor the professionals they met claimed that birth is completely risk free or always hazardous. Their accounts focused on a different set of risks, located in medicalized and institutionalized birth environments and practices:

policies and practices that are supposed to protect women from the risks of childbirth, have often created another set of risks to their physical and emotional well-being.[14]

Their concern was to avoid these risks during birth:

> *I'm less likely to be subject to unnecessary medical and surgical intervention in my own home. So that is the most important aspect of safety that I'm concerned with.*

The risks of medicalization and institutionalization

What did women perceive as risky?

Women's accounts aligned themselves more closely with the sociological than with the obstetric accounts of risk that I described in Chapter 3. Like women in other studies, these women identified risks to safe birth that included obstetric fear, impatience, coercion, facelessness, obstetric practices and technologies, inappropriate environments, and loss of control:

> *I think that the hospital environment imposes risks of its own which I find much more terrifying because I don't know what they are. I know the risks of the home environment, so I'm better prepared to cope with them whereas in hospital your risks are incompetent people or people who don't know you, or are not in contact with you, or are unwilling to listen to you and who maybe do things before it's absolutely necessary, and thereby create a whole series of problems. There's less risk of infection and you're just cared for much better at home.*

Echoing other research,[15] the women's descriptions of real or imagined hospital births included loss of autonomy over their concerns, their bodies and their babies. Like other women,[16] the thought of transferring to hospital and all that this entailed induced a feeling of fear rather than safety. This was sometimes exacerbated by bullying attitudes:

> *The consultant said to me, 'You don't need to bring a birth plan because if you come into hospital it won't be taken into consideration'.*

Planning home births was a way of reducing the impact of obstetric ideology. So while women believed that there are legitimate reasons for transferring to hospital during labour, one of their greatest fears was of being persuaded to transfer to hospital for inappropriate reasons, such as flawed hospital policies, or the midwives' insecurity, lack of skills, allegiance to colleagues or fears of litigation. (Indeed, where there is hostility towards home birth, women's or midwives' fear of transferring to hospital has been cited as a possible reason for adverse outcomes at home.) They described how risk could be located in the ideology and institutions of obstetrics with its focus on risk, generalities, routines, time limits, invasive procedures, life at all cost, and compliance.

The risk of focusing on risk

While an obstetric model of birth relies on relentlessly searching out signs of risk, the women believed that focusing on risk during pregnancy and birth generates unsubstantiated fear that undermines their confidence and paradoxically increases risk. This fear reduces their abilities to give birth safely at home:[17]

> *There's this big sort of worry that seems to surround it [birth] most of the time. Oh, something could go wrong. But it seems to be all pervasive. Most people seem to have that attitude to it most of the time. And I suppose you get into that yourself.*

> *There seemed to be this big emphasis on prevention – well, it's better that you take this drug in case this disaster happens. Or it's best you come in hospital cos we don't want a tragedy, was a quote from the consultant. It was like their focus was very much on fear, which I found completely disempowering. It made me think well maybe I can't deliver a baby. And I just found myself with a very weak attitude. So when I spoke to my sister or to my antenatal teacher and then to the independent midwife, the confidence came surging back. It was like, no, this wasn't a figment of my imagination. It is possible to have a home birth.*

Women wanted to maintain an optimism based on the premise that if all is well, there is a need to be watchful but not fearful. As two woman explained:

I don't seem to worry about things that haven't happened really.

I view birth as something you do naturally, rather than a dangerous occupation, so why would it be dangerous?

They wanted midwives to increase their confidence in birth as a normal life process, rather than dwell on the pervasive rhetoric of risk that implies, as one woman suggested, 'disaster at any moment'. Yet, obstetric practices have decreased midwives' confidence and knowledge in birth to the extent that some women felt that their midwives were 'so much more comfortable in hospital than they were at home'. Thus paradoxically, some women felt that they had to inspire their midwives with confidence rather than the other way round. The following quotation is from a woman whose long previous labour ended with a forceps birth:

I always feel they should be more confident and they should make me not have any doubts myself. But I always feel I end up trying to encourage them to think it's going to be all right. And this time round, I suppose it's harder, given the experience I had the first time.

Another woman commented that:

My experience of antenatal care was that they make you anxious and then try to reassure you.

This general fear and anxiety in the context of medicalization and fragmented care makes it difficult for women and midwives to distinguish between *peurs normales*,[18] and the kind of 'announcings' described by Elizabeth Smythe (1998), where women were indicating that all was not well.[19] Indeed, competent and confident women and midwives who practise holistic approaches to birth may be perceived as a threat to obstetric ideology. How often do we hear women say that they feel confident before antenatal visits but leave feeling deflated and anxious, even experiencing these as a 'slapping back down'.[20]

An inspiring antidote to this fear was a story told by Irish midwife, Philomena Canning, at the European Midwifery Congress for Out-of-Hospital Births in Aachen, Germany (September 2000). A woman expecting her sixth baby with an unstable lie and low-lying placenta at term went into hiding because her obstetrician had called the police, with a view to forcing her into hospital. The woman contacted Philomena, who felt that there was no reason to intervene and agreed to attend her at home. Initially she felt unable to document her opinion in the woman's notes, because she felt diffident about openly challenging the view of her medical colleague. On reflection, she realized that midwifery knowledge is as authoritative as that of obstetrics and that midwives must document their knowledge, for the benefit of women and midwifery. The woman gave birth safely at home as planned.

While all remained well, the women's focus was on the potential of birth. If they or their baby seemed unwell, this would take priority. This did not mean that they thought that other aspects of birth should be ignored. As Elizabeth Smythe (1998) observed, it is crucial to maintain what matters to women as far as possible. Responding to complications need not mean ignoring women's concerns, and imposing others. It is this separation of concerns and the assumption that obstetric concerns should take priority that troubled women.

> *What I feel is, just read the signs and stay with what's happening and try and deal with each moment at a time. I suppose 'safe' is that you can trust in the moment and deal with it appropriately and that if there was a need for medical intervention then that choice would be open.*

Women's optimism is frequently pitted against obstetric's pessimism, with obstetrics suggesting that women's optimism is a sign of lack of morality and responsibility. From the above discussion it is clear that on the contrary, women's focus on optimism is a responsible moral position. This position is based on their concern to promote safe birth in a way that reduces the likelihood of requiring potentially harmful interventions, in the knowledge that birth usually unfolds straightforwardly.

While dwelling on risk was seen as counter-productive, being ready to respond to complications was seen as necessary. Women considered the presence of midwives, the availability of flying squads in some areas and the ability to transfer into hospital as the main 'safety-net' available. However, there were few indications that women were able to engage with the complexities of uncertainty in discussion with their midwives. Most discussions focused on the risk of the baby not breathing at birth or the woman haemorrhaging:

There's basically only two big things that can happen. The baby won't breathe or I would bleed.

In response women felt that these were unlikely to occur, and if they did, that they could be dealt with at home sufficiently well to resolve or stabilize the situation before transferring to hospital, a view that skilled midwives endorse.

Living with uncertainty: 'There's nothing in life that doesn't come with a risk'

Women understood that babies and, very rarely, women do still die during birth in Scotland. But they rejected the conflation between catastrophic incidences which occur in parts of the world when enforced 'natural' birth takes place in the context of poverty, long-term ill health and lack of access to equipment and expertise, and their own circumstances. As reports into maternal and perinatal deaths suggest, they believed that death could lie outside obstetric knowledge and expertise and that uncertainty exists wherever babies are born, whether or not it is acknowledged. This was exposed in a paper examining the number of 'near misses' in hospital.[21] The women's acceptance of living with what they considered to be unavoidable uncertainty was in direct contrast to what they saw as the medical attempt to remove uncertainty (despite the fact that its ongoing quest to predict and detect complications has been so unsuccessful that all women are considered to be at continual risk):[22]

> *I suppose for me, I thought, well, you can't guarantee anything in a birth. In a way, you take a risk every time you enter into it.*

They shared Elizabeth Smythe's view that "[b]eing safe" is more complex than any risk management is ever likely to be able to accommodate'.[23] They believed that risk management could potentially reduce the creation of safe birth by focusing on generalities and routines rather than the women's individual and changing circumstances. They were aware that uncertainty crosses the home/hospital boundary and saw the attempt to empty hospital of risk and locate it in the home, as misleading:

> *Everyone kept saying, it's safer to have a baby in hospital, which I thought was disputable, you know. And I thought, there's nothing in life that doesn't come with a risk. Driving to the hospital*

itself is a risk, and crossing the road is a risk and for them to try
and imply that a hospital birth is no risk was misleading.

Women's accounts of uncertainty created a crucial space between
obstetric 'certainty' and impending 'disaster'. It was difficult for
women to articulate this space through the pervasive language of risk,
but in the quotation below, the woman attempted to move beyond
unthinking definitions of risk, to the potential and possibilities of
birth attended by skilled midwives:

Nadine: Can I ask you what you think about safety and risk? Is
that something that you've thought about?

Oh it is. I mean, I have the feeling, like with the midwives, that
their risk levels were very low. And I'm not saying that I wish to
harm myself or the baby, cos obviously I wouldn't. But I just feel
that there are some things in life that happen, that we can't
always make the way we want them to. And like a birth is a
risky thing, and sometimes, I wish that they would feel more
willing to take more risks than they do. Because I still don't
know if we were all being prudent last time [transferring into
hospital during labour] or if we could have pushed me further. I
still don't know that. And what the real limitations and bound-
aries are. I mean my friend has had the experience where she felt
people were taken into hospital prematurely. Things could have
been handled at home. Even having a cord wrapped round the
baby's neck doesn't necessarily mean a death. So I wish that they
would have confidence to deal with things that are risky, cos
they are risky in their nature.

It was in this space between risk and potential that so-called 'high-
risk' women might plan home births in the context of previous technological births that they felt impacted negatively on their own and
their babies' well-being. Because of the lack of support for this, often
these women demonstrated the 'splitting' discussed by feminist theorists,[24] seeing themselves through both medical and social lenses, and
being compelled to negotiate the risk of invasive obstetric procedures
and the need to protect their and their children's well-being. As one
woman observed:

That's probably my biggest risk – that I have had small babies.
I still smoke. I'll have another small baby. You know statistically,

I'm in the social class – I'm more likely to have dead babies and things, whatever that means. So I'm aware of like, how they're [doctors] looking at me.

But despite seeing herself and her circumstances through the gaze of medical ideology, her experience of hospital birth and its disruption of relationships between herself and her previous babies, made her feel that she and her baby would be safer in her own home.

The risk of subjecting individuals to general rules

So, women did not feel that the uncertainties and complexities they faced during pregnancy and birth could be solved by statistics. Nor did they think that they could be safely met by the generalities and routines of obstetric procedures. It was a striking feature of the interviews that wherever women positioned themselves in relation to birth ideologies they stressed the desire to be treated as individuals and to avoid general policies and practices. Their suggestions that decisions should be made using experiential as well as theoretical knowledge, rather than the questionable generalities of obstetrics, had echoes with Brigitte Jordan's (1993) analysis of decision-making processes among birth attendants in other cultures. Like the critiques of knowledge I discussed in Chapter 2, women pointed out the limitations of obstetric knowledge as well as the problems of generalizing from populations and trends, to individuals. Essentially, the women felt that the rules and routines of obstetric practice were too general, medicalized and formulaic to create safety for the individual woman and her baby and work with the complex interactions between body, mind and spirit:

I can't help thinking that giving birth is not just a physiological thing. It's a psychological thing and I don't think that's taken into account.

Their accounts concurred with Maggie Banks's (2000) observation that:

When the labouring woman is supported by patient attendance, the time frames and experiences of physiological labour for individual women teaches us that there is only one rule that can be taken with any certainty. That rule – there are no rules![25]

Indeed, seen in this light, standardized policies or rules prevent rather than promote individualized care. As the women's accounts demonstrated, individualized care is a misnomer for care that is filtered through a set of rules designed to normalize rather than respond to the individual progress of labour and birth. It would be more accurate to suggest that individualized care in obstetrics refers to attempts to improve and humanize it through standardization of good practice and better communication. This does not amount to the kind of care in which each woman's circumstances and beliefs are a meaningful part of that care. Furthermore, set rules lead to pathways of care: the 'cascade' of interventions that preclude the development of alternative skills and practices.[26] Women whose labours needed help became particularly aware of this. As one woman attempted to explain, had she had access to more skilled practitioners it may have been possible to avoid a caesarean section, or make the decision to proceed to a caesarean section without moving though '*all* of the steps' of actively managed labour:

> *I think I maybe went in [to hospital] too early. If I'd have had an expert there saying, you can do this, then that would have made the difference. But because they [midwives] were being anxious, I became anxious. But I don't think it would have done any harm if I'd spent a few more hours at home. I do believe there wasn't any great time limit on the whole thing until they started intervening. I don't know whether if they'd left me longer they wouldn't have needed to go through all of the steps – having to break my waters, give me all these things to induce me and have all the monitors and everything that they did in-between – put me on a drip. And if I really needed a caesarean they maybe should have made that decision earlier.*

So while clock time and urgency are of essence in obstetric ideology, to ensure that labour progresses according to its designated timeframe, in the women's accounts, patience is of essence for women to birth their babies in their own times and ways. Interestingly, as services become more stretched, so does clock time: I hear more stories from women who had been prepared for forceps births or caesarean sections but had spontaneous vaginal births during the wait for medical staff or theatres to become available. While clock time has come to represent the boundary between risk and safety in obstetric management, in the women's accounts feeling safe and relaxed was the key to safe birth. In this way of thinking, clock time is not the main basis for decision-making. Thus, from the women's perspectives, imposing obstetric time on women's time posed yet another risk to safe birth.[27]

Is clock time the answer to risk?

As I explained in Chapter 3, the relationship between time and safety is far more complex than obstetric policies and practices account for. For example, the assumption that home birth increases risk because the woman is not in close proximity to doctors and technology ignores a whole set of different risks imposed by institutionalized birth and assumes that complications can be safely dealt with only in hospital:

> *The midwife really hammered it home, you know. You do understand that this may well be a small risk, but it's still a risk. And if something happens, it's ten minutes to get somebody here and less than thirty seconds or whatever in hospital.*

Because of the assumptions about time, women who lived close to hospitals often appealed to this fact as an additional lever to support their plans:

> *I think one of the main things was that we were in [city] and to get from here to the [hospital] in an ambulance would take you probably about fifteen or twenty minutes at the very most. And then somebody said, you know, to get the theatre done for an emergency section takes fifteen minutes anyway.*

Women who lived further away from hospitals were obliged to engage with this assumption more overtly. These women resisted the assumption that emergencies usually occur without warning and are catastrophic. They were aware that in the event of complications, protecting women and babies' safety depends on the vigilance and skills of the practitioner, and that speed alone does not usually confer safety:

> *I mean, if it does go wrong, and something happens, how am I going to deal with it. I mean, that's something I have to think about. If I don't get to the hospital in time.*
>
> *Nadine: What have you thought?*

I'm just too confident that it won't happen. And I'm just too confident that we'll detect anything really serious beforehand.

If there was any difficulties with the baby, all the equipment's in hospital, but at home you've got nothing was their attitude. But I mean, you have the oxygen and the midwives are very good. I mean a midwife in hospital's no different to a midwife at home who's going to cope with the cord round the neck or any of these problems.

Imposing obstetric time may lead to the 'semblance of safety' Elizabeth Smythe (1998) describes where the woman is not listened to. The Dunne case in Ireland demonstrated this: a woman in labour knew that all was not well with her twin babies. She was not listened to and consequently nothing was done to help her babies until it was too late.[28] The women I interviewed described similar experiences:

In the hospital they leave the room, or they put you in the room and leave. So to convince them that there's something going on takes a little while. And even if they're there with you, they're still not always listening, cos they're busy doing all sorts of other things as well. I'm not criticizing them, but they're not listening to what you are feeling or what you think's happening. So it could be twenty minutes before anything's picked up.

Time limits are risky

Basing decisions on the passage of clock time alone seemed illogical to women. For example, women were told that after forty-two weeks of pregnancy, they would no longer be deemed 'normal' and would have to give birth in hospital. To the women, these arbitrary time limits seemed too restrictive, and based on inappropriate, preconceived generalities rather than individual circumstances:

She [midwife] explained that they would be basically available for me for the two weeks before the birth date and two weeks afterwards. After that time, I was in hospital. That is what I was told.

Nadine: Right. What did you think about that?

No, that sounded a bit sort of like cut-off time, you know. Doesn't it depend, surely, on how I feel and what's happening with my body at that time. Cos, I mean, some babies just don't want to come out on time. It made you feel like you were on a tight schedule.

The risk of rushing

Confirming the sociological commentaries on time, a sense of urgency featured strongly in the women's accounts of maternity services. Midwives were frequently described as lacking time, 'rushing' or 'running about', and babies were 'whisked away'. There was talk about things happening 'quickly' and 'suddenly'. The prominent 'clock on the wall' (with little else to focus on) was the symbolic visual reminder that birth takes place through clock time rather than women's time. The attitude was often that, 'there's nothing to be gained by waiting – it's almost like wasting time'. It is difficult to capture in words just how this impacts on birth, the way practitioners respond to women, the pressure women feel under, and the anxiety this causes. There was a sense of time 'run[ning] on and out',[29] leading to the inevitability of obstetric interventions despite women's concerns about this:

> *Well, we sort of were in early labour for about four hours and only sort of went about a centimetre which was a bit depressing. And then the clock started ticking and, well by 12 o'clock, if we haven't gone a bit more we've got to do something about this. Which is, I mean, (sighs) exactly what happened last time. And it's just such an arbitrary thing. It's like they take this four hours out of the air and, you know, dangle it in front of you which just makes you anxious, I think. So I was really, really anxious. I did not want to go on this drip.*

The management of birth through time was particularly confusing and disturbing when the institution's time meant that the stated urgency of a situation was met with inaction until the institution found time, while ignoring the woman's time and knowledge:

> *I think the thing with my instinct was that he was all right, but he wasn't terribly comfy, and I really needed to do something about it. But I wonder if I could have done something about it at home if I'd been given a bit more time, and felt that there wasn't such a time issue around it. Which, in fact there wasn't when it turned out. There was a big time lapse in hospital. Cos*

I hadn't really wanted to do that [have an oxytocin drip] and I suppose looking back on it I think I should have just said, no, I'm not doing that, I'm just going to let it happen itself, cos it had started. It was just not quick enough.

So while women and professionals might share similar concerns, there could be profound divergences between them about how to respond to these. As the quotation above suggests, divergences often centred on the role of time and on the level of intervention needed. While obstetrics may believe that 'there's nothing to be gained by waiting', women might believe on the contrary that there is everything to be gained.

The risk of a limited timeframe

The notion of nature's time, women's time and cyclical time extended beyond birth itself.[30] It is the 'ongoing experience of being a mother to a child' that most radically differentiates the concerns of obstetric ideology from those of women.[31] The linear, fragmented time in dominant birth ideology muted how women connected birth to the rest of their lives. While pregnancy and birth are frequently disconnected from parenting, for women, the ongoing decision-making during pregnancy and birth brought them into a relationship with their babies as part of the process of becoming parents. In other words, fragmented obstetric time risked undermining the woman's relationship with her baby:

My responsibility is to form a relationship. It's almost like that the birth is a rite of passage and by the end of it, you've been through it together and you're in relationship to the baby. The baby is what comes at the end of the process of giving birth, and I think the more connected I am with the birth, the more connected I am with the baby and maybe my responsibility is to be open to having that connection with the baby.

This focus on relationship contrasts with the relatively new 'bonding' rhetoric where the complex process of relationships has often been reduced to the woman and baby spending a short time together after birth with a focus on 'skin to skin'. Even at home, women were sometimes distressed that the checking, weighing, measuring, cleaning and dressing of their babies prevented them from having the peaceful, unhurried time together after birth that they felt was so important. In fact, some women noticed that their focus on relationships was very much at odds with society's focus on separation rituals. They felt that relationships had to be thought about and nurtured by them:

The bonding is an individual thing it seems, whereas separation is a social thing. I mean, if you want to bond with your infant, then it's probably your own responsibility and you've got to work at it yourself.

The baby's relationship with its siblings was also considered to be important:

For me to come home with this strange little person, that she'd [daughter] then have to get used to. It seems to me unnatural to split up a family when there's something so important happening and such a natural event happening.

Paradoxically, by not recognizing birth as part of a network of family relationships, when parents do attempt to create what they believe to be safe birth, they are often accused by practitioners and others of not seeing beyond birth. Yet women's accounts were filled with examples of how they were thinking about the hours, days, weeks, months and years ahead of them, by focusing on birth as a rite of passage from which they needed to emerge physically and emotionally well in order best to nurture their babies:

I think it will probably be safer for me not to have the drugs and too much medical intervention. Even though it'll be much worse at the time, it'll be safer in terms of all kinds of knock on effects and the catheter and all that stuff that goes with the epidural. They make you feel ill afterwards.

Their accounts provide compelling reasons to rethink obstetric time and to consider the long-term qualitative and social implications of birth as well as the more immediate physical outcome of birth, so that safety can be seen in much broader terms:

I think it [home birth] has contributed to the sort of seamless-ness of a new baby coming into our family, and it's probably affected the way we've been with him since his arrival. We've somehow been able to accommodate him very easily and very confidently. I remember close to the time having a feeling of like, if we can do that we can do anything. And so there was a sort of sense of confidence in our abilities to look after him because we'd brought him into the world at home.

Some women felt that the experience of home birth impacted positively on their journeys and abilities as mothers:

I feel I've got more into mothering this time, and being with my family, with my children. I think it's because I'm finding a sort of satisfaction that I'd like to get into more and have more time to get into. And, I mean, that also seems to fit in with a feeling of getting something natural that I've maybe got into more deeply through the home birth, through feeling more confident this time around. It's almost like, ah yes, I can see what this is about, and I'd like to go further into it.

In essence, imposing time restrictions was identified as risky by the women because it diminished the likelihood of them being able to birth their babies in their own time and increased the likelihood of invasive procedures being imposed on them. These obstetric interventions presented not only physical risks to their bodies and their babies, but emotional risks to their integrity and family life.

'Looking at surgical intervention as a violation of women's bodies'

Like women in other home birth studies, these women talked a great deal about avoiding the dangers of interventions to the birth process. Their definition of intervention varied but tended to mean the avoidance of what Alice Adams (1994) described as 'the machine/physician [entering the woman] by way of needles and monitors'.[32] While women acknowledged the potentially life-saving attribute of obstetric knowledge, procedures and technology, they felt that their overuse compromised their own and their babies' safety. They described the simultaneous reduction of midwifery support and the increased reliance on technology, making interventions more likely. They needed:

Freedom from the technology in hospitals. I'm wary of hospitals. I'm wary of their dependence on technology unnecessarily. Technology is good if you need it but it's wholly unhelpful if you don't. I think one of the reasons is because their [practitioner's] attention is divided. You don't get their attention because it's with the machines. And I didn't want to be at risk of being strapped up or being injected with anything.

Women redefined obstetric technologies as invasive rather than benign: the material means to appropriate their bodies, control, restrain and work on them, in ways that could impose physical and emotional pain and harm. A number of women talked about the feel of 'gleaming, metal' instruments against flesh and the 'hardness' and potentially 'hurtful' nature of obstetric instruments and interventions. So while obstetrics considers birth to be risky and has developed a series of practices to make it 'safe', women not only defined these practices as a risk to birth going well, but also talked about the risk of violation:

I don't believe that one is less safe in one's own home. On the contrary, I feel that there may be a case to be made that home births could be considered safer, if you want to start looking at surgical intervention as a violation of women's bodies.

Women were not afraid of technology itself. Like those in other studies, they were attached to their babies and families rather than ideologies and had no intention of 'chasing after an ideology'.[33] There was a general consensus in this study, as in others, that prioritizing the baby's safety may become inevitable if complications occurred:

I mean, if the baby's distressed and they say, well, look, you know, we really think we'll have to go in, I'll just go in. I'm not going to risk the baby or myself just because I'm so determined to have a home birth.

They felt unsafe, however, if they felt they might become the unwilling objects of obstetric practices and technology and have their autonomy undermined. Individual women had different views about how far the environment and artefacts of obstetric birth are threatening and dangerous. This depended on how far they felt that their midwives shared their concerns, and how far they subscribed to obstetrics' 'life at all costs':

But, you know, I think this equipment can frighten you, if you're in labour. It's daunting. Perhaps contrary to some other people, I don't find those things at all reassuring and when I first saw the rooms in which women are in labour in hospital, that really brought it home to me. These gleaming sort of instruments. I mean, I would just be so frightened of what they might be for – just fixed to the wall for drips or whatever. Some kind of tubing and dials and knobs, and I wouldn't be able to tell you really what they are. And just the way the bed looks and the room is very small. It's like a cell. I mean, it's really like going to jail or something. You know, you can't just walk about.

While their homes reflected their own beliefs about birth, some women felt that the community midwives' equipment symbolized moving the hospital, with its emphasis on risk, into the home, whereas others saw it as part of creating safety. Whether or not midwives and their practices and equipment were experienced as providing safety, largely depended on where women placed midwives on the obstetric–holistic continuum and the level of trust between them. Given the views of some women, that midwives' skills to support normal birth at home are underdeveloped and their policies and practices too closely aligned with medical ideology, there was some ambivalence about just how far they could provide the kind of safety women wanted:

I mean, I really don't see how the equipment and the professionalism and the training really adds in some ways. I mean some people talk of it as a safety net and that it's reassuring. But I don't really see it that way. I mean, I find it quite sort of frightening that this possibility that things are going to go wrong, that you need a big oxygen tank or something. And would it really help if something did go wrong?

When the midwives leave the packs and things, they leave an entonox cylinder. They leave a little oxygen cylinder in case the baby needs some oxygen after it's born. So they bring all the things with them. They also bring – if you do want pethidine or anything like that – they do bring that with them as well in case you want it. So I mean, they really have everything that you could need at home.

The risky 'immortality' strategy: 'All you want is a healthy baby, don't you?'

Behind the discussion about home birth and the potential introduction of obstetric ideology into women's homes lies the issue of 'life at

all costs'. Discussion about death at birth and the possibility of negative consequences of preserving life is particularly difficult and threatening. Yet, for some women the ongoing impact of birth made the
obstetric assumption that saving life is an unmitigated success and
that not preventing death is an unmitigated failure, less clear cut.
Some women worried about having little control over decision-
making about life and death and thought that being at home might
increase their control over this, unlikely though this is.[34]

> *If the baby would naturally have died then it should naturally die
> rather than having it on life support systems and whatever for a
> long period of time. So I would want to make that decision.*

They were aware that in the same way that qualitative aspects of birth
are systematically emptied out of obstetric concerns, so too are the
qualitative aspects of death. They questioned the categorical 'no' to
death that is implicit in obstetric ideology and the impact of this on
themselves, on their relationships with their babies and on their
babies. Women clearly shared the view that the preservation of their
babies' lives was of ultimate importance:

> *I've made it very clear to them [midwives] that I'm not rigid. I'm
> really flexible about anything. If there's good reasons for any-
> thing then I want to talk that through, and I'm not going to say,
> absolutely not. Never say never. I mean, I may have to transfer
> to hospital and have every medical intervention known to
> woman. And if I do, that's just the way it is. And it won't be the
> end of the world, because ultimately all I want is a healthy baby.*

However, they did not want the focus on life itself to overshadow the
quality of that life. Women understood that difficult relationships
with their children, or postnatal depression for example, have complex causes, but felt that having their feelings overridden and losing
control had a strong impact on them. Indeed, Jo Green and colleagues
(1998b) noted that the women most adversely affected by birth experiences were those who had felt they had had unnecessary interventions. One woman explained how she felt after following obstetric
advice to have a planned caesarean section for her breech baby:

> *All you want is a healthy baby don't you? I didn't realize that it
> meant feeling . . . I didn't realize any of that. I thought it would
> just be the same. I thought, like, it didn't matter if you got one*

off a supermarket shelf or something. I mean, it was just the
same wasn't it? If you wanted a baby, you had one. But it's not.
It's definitely not. You know, even now, my relationship with my
daughter [born by caesarean section] is totally different. I just
can't get on with her. That's how I feel. I just can't get on with
her.

In other words, the very real costs of obstetric ideology and practices
need to be brought into the debate about birth, because otherwise
women remain at risk of having their bodies abused by an attitude of
'anything goes' in the quest for a live obstetric product (the baby). In
essence, the obstetric view of life at all costs may involve loss of
autonomy and aggressive/invasive techniques which may or may not
preserve life and if they do, may have long-term consequences for
parents and their babies.

The risk of losing autonomy over death

Women's need for autonomy covered two areas: the importance of the
quality and dignity of death as well as life, and the burden of keeping
babies alive that would have otherwise died. While the death of a
baby is devastating, women talked about the importance of being able
to hold and cuddle their babies. As in other birth accounts,[35] this pre-
cious time with their babies could comfort and integrate the experience in a more tolerable way. Many women felt that if their baby was
going to die, they would prefer to be at home, where the baby would
be less likely to be 'whipped' away and subjected to harsh, invasive
treatments, and kept alive when it should have been enabled to die
with comfort and dignity:

I think if anything really was seriously wrong, I think it would
be so much nicer just to let the baby die in your arms. I mean I
can't think of anything worse than your baby being rushed away
and its body battered to try and bring it back to life, and it may
be severely handicapped or whatever. Well, we don't agree with
that. We're quite keen that if anything is really wrong, we don't
want any intervention. If the baby's going to die, well, it will do
it in its own house.

We talked about if the baby – cos I suppose it's something you
have to talk about if the baby was born very badly handicapped
or died shortly afterwards, how we'd feel about it. And I said,

well, I'd probably prefer to have a baby at home in that situation because you can be with the baby. The baby's not whisked away to special care or to resus or whatever, where you're suddenly separated and you haven't got those few minutes. And also if the baby is very badly handicapped and isn't going to survive, do you really want someone to intervene and keep the baby alive when it really shouldn't be alive. And we discussed that and we both felt that we were happier at home in that situation.

Having little or no control over life and death decisions threatened women's values about how a baby lives or dies and the impact on them as mothers. As the quotations above and below suggest, the burden of care arising from a view of life that sees death as a failure would fall on them. The woman's sighs below suggest how difficult this is to contemplate:

I did think the other day, that if I had a difficult birth or something went wrong (sighs). You know (sighs) it would be nature taking its course in a way. That might sound really hard but perhaps too many children are actually born and live that maybe shouldn't. I mean, if it's taken out of your hands at some point and they give the baby oxygen that is not doing well, or not thriving or something. Then (sighs) as a parent you maybe feel afterwards that you have a burden that otherwise you wouldn't have had.

Thus women were not questioning a focus on babies' lives, but questioning how we balance other ethical concerns, such as treating the woman as a person, the quality of babies' lives and how dying babies could be treated with love and respect rather than with unthinking, aggressive procedures. The quest to erase death from birth that dismisses all other concerns not only attributes blame to parents and practitioners who deviate from obstetric beliefs and practices,[36] but also introduces a potential conflict of interests over the life and death of a baby. While women's narratives posed the question: has the preservation of life in modern obstetrics overridden other legitimate moral positions, practitioners have little choice but to bypass the moral dilemma of obstetric uncertainty and do everything medically possible to preserve life, with little consideration for the quality and dignity of that life, or implications for living family members. Mostly, the kind of safety that Elizabeth Smythe (1998) describes as 'a paradox between doing and not doing, and knowing which to do when',[37] is replaced by doing everything possible all of the time. Fragmented and time impoverished relationships between practitioners and parents meant that discussions about uncertainty could not arise. As an experienced midwife commented:

> *I think this has a lot to do with the relationship between the woman and the midwife. It was a subject frequently raised by women when I worked independently. It was rarely raised by women when I worked in the NHS and I don't think it was simply because of the changes I underwent in the process.*[38]

Thus in the day-to-day course of events, life and death decisions are removed from the agenda and the immortality strategy prevails. While women may have different views about how much should be done to save life, their accounts suggested a need for practitioners to reject the myth of immortality and move towards some acceptance of uncertainty. The attempted erasure of death from birth creates the context in which the practitioner cannot engage with women's ethical concerns and can thus objectify women and their babies and subject them more easily to painful interventions. Otherwise they are blamed in the same way that parents are blamed. So while death at birth is a devastating tragedy, it is not the only potential tragedy. Defining safety and tragedy in limited ways is endemic to dualistic thinking, but does not necessarily reflect the views and experiences of all women.

The risk of being blamed

But the women's acceptance of uncertainty and their courage to follow their beliefs was not without its costs, in the face of the persistent dominant message that desiring a home birth means prioritizing their experiences over their baby's safety. Although women planned home births because they believed them to be safer for their babies, themselves and their families, this powerfully blaming message meant that 'if anything did go wrong, you'd naturally feel guilty'. Parents are forced to come to terms with the powerful but usually erroneous view that death or injury at home could have been avoided in hospital and that even problems after birth might be attributable to home birth:

> *I mean, with [son] the first thing I wanted to know was did he get ill [several days after birth] because I wasn't in hospital [for the birth]? But that is a guilt which I get because society's con-*

ditioned me to have my children in hospital. Or is it because generally it's more safe in hospital? I think the statistics say it's actually not safer in hospital but I don't know. It's difficult to say.

The destructive nature of our blaming culture means that parents are obliged to negotiate between doing their best for their children in the knowledge that if anything untoward occurs they will experience an overwhelming sense of guilt as well as loss:

I feel that people can't understand. You know [they think] I'm taking a big risk mentally with – if this baby was to die, I'm going to feel responsible because I had a home birth. And well, you know, for me, it's like, I've had a baby die, it doesn't matter how they die or what they die of, you've still got that – if only I hadn't done this, if only . . . Every person that's lost a child has got to go through the – was it my fault? And people even blame themselves when it's a straightforward. I just can't believe that it's [home birth] any more dangerous because I don't think I'll have the same fears.

The obstetric attempt to erase death from birth by any means evokes and reinforces a culture of fear, blame and guilt around birth. Its own profound fear and lack of tolerance of death makes it unable to address social, structural and relational circumstances surrounding death. When death occurs, negligence and blame have to be apportioned to individual parents and/or practitioners, when it happens at home or outside other obstetric norms. The ideology and the structures of care, training and skills developed by obstetrics remain relatively unexamined and blameless. Thus compliance (through bullying if necessary) becomes a priority,[39] and deflecting blame onto others becomes a necessary survival strategy for practitioners.[40] Some women suggested moving away from blame towards doing one's best in the context of what they believe is right:

There's risk. I mean, women still die in childbirth and that can still happen, but it doesn't put women off having babies, does it? I think you can just sort of try your best really. I don't feel particularly scared by it and I wouldn't do anything to risk damaging my unborn baby obviously. But I'm doing what I think is right.

But given the hostile climate for midwives, while they might want to support what women think is right, they were fearful of moving outside their local policies and attracting blame and censure. This fear might lead midwives to persuade women to abandon what they (the women) thought was right.

The risk to women's integrity

Even when women knew their rights and were well informed, the power of the institution over the individual is immense.[41] They knew that in a hospital setting they would be more likely to comply with, and less likely to stand up for themselves and resist obstetric ideology and practices. One woman described 'falling into that infantilized position' where one obeys authority figures. This can decrease women's self-esteem.[42] Very similar quotations from Kirsi Viisainen's (2000b) work and my own study exemplify how expectations on women to conform put their integrity and thus safety at risk in an institutionalized setting:

> I do not want to go into hospital because of what happens to me there. I am such a good person. I do what they ask me to. And they will ask a lot. 'Let's have an enema, let's examine, all right lady, let's stay still, we'll listen to the baby's heartbeat, we'll put this strap here and this string here, and let's break the membranes.' I do not want that. I want my birth to progress in peace on its own ... I have to relax and concentrate: I cannot fight with them at the same time.[43]

> I really thought I'd rather just stay at home and remove the temptation to do it the hospital way and have the epidural. Which you do, you know. It's so overwhelming, you sort of forget how painful it is, and you do suddenly want anything that's going to stop this pain, and defocus, and not rely on yourself. So I wanted to remove that temptation and try and help myself get focused in my own system, my own environment, and not feel that I had to give myself to someone else's system. It's very much if it's someone else's house, you do what they do. And if you're in the hospital, you do what the hospital does. And you try and fit in and be very polite and obliging everywhere you go. But in your own home you can just do your own thing.

Women explained that institutions influence how people relate, because institutionalization requires ideological and professional allegiance and develops an unstoppable momentum of its own. This makes it difficult for it to respond to the individual and therefore generates impersonalization and compliance:

> *In hospital they're relating to you on a different basis. Here, they're relating to you as a person in their own home who's quite relaxed and comfortable. I definitely think that people working within a hospital environment, especially where there's a lot of teaching going on, have a completely different attitude towards you – you're somebody that they're learning off or that they're teaching off or whatever. So in a hospital it wouldn't matter if I was assertive or not, the hospital couldn't change their procedure just to suit me.*

There was a sense that the institution could distance the woman from her baby in ways that are not immediately obvious:

> *I think I probably just had a sense that having it at home would be nicer in lots of ways. But it's not till it's happened that I'm clear about what those are. And actually they're much more about positive things than just avoiding hospital. And I'm much clearer about how awful hospital would have been, I think, for me. I just think it feels more like you've given birth and so it's your baby. Whereas if you feel that you couldn't have done it without this huge building and all these people and instruments and drugs then it's almost not so much yours is it? But I did feel she was very much mine.*

Powerful stories about personal integrity being breached circulated here and there. The narrative below demonstrated both the difficulty of protecting women's safety and exerting any kind of autonomy in the context of obstetric ideology, and the consequences of breaching women's integrity:

> *I do know somebody who had really, really been wanting a home birth and had ended up having to go to hospital. And she was recovering from it two and a half years later. And it was almost like a rape really. It was so devastating. And she couldn't equate those two experiences of having had a hospital birth – which is a normal thing – and her feelings of complete violation. Everything that she had wanted had just been swept aside and she was left with a whole lot of feelings that she was still really dealing with two and a half years later. I find it quite*

shocking. Just the kind of strength of her feelings and how long they'd lasted and also the fact that she had been so disempowered.

Women challenged the view that safety is a priori located in hospital, technology and obstetric expertise and that home birth is risky and relies on luck. A view that women observed less confident midwives subscribing to:

My midwife's the first to admit that she hasn't done a home delivery for four years and although she did quite a lot in training she's not up to date and doesn't feel that it's something she does often enough to feel particularly confident in. And her reaction's been that anybody that delivered a child at home would then go away and breathe a sigh of relief if it all worked out well.

To sum up this section on women's definition of risk, from the perspective of obstetric ideology the woman's home seems emptied of all that contributes to safety because the attributes of home birth that increase safety and decrease risk are invisible to it. Yet, for the women, their homes embodied all that is safe. Like other women, from their perspectives,[44] the potential of home birth and the risks of hospital birth were many-fold and decisions to plan home births were accompanied by a sense of moral rightness and a belief that research supports this. They did not believe that all complications are better dealt with or amenable to treatment in hospital, so did not shy away from the inherent uncertainty of pregnancy and birth. For the well-being of women and their families it is crucial that the meaning of safety be expanded to include their concerns, so that those aspects typically attributed to a 'nice experience' in obstetric ideology become understood as the crucial contributions to safety that they are.

Women's weave of safety

What do women believe makes birth safe?

For women, every aspect of their environment and how they felt as they approached and then journeyed through birth could contribute or detract from their sense of safety and confidence. Unlike the rigid, but fragmented safety of obstetric ideology, women's meanings of safety formed a weave of interrelated attributes. Seeing birth in its social context, as a powerful but fragile rite of passage, gave them a profound understanding about how it is influenced by complex inter-actions between psychosocial, physiological and environmental fac-tors. Thus women focused on creating safety that connected physical, emotional and often spiritual security.

Safety was not seen by women to exist either at home or in hospi-tal as a predetermined, pre-packaged entity. In the same way that Elizabeth Smythe (1998) described, they saw it as a process that depended on developing confidence over the course of their pregnan-cies. They saw safety as a process that depended on competent, holis-tic care during pregnancy and birth based on watchfulness that neither looks for nor denies danger, but attempts to be open to recog-nizing it if arises. And they saw it as a process that depends on trusting relationships with midwives and being in a familiar, safe environment. The following quotation discusses some of the interconnectedness of different facets of safety:

> *Well there's the environment, being at home with people that I care about and who care about me is very positive. Labour is quite an emotional time or a trying time. It's a time when you need supportive people and an environment that you know and like. And that makes such a difference. I think, it certainly makes a difference to my labour because I have freedom from limitations on me during the labour, limitations on time for the first, well, for all three stages really. Limitations on my freedom of movement. My second child was occipito posterior (when the baby's back is lying against the woman's spine, so the baby is facing out) and so I spent a lot of time in different positions and finding comfortable positions and helping him to turn. And I felt far more at ease choosing these and getting into these without strangers about, without people seeing what I was doing, and I think that that really helped the labour progress.*

Perhaps because women were unable to get to know their midwives and were aware of the constraints their midwives faced, being at home in their own environments was seen as particularly important. Feeling safe and relaxed in their own environments that they could control, compared to the impersonal, often disorienting hospital environment over which they had little control, featured in all the interviews. The 'uneasy compromise of flowery wallpaper is the inadequate surrogate for the constellation of factors, comforts and rhythms women have at home',[45] and cannot provide safety:

I think a lot of feeling safe is to do with security and feeling comfortable in your environment. And if that can help things to go well then that's you actually creating a security and a safety for the birth, just by making sure that your environment's right.

The women were convinced that feeling positive, confident and above all relaxed during pregnancy and labour would contribute significantly to how birth unfolded. 'Relaxed' could refer to reducing physical tensions, but usually meant creating a sense of emotional security and safety by having comfortable physical surroundings, and being able to completely trust those around them. Feeling 'relaxed' meant not having to worry that their integrity might be at risk in any way, and feeling at home and trusting enough of those around them to be themselves, to be able to 'let go'.[46] 'Feeling relaxed' was how women felt they could reduce risk and increase safety. Knowledge about hormonal activity during birth supports this view and as Maggie Banks (2000) observes: 'The sensual nature of birthing demands a birth scene that resembles the intimate environment in which the baby was conceived. It is this environment, which frees the woman from her need to be vigilant and ensures her maximum relaxation'.[47] Of course not all babies are conceived in intimacy, but this does not detract from the need to give birth in an intimate environment. This view is not widely accepted, but women resisted the currency of luck I referred to earlier that suggests that women and midwives have nothing to contribute to safe birth:

I knew this was the only place for me, definitely. It's just the way birth is meant to be. And I suppose you could say, well, I was lucky because my birth went well. But on the other hand you could say well, I'm sure it went well because I was so relaxed. I had nothing to do except [give birth]. I was in my own house, you know. To me, it was just perfect.

While there were many aspects to safety, women located a major part of it in midwives. The midwife's experiential knowledge and competence, her trust in the woman's ability to birth her baby, and her ability to focus on the individual woman, were seen as the bridge that could unite feeling and being safe.

The focused presence of a skilled, trusted and experienced midwife

On one level, many women felt that having the continuous, undivided attention of a midwife would provide greater safety:

> *I mean anything can go wrong anywhere with anything. And it can go wrong in hospital, and as I said before, you might not have the attention you might get if you've got a midwife with you, your own personal midwife at home with you.*

On a deeper level it is much more than this. It is about the quality of the attention, the nature of the relationship between the woman and midwife and the level of engagement, trust and skill. From this perspective, the important contribution of relationship to safety that is separated by obstetric ideology is reunited:

> If a relationship is such that the practitioner does not listen, does not come to know the hopes and fears of the woman, does not respond to her anxieties, then the mode of care can only be one of leaping-in, and can only be based on the semblance of what the practitioner thinks should be happening. It lacks attention to the things that are 'mattering'. It traps the woman into a passive role of accepting inappropriate, unsafe care, rather than freeing her to involve herself in the accomplishment of personalized care that promotes all that is safe.[48]

This approach makes it possible for the midwife to extrapolate from a broad range of experiential and intellectual knowledge, to develop the sort of 'wisdom [that] melts down all the moments of understanding and blends them together to become something more, something deeper and something more open to new understandings'.[49] But as the women observed, obstetric ideology relies on abstract generalities and fragments relationships between women and midwives in a way that reduces midwives' knowledge, practice and confidence. Its limitations limit the potential for increasing midwives' abilities to extend and generalize from their own experiential knowledge:

> *The midwives should be confident. Even my midwife who'd delivered loads [of babies] had never delivered first and fourths. So she was confident in delivering babies, but not firsts. And when she was saying, 'I think maybe we should think about*

*going into hospital' I thought, she's not confident in doing this.
She doesn't know. She saw it as going on unmapped territory.*

Women wanted midwives to be able to:

*Guide me through a safe birth process and to give me the benefit
of their training and wisdom.*

But there are few places in Britain where midwives are able to develop
this kind of competence and confidence that comes from seeing home
birth unfold safely again and again, so that it becomes her 'birthing
culture – her reality'.[50] Without this 'reality' it is difficult to see how
changes in birth ideology and culture might come about.

Broadly speaking, women identified two interrelated spheres of
competence: the skills to facilitate birth at home, and the skills to safeguard the woman and her baby if danger arose. They needed their
midwives to be able to discern the boundary between danger and
safety from a position of knowledge rather than fear and from a perspective of holistic midwifery care rather than obstetric ideology, so
that they could support them when birth was difficult but not complicated, and respond appropriately to actual complications. They
accepted that there are degrees of safety and danger and needed midwives to be able to work with uncertainty and to be able to think
through their individual circumstances on an ongoing basis. For
example, a woman with diabetes, planning a home birth, continued to
gather information and reassess her plans throughout her pregnancy.
Some of the practitioners she engaged with found this procedural
approach to safety alien and disconcerting.[51] While many women dis-
cerned a lack of skills to keep birth normal, unless the midwife herself
questioned her competence, the women assumed that the midwife
would respond appropriately to complications. The women who were
most concerned about their midwives' lack of skills to facilitate birth
understood the impact of this on the likelihood of them being
transferred into hospital for less than necessary reasons.

*I wish that they have more confidence themselves, so it isn't a
risky thing to have baby at home, I don't always get that feeling
that that's the case. There's always at the back of the mind, this
back drop of the hospital.*

*I think that the midwives should have much more experience of
it [home birth]. And I think that they should be much more con-*

fident in their own abilities. And that's most of the problem really.

Because of this they considered not calling midwives during labour, but did so (usually late in labour) because they wanted someone present who could protect them from the danger of a serious complication if it arose. Ironically, they knew that calling a midwife might, at the same time, reduce the protection from obstetric practices that they had hoped to create in their own homes. They understood that while home birth can *attenuate* obstetric policies, practices and allegiances, some of these almost inevitably cross the threshold with a midwife who is employed by the NHS.

I have mentioned the question of changing allegiances earlier and one of the cultural changes in industrialized societies, that women commented on, is the fact that midwives are no longer necessarily women with grown-up families who are part of the communities in which they serve.[52] Yet, for some women, feeling safe enough to give birth entailed the presence of a woman who had given birth herself: the 'motherly' figure described by Michel Odent (1999) and Sheila Kitzinger (2000) – the 'living proof that it can be done and that it'll be all right'.

> *Some midwives who are a bit older and who have had several children – I suppose it's that sort of a role. But I mean, again because [birth supporter] was there, I felt that she could provide that in the way [that she was] someone who'd been through it. I did feel that, looking back, when she came that I could relax. Like now I could give birth. Whereas if I had just been alone with my husband, I wouldn't have felt nearly so confident or comfortable about actually letting go and giving birth. I think it really does help to have someone there who's been through it before and who has children, who knows.*

As women talked more about their hopes, their fears and about their midwives, it became clear that for many women, being and feeling safe needed to be woven together through the competencies and attributes of their midwives. I discuss more of the detail of these relationships in Chapter 5. Meanwhile, contrary to obstetric ideology which locates risk in the body, women identified their embodied knowledge as another potential source of safety.

Women's embodied knowledge as an (unacknowledged) source of safety

I began Chapter 2 by posing the question 'Who can know what?' and then developed a theory of knowledge that suggests that it can arise from a much broader base than from reason alone. Yet many of us have internalized the dominant view that knowledge is produced only through our intellects. For example, Robbie Davis-Floyd (1992) suggested that the women in her study equated knowledge with intellectual information rather than with intuition, emotional, or bodily knowledge.[53] They also assumed that intellectual information would give them control. I found that the women I talked to drew on different forms of knowledge when challenging assumptions about how mothers protect their babies. Current ideology is rather confused about women's knowledge in this area. Mothering is frequently said to be innate, yet at the same time it is assumed that women know little about their babies' well-being before or during birth and might even be a danger to them. Once they have given birth, they are expected to take professional advice on how to raise their children.[54] So on the one hand they are expected to 'know' if knowing suits patriarchal ideologies about women's innate abilities to nurture. On the other hand their knowledge is frequently discounted:

> *My experiences have always been that they know best. And I just think it's a great contradiction that paediatricians and health visitors and people like that – they're always told that the mother's instinct is great in making any sort of diagnosis or considering any complaint. So* why, *when you go into [hospital], do they think that you don't? They can't seem to think it starts before. When it comes down to it, really mothers don't know. That's how they put it across to you. And as I say, I find that it's all very contradictory.*

In practice, women drew on experiential, intuitive and bodily knowledge, but they tended not to share this with professionals because of the perceived illegitimacy of these knowledges.[55] The problem with obstetric knowledge is not that women did not find it useful, but that it ignores other valuable (and sometimes contradictory) knowledge. As Barbara Duden (1993) pointed out, gestation is measured by ultrasound, and the woman's experience of 'quickening' (the baby's first movements) is discounted. There are countless similar examples.[56]

Women commented that their knowledge was often unwelcome, belittled or silenced in the face of 'expert' knowledge:

> *It really, really annoyed me when you go to your GP and you're pregnant and he says, 'What's the date of your last menstrual cycle?' And I actually know the day I conceived. Would you like to know that? 'No, no, no, the date of your last period.' And actually my GP had the nerve to say, 'How do you know you conceived on that day?' And I just thought that is so incredibly patronizing. I know that is the day I conceived. It's just so disregarding.*

While they observed that their knowledge was often discounted, they felt that it was valuable and should be recognized. In Kirsi Viisainen's (2000b) home birth study, one women described professionals as having 'such authority that I get the feeling I can't know anything myself'.[57] Some of the women in my study had similar experiences and described these as humiliating. One woman had regular contractions a month before she expected her baby to be born and contacted a midwife. 'She made me feel so foolish', by completely discounting her experience because of the ultrasound date. This unnecessary humiliation resulted in a woman, already distant from her midwives, withdrawing from them even more. Because of the predominant cultural overlay of our bodies with technology and technological understandings of bodily processes, women had different levels of knowledge about their bodies, and made no claims that it is always more accurate than other knowledges. But they wanted opportunities to share and discuss the knowledge they had, rather than be discounted. Some also felt that women could increase their own experiential knowledge by being more exposed to birth before becoming pregnant and giving birth themselves. But as Jo Murphy-Lawless (1998a) pointed out, one of the ways in which obstetrics exerts and maintains its knowledge and thus power over women is through the separation of birth from women's day-to-day lives. Some women felt that if birth could be a part of their lives, this would enable them to be more knowledgeable and make them less susceptible to the pressure of obstetric knowledge.

> *I think what would really help women having their first babies, more than anything else, would be to actually attend a birth at home.*

Jo Murphy-Lawless (1998a, 1998b) and Elizabeth Smythe (1998) discuss how alienating women from their bodies – because of the influence of technology – and excluding their experiences mutes a primary source of knowledge and thus decreases safety. Like the women in Smythe's study, many of the women believed that their own knowledge of themselves, their bodies and their babies would interact with and contribute to the knowledge of those involved in their care and thus contribute to safety. One woman commented that the woman in labour:

> *Is the best source of information about whether things are going okay or not. She knows best if her body is working right more than anybody else.*

Another said:

> *I might know first if something was going wrong.*

Another woman commented:

> *I think if anything's going to go wrong, I think you're aware of it or I'll become aware I think before any kind of major danger. Maybe that's not true, but I think I would feel it within myself. If I really suddenly felt things don't feel right and I want to be somewhere where they have got lots of equipment and they can do things then I would bring it up.*

Many women also knew that their bodies would be more able to give birth at home where they would be more at ease and in tune with them:

> *My experience of me in hospital is that I'm much happier out of it, and that my natural body processes happen much better when I'm not under stress. So for me, I see it as, in that respect, a safer option because, I mean it's a funny process giving birth. I really believe that the more in tune people are with themselves and particularly with their bodies and what their bodies are needing, the more healthy they're going to be and I would hope in my labour that I actually am really able to listen to my body and almost just do what it's telling me to.*

And that if they could feel relaxed and focused on the process of birth, they might interpret bodily sensations more accurately than practitioners:

You know, I said to her [midwife], I mean, it was a few minutes later, I said, I feel the baby really low. I said, I feel like I want to push, and she's like, 'You're only five centimetres'. And she had a look and his head was there, and a few good pushes and out he came.

They were also aware that in the context of contested definitions of safety and the societal alienation of women from their bodies, they could not always rely on their bodily knowledge and intuition and thus valued the interaction of knowledges between themselves and their midwives, as well as reassurance for their general anxieties:

I think there are times when I know and there are times when I don't know. I can see that I have got limitations. There are ways in which I'm in touch with myself physically and there are ways in which I've become more in touch with myself physically, but some of the time, I'm not. But I certainly think that that should be listened to.

It's so hard to separate your intuition from your fears. Like everyone has fears that things'll be wrong.

The notion that women are able to provide crucial information about themselves and their babies and may be more able to develop their knowledge in favourable circumstances is significant in terms of how women are listened to and thus how safety and continuity are inextricably linked. In this scenario, trusting relationships form the basis for safety, and medical ideology poses obstacles to this through its imposition of rules (which disregard individual women), and its structure of fragmented care. In essence, many women experienced a rhetoric of safety that was more akin to a 'semblance of safety'.[58] A misplaced faith in the inherent safety of institutions along with impersonal services, staff shortages, adherence to risk-based policies and discounting women's abilities to care for their babies all contribute to practitioners disengaging from women and unthinkingly relying on rules that may in fact reduce safety, as one woman explained:

Now let me think to get this right. My [community] midwife got us set up [in the postnatal ward]. She went away and suddenly, I was sort of half asleep and this nurse appeared and I saw her wheeling out my baby. And I said, where are you going? I mean, obviously people steal babies and things as well. I mean, it could have been anybody with a nurse's uniform on. And I mean, you've just had a baby, you're so protective against this baby as well. And she said, we're taking the baby to the nursery. And I said, well, I don't want the baby to go to the nursery. I want the baby beside me. That was one of the reasons I wanted a home birth because I don't really believe in a mother and baby being separated after birth. So she said, oh no, we'll have to take it away. And I said, well, no I don't want you to take the baby away. And it was going to get to the stage where it was like, yes I am, no you're not. And I said, no. You're not taking the baby away. So she sort of huffed away and went away out. And then some more senior nurse appeared and said, well, really because of the meconium, we really feel that the baby would be safer in the nursery, just so that it's got somebody constantly looking after it. And I thought, ooohhh. I didn't want to put my baby – I didn't want to wake up and him to be sort of struggling for breath or anything. So I said, right, okay, fair enough. But as soon as the baby wakes up, I want somebody to come and tell me, or somebody to bring the baby back to me. Well, of course I couldn't sleep. You know what it's like. And I didn't have my baby beside me and it was really getting me down. And I thought, well, I can't sleep, I might as well go and sit in the nursery myself. So I went to the nursery and there was no staff in the nursery. And I thought, well. You have just told me that the reason the baby couldn't be beside me was because I would be sleeping and there would be nobody looking after him. And yet he'd be safe in the nursery. I walk into the nursery and all the staff were obviously on a wee break and having cups of tea and there's nobody in the nursery. So I just got him and wheeled him back through to me, and nobody came back and said anything. I mean, I suppose there was staff in and out, but it just so happened that when I was in, there was nobody there and that was the whole point that she persuaded me to take him into the nursery.

Women's and midwives' knowledge is disregarded if the system of care relies on the rules of risk management. And the intended goal of increasing safety may not easily materialize when policies take the place of thoughtful engagement between women and practitioners where safety is a shared concern.

Obstacles to safe birth

Limiting midwives' skills

From the women's perspectives, one of the most intractable barriers to safe birth was the way in which obstetric ideology and practices decreased their midwives' autonomy and ability to develop alternative birth skills. If their labours were not completely straightforward, they wanted their midwives to be able to draw on the midwifery alternatives to obstetric practices that they knew existed. They found that some midwives used birth pools, birth balls and breathing for example, but that few appeared to have a range of both practical and emotional skills that come from a deep, holistic understanding of how women give birth. While the women felt that midwives had positive intentions and empathized with their beliefs and decisions, they (midwives) might at the same time be powerless to assist them to birth their babies at home. Thus, some women believed that they transferred to hospital and received interventions because their midwives' skills remained underdeveloped, leaving little alternative but to fall back on obstetric solutions. As one woman explained:

> *They never sort of came towards me. They just sat all the time, and never said anything. And then they would just say we'll wait and see. Whereas I felt if they'd really come towards me as a person, it might have all gone very differently. And I thought they must see so many women and they must begin to understand people's characters a little bit and get more the feel of what I particularly needed. They wanted to be supportive, they certainly did. And I just always remembered thinking it was sad they didn't have more things included in their training that they could just feel more supportive. Cos they wanted to but . . .*

Women could see that restrictive policies disempowered their midwives, by preventing them from experiencing unusual or challenging, but nonetheless potentially normal situations at home. They also realized that the midwives themselves were not always aware of these restrictions on their practice. They commented that midwives might even comply with local policies because they mistakenly believed that they have some sort of legal standing. I too experienced this while I was supporting a woman during a planned home birth. The woman was in advanced labour when the midwife arrived. She immediately informed me that the woman would have to transfer to hospital. This was because she believed that there was a legal requirement for two midwives to be present at a birth and was concerned that the second midwife might not reach the woman's home in time because of snow. Similarly, women have been led to believe that midwives cannot attend them at home if their pregnancies last more than forty-two weeks, or if their baby passes meconium during labour. This prevents women and midwives working together to support women's ethical decisions and their desire to take responsibility. One woman observed that:

> *Often when I speak to my contemporaries, their comment is, oh, you just want to get into hospital into a safe place and hand over responsibility. And you think, do you? Whereas to me, handing over responsibility is just not at all the way it's meant to be. I mean you have to take responsibility.*

When midwives are unable to practise autonomously and expand their knowledge and skills, they become anxious if asked to do so. Thus women are forced to weigh up their beliefs about safety with their midwife's anxiety. And even when midwives do have skills, it is difficult for them to use them – other than subversively, which as Sally Hutchinson (1990) suggests has its limitations – if they contravene local policies. For example, women were told that if their babies passed meconium during labour, NHS community midwives' policies required them to strongly advise immediate hospital transfer, and recommend that their babies' heartbeats should be continuously monitored and that their babies should be taken away at birth to be suctioned. The women who booked with independent midwives found that in the same circumstances, their midwives would discuss the best course of action with them at the time, as there are indications that meconium staining in labour need not always require hospital transfer.[59] If the woman and midwife decided that transfer to hospital was advisable, intermittent monitoring could be continued and the baby would be suctioned only if this was felt to be unavoidable. The contrast between the two following quotations from two different women show how autonomy, skills and mutual trust increase safety and how inflexible obstetric policies can be divisive, confusing and decrease safety:

> *I knew that she [independent midwife] would tell me if there was anything wrong and if she was ever really worried about the baby because it was a long labour and I did have meconium*

staining at one point and we carried on. Whereas, definitely it seems to me that with the community midwives – that's it – you're just into hospital. And she knew I didn't want it so she said, 'Mm the heartbeat's fine, I think we're okay' and I thought well we must be. I never thought that when I was in the bathroom that she would say to [partner], 'Look, another half an hour and that's it, we're going to have to go'. I never felt there was any subterfuge. I knew that she was respecting me and telling me the truth the whole time.

They [midwives] said meconium staining. They said the baby was in distress and that they were going to phone the ambulance and then they said that the heartbeat was a hundred and forty, which was as it had been from the very beginning. So it sounded as if they thought there was meconium, however the baby was well. So the two of those things don't seem to combine for me. But anyway they said that it would be advisable to go into hospital. They were very keen for us to make the decision immediately. [The midwife] came up to me and she was at the very most a foot away from me, and she was being very directive and saying that we should be going to hospital. And then she said at the end of all that, 'Of course we'd be very happy to stay here and deliver you at home', and I thought well if you are worried – in hindsight – if you are worried then surely you wouldn't be saying that. So although I felt that they'd tried to indicate that there was a sense of urgency, I felt that that particular thing that they said meant that they weren't all that worried.

In other words, birth may be responded to in different ways depending on the ideology through which it is viewed and the skills that have been developed and are thought to be appropriate within that ideology. For example, through the obstetric lens, high blood pressure during pregnancy may require hospitalization, frequent monitoring and induction. Through a different lens it may require supportive watchfulness at home, as it can be exacerbated by the stress of hospitalization, frequent monitoring and induction. So while women appreciated that practitioners were 'doing their best', they also commented that they were not always able to meet their needs.

The lack of midwifery autonomy and skills decreased one of the most important ingredients for safe birth – that is, trust between women and midwives. Indeed, the initial discussions about risk that I described at the beginning of the chapter suggested that 'political tensions may dominate possible relationships and set up conflict before the relating even begins'.[60]

Distrust between women and midwives

Neither women nor midwives could create safety or feel safe when they were unable to find common ground. Differences in ideology reduce engagement, information sharing and dialogue. Both women and midwives found that attempting to move across incompatible ideologies, or mesh holistic care with obstetric policies created mutual confusion, distrust, fear and danger. The woman might attempt to make decisions based on one system of beliefs and knowledge about birth, with information from a conflicting one, and the midwife might attempt to support the woman without fully understanding her and without the knowledge and skills to support her decisions safely and confidently. The following excerpts exemplify the dangers of polarization and the difficulty of decision-making across ideologies:

> *If there was a good reason for me going into hospital, I wouldn't trust that it was for a good reason, because I wouldn't know that she [midwife] wasn't just panicking or plotting to get me away.*

> *If there seems to be a problem, I don't want to hold out and have a bloody natural childbirth and a dead baby, or a really unhealthy baby. I'm just really anxious that they'll kind of panic and want to take charge really quickly. If the baby's in danger, then of course, do anything. But I suppose it's just if I don't know I'm coming from the same value basis as somebody, then I don't know if they're going to be making decisions on the same basis as I would.*

'The climate of trust' is disturbed,[61] not only through discordant ideologies, but also by a system of care that devalues relationships. Even if midwives attempt to listen to women, lack of continuity may increase the likelihood of them listening to censored versions of women's feelings and knowledges. The fragility of relationships and the need for trust to enable women to feel safe enough to share some of their thoughts and feelings is clear:

Nadine: How easily do you feel you can raise any concerns you have?

With things that I feel will be disapproved of, I suppose I haven't necessarily felt comfortable about raising them as issues. I only want to raise things that make me out to be the model patient, and an easy, straightforward case, obliging and not difficult. I'd be more inclined to talk to [partner] a lot about it, or to read about it, or to find out from other sources, than risk the relationship I'm having with my midwife. You know, mostly I would wash my dirty linen elsewhere and that's all part of this need to be accepted. I'm sure a lot of women feel that. I'm sure that's why a lot of women end up doing exactly what the doctor wants or having the full medical thing because they don't want to cause trouble.

To sum up this section, if women cannot trust the ideology and practices of those accompanying them on their birth journeys, they experienced the irresolvable tension of two conflicting needs: the need to feel relaxed enough to give birth and the need to remain alert and on guard.

Devaluing women's knowledge

As I discussed above in the section on women's knowledge as an unacknowledged source of safety, devaluing this knowledge undermines the creation of safe birth. Elizabeth Smythe comments that:

> It is the woman who will be most sensitive to subtle changes in her being-of-pregnancy, yet she is the one least likely to understand what the changes might mean. Safe 'concernful' practice is open to announcings. It heeds the woman. It gets as close to the announcings as it is able, bringing the wisdom of knowing.[62]

When women are not expected to know,[63] and when obstetric practices and rules override women's knowledge, there is little room for the knowledge and experience that they do have to contribute to safe birth. This was clearly demonstrated in the Dunne case that I mentioned earlier, where the woman's awareness of 'tumultuous contractions' prior to her twins becoming compromised was ignored.[64]

Many of the women felt that there was little meaningful recognition or place for their knowledge within obstetric ideology. They were often unable to make their 'announcings' in ways that could be heard or acted upon. While of course there were fine examples of midwives encouraging women to draw on their own knowledge, listening to, and dialoguing with them (see page 185), this depended on individual women and midwives. An ideology that has no concept of knowledge being located in the woman herself systematically mutes this knowledge:

> *Like I was saying before about* feeling *him [baby] not to be engaged and* knowing *that he wasn't as other women had described it. They should have listened more to that because they constantly asked me if I felt this pressure and if I had an urge to push. And I kept thinking, well maybe I should, maybe this is an urge to push that I'm not really recognizing. I was questioning my own feeling which in retrospect I just didn't have. It wasn't there. And I think they should have listened to that and if they'd been more experienced they'd have known from that. Not just from internals, but they should have known from what I was saying that it wasn't happening. And there was no benefit to it [directed pushing] except to make me even more tired. Yeh, I think they should maybe talk to you more about how you're feeling at each stage. And they could maybe discuss it with you a bit more and that would indicate more to them.*

The impact of obstetric ideology privileging its own beliefs and practices, undervaluing and limiting midwifery knowledge, skills and autonomy, and undermining the possibility of trusting relationships between women and midwives had devastating consequences on women and the potential for safe, empowering birth.

Limiting women's autonomy over the creation of safety

Women became aware that the practice of safety takes place in the context of midwives being under pressure to coerce women to accept attenuated obstetric policies. They were expected to do this by emphasizing risk and implying that for women, 'taking responsibility' means prioritizing the safety of their babies in ways that obstetrics has deemed appropriate. Many women internalize these limits set on their autonomy in early pregnancy by signing up to the unwritten rule that obstetrics should have the final say:

They [professionals] feel responsible. They feel they have to point out the risks. But since everything went smoothly the other times, they had no qualms about my having a home birth. And also, I made it clear that if anything seemed to be going wrong, I wouldn't resist going into hospital.

Indeed women's discourses are heavily influenced by the deeply held, patriarchal view that women and unborn babies are separate entities rather than connected through a mother–baby relationship. In a separatist view, there are two separate responsibilities and the responsible pregnant woman is expected to prioritize her responsibility to her baby over her responsibility to herself. The woman who talked about 'a maternal–fetal unity' and the baby 'as an extension of myself, that I should have complete control over' described her view as 'aberrant'.

This meant that there was an assumption that decisions about safety and risk would be made by professionals rather than women. Many women assume this to be the case.[65] At home this usually focuses on hospital transfer, where women are told about predetermined risks and advised to go to hospital if these arise. Dialogue tended to be explanatory, with an expectation of compliance, leaving little scope for any kind of dialogue that might question the construction of risk:

They [midwives] said that what generally happens is if they think that there's any risk at all, then they'll ask you if they can take you to hospital. I said, oh that's fair enough, if there's any risk I'm quite happy to go into hospital. But on the whole if there's no risk I'd rather be here.

For those women who held different views about safety and risk and therefore needed to retain control over decision-making, this assumption undermined the ethical responsibilities they assumed for their babies and the means to fulfil these moral obligations:

I feel like maybe I'm losing control over my responsibility to the baby. I don't feel able to exercise that because I don't really know the situation and I don't know how far to trust the midwives to be doing or understanding what I want.

Yet as Mary Cronk (2000) suggested, if professionals do not trust or encourage women to retain responsibility during pregnancy, birth and postnatally, the opportunity for women to develop the abilities and skills needed to care for their babies and children is undermined.

There is a curious irony about obstetric ideology's focus on risk. It claims to best represent women and babies safety and assigns itself the moral high ground. Yet in doing this, it alienates women and midwives from each other and prevents women from putting in place all they believe is necessary for safe birth. It leads to women disengaging from practitioners who they believe might mislead them, and forces them into the powerless position of 'hoping for the best' when they have no idea whether or not the best is likely to happen:

> *It's either been like, no I don't want to hear you, I don't want to hear this stuff because it's been just designed to make me say yes, yes, I'll go to hospital. Or I've just been trusting that everything will go okay and I won't need to worry about it. And there's something that is unresolved between me and them [practitioners].*

Of course, birth is likely to go well, and 'care may be safe if there is nothing to make it unsafe (just as the day is fine if it does not rain)'.[66] But the idea that safety should be taken out of their hands, and left to chance seemed anathema to women. And yet women who attempt to influence the creation of safety are frequently hampered by bureaucratic constraints.[67] The following woman illustrates this:

> *Like they [senior midwives] don't like the system. They're trying to change the system [to improve the skills and confidence of community midwives] so they obviously feel the system doesn't work. Yet when I say my worries, they say, we can understand, but they are qualified midwives. And it's like, well, I know they're qualified. They do understand why I'm pissed off and they want to change it, but somehow they're not prepared to do anything to make it slightly better. I don't see why they couldn't have a midwife from the hospital come out, except that it's not procedure. It's just the bureaucracy thing. It's like you've got community midwives on a rota for you and you should be happy with that. Even though we're not happy with it, you should be, which isn't really making much sense.*

But they are still deemed to be (and indeed feel) responsible for any adverse outcomes:

There's quite a few women around here who have had home births, and I think they've had the local midwives and it's all been fine. So I sort of thought I'd just trust to that. But it would just be like giving up in a way, because I'm not completely happy about it. So then I guess if something did go wrong, I would feel like I hadn't maybe done my full responsibility towards the baby, cos I'd sort of been overwhelmed by all the difficulties.

In addition to the problem that women in patriarchal societies are often expected to take responsibility without the means to do this,[68] there is little understanding that safety depends on autonomy, and that autonomy is usually relational.[69] It develops over time through trusting relationships that enable a deep, ongoing, open dialogue. But the structural underpinning of relationships between women and midwives builds in separation rather than connection. Safety is said to be unpredictable, but depends on women following their midwives' advice and midwives following correct local procedures. This encourages practitioners to focus on surveillance and management rather than engagement, leaving women isolated rather than supported:

She [midwife] explained that if there was an emergency, she said, you really would have to psychologically gear yourself up, thinking – you're on your own. You've got to cope. Although we would obviously, do everything we could to get you both to the hospital safely.

Expanding definitions of safety and risk

Valuing women's definitions of safety

These women's narratives underscore a number of crucial issues. First, they are the people most concerned about their own and their babies' well-being. Everything they talked about was to do with protecting their babies and themselves in order to begin the parenting relationship from the best possible place. In this sense women who plan home births, elect to have planned caesarean sections, or plan to have unassisted births share the commonality of desiring to be autonomous and able to minimize emotional harm in order to become the self-confident women and mothers they need to become. Safety was described by them as integral to the quality of their lives and those of their families. Thus, women cannot be safe if their concerns are of no concern to those attending them, and if these concerns are likely to be overridden. They need to decide what safe means for them and receive support to promote this wherever they give birth. Being safe needs to be more than the precarious hope that they will be able to avoid transfer to hospital during childbearing.

Second, they concurred with the view that safety is not an absolute concept and cannot be guaranteed.[70] Their experiences described those principles that contribute to safe outcomes and the constraints that limit these. As Smythe (1998) suggested, safety is an ongoing process affected by current ideology and knowledge, physical health of the woman and her baby, emotional feelings of the woman, women's and professional's knowledge, localized policies and practices, resources, levels of support within the general system of care, the presence or absence of trusting relationships between women and carers, and undoubtedly other influences. Imposing obstetric knowledge and practices while ignoring many of these other crucial aspects of birth does not ensure safety or eliminate risk. At the same time, moving from risk criteria and management to a more procedural account of safety is far from obvious and demands renegotiating autonomy, risk and potential, the definitions of normality and abnormality, and decisions about whether to act or wait.

Third, the women's beliefs aligned them more closely with holistic approaches to birth, than with technological models of birth. One of the most important challenges to current birth practices they posed was whether or not there are safe, less invasive midwifery alternatives to invasive obstetric procedures. Their ethical concerns to give birth in their own ways as far as possible suggested that they need high levels of midwifery skills. Skills that reconnect the physiology of the birth process with the emotional needs of women. Skills that have largely disappeared in a culture that has lost its birth wisdom. The women's definitions of birth suggested the need to draw on wider knowledge pools than on the limited knowledge relied on by obstetrics. Even though midwifery skills remain underdeveloped and we know that poverty, lack of support, and location, for example, continue to impact on the safety of childbearing, a growing body of literature suggests that when midwives respond to women's circumstances, even those most vulnerable to complications remain healthier.[71] We also know that dominant knowledges mute other knowledges,[72] making alternative birth practices elusive. Ironically, the move towards evidence-based care, audit and review can further undermine alternative ideologies, where 'best practice' encourages compliance rather than providing woman-centred care (the immunization debates provide an example of the conflict between choice, autonomy and what medicine 'knows' is best).[73] All too often women fear that their integrity will be breached by those who are unable to provide the skills they need and midwives fear that women will want support for situations for which they have been unable to develop adequate skills. Yet anecdotal stories suggest that midwifery skills may provide greater safety than technocratic solutions while avoiding harm, and that changing the balance between midwifery and technocracy would enable women and midwives to be supported rather than dominated by technology. For example, a woman who had experienced complications because of obstetric cholestasis (a condition that can result in a baby being stillborn towards the end of pregnancy) in a previous pregnancy, used a dietary approach monitored by blood tests to stabilize the condition in her next pregnancy. This use of obstetric knowledge and technology to support a means of avoiding complications and the need for induction of labour moved beyond the technocratic and holistic boundaries to protect the woman and her baby and support her concerns and beliefs. An independent midwife facilitated the autonomy of the woman by integrating different knowledges, the woman's concerns and her own midwifery skills.[74] This is very different from the uneasy attempt to merge ideologies with conflicting views on safety where risk criteria and rules undermine midwives' autonomy.[75] Women's autonomy depends a great deal on midwives' autonomy and skills. Without these women feel they have no option but to follow obstetric advice in the absence of any alternative, even if they believe it to be unnecessary or harmful. The responsibility heaped on women and midwives without the autonomy to meet that responsibility is dangerous and leaves them wide open to blame.

Fourth, the women described the rhetoric of choice and control, based on rights as an inadequate obstetric substitute for trusting relationships between them and their midwives (I discuss this further in Chapter 6). Like other women,[76] they accepted uncertainty, but believed, as others do,[77] that trusting relationships with midwives is fundamental to safety. But, as the women observed the impact of obstetric ideology on the system of community care formed a formidable barrier to women and midwives creating a broader and deeper safety based on women's concerns and needs. It had a devastating effect on the relationships between them. Yet, despite this, women believed that home birth offered at least some protection from the full impact of obstetric ideology and relied on their midwives to do the best they could to help them give birth at home. In the next chapter I elaborate on these relationships, and how women described and negotiated them.

Notes

1 Department of Health 1993: 10.
2 Scottish Office Home and Health Department 1994.
3 Mavis Kirkham, personal communication, 2001. Mavis Kirkham is Professor of Midwifery at the University of Sheffield.
4 Beck 1992.
5 Murphy-Lawless 1998a.
6 Mauthner and Doucet 1998.
7 Douglas 1992.
8 Jordan 1993.
9 Kuhn 1970.
10 Maynard 1994: 13.
11 Smythe 1998.
12 Davis-Floyd 1992; O'Connor 1992; Viisainen 2000a, 2000b.
13 Rutanen and Ylikorkala, in Viisainen 2000b: 796.
14 Aspinall et al. 1997: 3.
15 Green et al. 1998b.
16 Viisainen 2000b: 804; Walker 2000.
17 Lemay 1997: 85.
18 Lemay 1997: 95.
19 Smythe 1998; see also Daviss 2001: 170; Woolford 1997.
20 From unpublished interviews carried out by Nadine Edwards and Cathleen Sullivan in 1994.
21 Waterstone et al. 2001.
22 Strong 2000.
23 Smythe 1998: 257.
24 Belenky et al. 1986; Debold et al. 1996; Gilligan 1985; Hamer 1999.
25 Banks 2000: 145 (original italics).
26 Inch 1984.
27 Murphy-Lawless 2000.
28 Murphy-Lawless 1998a: 214.
29 Adam 1992: 161.
30 Gregg 1995; Murphy-Lawless 1998a.
31 Murphy-Lawless 1998a: 47.
32 Adams 1994: 57.
33 Lemay 1997: 92.
34 Murphy-Lawless 1998a.
35 Banks 2000: 179; Noble 2001; Wesson 1990: 184; Women's Health Information Collective (WHIC) 2000.
36 Viisainen 2000a.
37 Smythe 1998: 40.
38 Helen Stapleton, personal communication, 2000. Helen Stapleton is a Research Midwife at the University of Sheffield.
39 Hadikin and O'Driscoll 2000.
40 Leap 1997; Stapleton et al. 1998.
41 Belenky et al. 1986.
42 Griffiths 1995.
43 Viisainen 2000b: 805.
44 Lemay 1997; O'Connor 1992; Viisainen 2000a.

45 Erin McNeill, personal communications, 2000. Erin McNeill was a Senior Reproductive Health Adviser with Family Health International, but very sadly died on 31 January 2003.
46 Anderson 2000a.
47 Banks 2000: 147–148.
48 Smythe 1998: 202.
49 Smythe 1998: 226.
50 Banks 2000: 132.
51 Lawson 2000–2001.
52 Allison 1996; Donnison 1988; Leap and Hunter 1993; Marland 1993b; Towler and Bramall 1986.
53 Davis-Floyd 1992: 31.
54 Cronk 2000.
55 Belenky et al. 1986; Jordan 1977.
56 See, for example, Duden 1993; Gregg 1995; Jordan 1997.
57 Viisainen 2000b: 806.
58 Smythe 1998.
59 Page 2000.
60 Smythe 1998: 184.
61 Smythe 1998: 188.
62 Smythe 1998: 195.
63 Belenky et al. 1986; Jordan 1977.
64 Murphy-Lawless 1998a: 214.
65 Green et al. 1998b.
66 Smythe 1998: 233.
67 See, for example, Anderson 2004; Mahoney 2004.
68 Benson 2000.
69 Mackenzie and Stoljar 2000.
70 Department of Health 1993; Smythe 1998: 249.
71 Davies 2000; Evans 1987; Rooks 1997.
72 Davis-Floyd and Sargent 1997; Kuhn 1970.
73 Bedford and Elliman 2000.
74 Jane Evans, personal communication 2000. Jane Evans practised commmunity midwifery within the NHS for many years and now provides skilled independent midwifery care to women in the North London area.
75 Clarke 1995.
76 Lemay 1997; O'Connor 1992; Viisainen 2000b.
77 Lemay 1997; Smythe 1998; van Olphen Fehr 1999.

5 'What I really need is support'

Relationships between women and midwives

With Woman

Will you be 'with me'?
No, I mean 'really' with me?
I can feel this power, rising up within, sweeping along on
                                                    huge waves,
I need someone, you see, because I am frightened.
I am also exhilarated to be on such an ancient journey.

I am tired to tears of people who will not listen and
              I barely have the strength to protest
At their formulaic phrases and litanies of self comfort.
I cannot bear to be reduced, a product of tunnel vision.
Not now, not when I am at my most powerful, my most
              dangerous, my most
                            beautiful.

I am incredibly sensitive. Your body does not lie and
When you touch me
              I will now if you are not really 'with me',
                            if you do not respect me.
Do not insult me with platitudes
              or falseness for convention's sake.
I would rather be alone.

Sanctify me. We are equal.
Do not collude with those misguided,
              or more sinister still, those who would masculate me.
You are powerful and so am I. Touch me gently.
Share the power of life with me honestly, let me be.[1]

This chapter focuses on the relationships between women and midwives during the childbearing period. Once again, issues of connection and separation emerge. Focusing on relationships between individual women and midwives in the context of obstetrically dominated maternity services poignantly demonstrates the inevitable distancing of women and midwives in a collective sense too. It shows the difficulties women experience in getting to know midwives, communicating, getting information, developing trust and asserting their desires. Because relationship has been largely discounted by modern health care, its concept of 'continuity' does not include the level of engagement that women describe as crucial: as one woman commented,

> *There's so much potential for it [the relationship] and for whatever reason, it's not being realized.*

The complex ways in which women and midwives attempt to negotiate a system not designed to foster relationships, or to support midwives to support women left some women feeling:

> *There's quite a cultural gulf between the women who are choosing home births and the women who are providing the service.*

This led to a continual tension, oscillation between, or suppression of women's understanding about the potential of birth in their lives and the realities of a service that has eliminated much of this potential. Thus theories about relationality and power enabled me to examine how women negotiated conflicting ideologies and how they:[2] incorporate, reject and accept these, in their attempts to reconcile the inevitable fractures caused,[3] and yet maintain emotional, embodied and spiritual integrity.

By examining relationships between women and midwives empathetically rather than judgementally through the social context in which they occurred, I attempt to make the personal political, in such a way that is empowering and plausible to women and midwives, rather than blaming. By acknowledging coexisting belief systems,[4] and the authenticity but instability of the feminist postmodern subject, I attempted to listen to and understand the accordances and discordances women described between them and their midwives without ascribing fixed identities or beliefs to them.

Relationships between women and their midwives were one of the most significant determining factors on how women experienced planning and having home births or transferring to hospital. It was within these relationships that women developed their knowledge about local maternity services, about how their ideals fitted or challenged the midwives' practices, and about how far midwives could and would support them if their ideals challenged local obstetric beliefs and practices.

I have already observed that home birth is viewed by many lay people and professionals as unnecessarily risky and irresponsible, and that women were transgressing contemporary cultural norms by planning home births. I have also observed that women approach home birth from multifaceted positions.[5] Thus relationships with midwives were set within a complex network of influences before they even met. The crux of the matter seemed to be that women needed midwives to be on their side, to understand them as individuals, and protect them from the routine obstetric practices that they wanted to avoid.

On the basis of previous experiences, stories from friends, and birth accounts in books on home birth, many women approached community midwives with anxiety as well as hope. They hoped that midwives would respond enthusiastically to their plans to have home births, be able to support their ideals throughout pregnancy and birth and be able to give them reliable information if problems arose. They were anxious, however, that midwives might instead lack the skills and confidence women needed and would therefore suggest transferring into hospital unnecessarily. The paradox was that while the women needed midwives to be powerfully and resolutely 'with' them, midwives are located in a context that vigorously prevents this.[6]

Constraints on midwives

While the catalyst for this book was the struggle over home birth, midwives are engaged in a parallel struggle for survival and autonomy that I described in Chapter 3. While midwifery improves outcomes for women and babies,[7] it lacks the cultural authority described by Robbie Davis-Floyd. It is continually under threat from obstetrics, nursing and employment regulations.[8] Because of this it carries features of oppressed groups.[9] That is, it adheres to obstetric-based policies, victimizes those who challenge this,[10] and holds conflict within its own ranks rather than externalizing it.[11]

At present, in Britain, only independent midwives work relatively freely of restrictive obstetric rules, but the hostile environment in which some work infringes on their autonomy all the same.[12] NHS midwives are in the unenviable position of attempting to work from a woman-centred perspective (a perspective systematically denied to them), empower women from a disempowered position,[13] respect when they are frequently disrespected, nurture without being nurtured themselves, offer choice when they have few choices, and provide 'unbiased' information (as though this existed) that they cannot then act upon because of local policies which constrain them.[14] The NHS midwife has become the 'piggy-in-the-middle',[15] caught between policies, employers, colleagues and women.[16] She is expected to carry out the impossible task of bridging women's diverse needs and obstetric hegemony. The 'steering' she engages in,[17] and the attempts by women to assert agency frequently led to a muted power struggle (carefully avoiding open conflict), marked by fear and anxiety.

The prevalent lack of continuity in maternity services ensures that while women attempt to align themselves with midwives in an effort to establish relationships, midwives are likely to align themselves with each other. Women reported that midwives were reluctant to cause conflict within their teams, even when women felt strongly about not being attended by a member of the team. The following was the only example of a midwife informing a woman of her rights in this area:

> *I think she must have realized because she did say to me, a lot of women do find her bossy, but you can ask for her not to be there. So I didn't realize that you could actually request, that I don't want this midwife in the house or whatever. But I wouldn't do that. If it comes that she's here, well, fair enough, you know.*

But as I explain later, women's ways of relating and decision-making were more akin to the ethics of care and relationality that I described in Chapter 2. They balanced their own needs with those of their babies, partners, other family members and the midwives involved in their care. So pointing out women's choices and rights was not always experienced as truly supportive, if women felt unable to assert these.

Perhaps one of the most invisible, yet constraining aspects of the woman–midwife relationship is the assumption that it must exist and that women and midwives are usually unable to select each other on grounds of ideology and personality. In other cultures women have more autonomy about if and when to call an attendant, who that attendant will be and this person's role.[18] For example, the only task assigned to the dai (the traditional birth attendant) in Pakistan is the removal of the placenta. All other tasks are negotiable, depending on the knowledge and abilities of those with the birthing woman.[19] This potentially increases women's knowledge and autonomy around reproduction. With few exceptions,[20] professionalization has defined a less negotiable role for the midwife, which largely excludes women's family and friends and increases women's dependency on 'experts'. This relative inflexibility of relationships with midwives inevitably and profoundly affected women's experiences.

Focusing on women's definitions of supportive relationships

As I described in Chapter 3, there is no agreed definition of support, but a general acceptance that support is a good thing. Listening to women talk about their relationships with their midwives begun to unpack the different facets of support and the diverse needs of individual women. I have described how women experienced their first meetings with midwives in Chapter 1 and how this gave them some understanding about the midwives' beliefs, policies and practices. Their ongoing meetings shed further light on how women define their own priorities and explains why obstetric ideology cannot easily respond to these priorities. One of the first issues to arise was the fact that support is best provided within the context of meaningful relationships.

Getting to know midwives or recognizing a 'familiar face'?

Having met their midwives for the first time, and having been told about some of the perceived risks of home birth, women were then usually given basic information about how their antenatal care was likely to proceed. One of the first issues that many women commented on was the number of midwives allocated to their care. The idea was that the woman would meet a different team midwife at each antenatal visit so that she would have a 'known' midwife with her during labour and birth. But the women reported that meeting someone briefly once or twice does not correspond with getting to know that person. However, women's assessments of the community services were often tempered by their knowledge of hospital services, so a typical view was that it was paying lip service to continuity, but was still an improvement on hospital services:

> Continuity will have to be better because in hospital there's a never-ending stream of trainees, students – anybody and everybody.

I mean six is a lot, but it's better than just going up to the hospital and not knowing who you might get.

A realistic assessment was that they may be attended by a 'familiar face' rather than a known midwife:

You know who they are and they've been in your home and I suppose that helps. But it's not like you've been able to talk through it all and explain exactly what you want – or how they felt about things or whatever, or what their experience was. You know, it's a bit half-hearted really.

So what they try and do is get you to meet all of them before you actually have your baby, so obviously they've got faces that are familiar, even if you don't know them very well – but they're faces that are familiar.

The need to get to know a midwife increased rather than decreased during women's pregnancies, but even in early pregnancy, nearly all the women expressed concerns about the lack of continuity. Some felt very strongly:

It's anathema to have someone you don't know and if you're lucky it might be the person you like. I wouldn't do that to fix a car.

Any number would be horrible, because you still wouldn't know who's going to come. That's the point.

They observed that most meetings with midwives were in fact first meetings and challenged the implicit assumption that meeting midwives is the same as getting to know them:

You just get a faceless professional really, pretty much faceless because, you know, even in the community midwife system you're pretty well talking about seeing them cold. You've seen them, but that's pretty well it.

Inevitably, in the face of no obvious alternative, the emphasis on meeting all the midwives on their team became a preoccupation for women. Given the women's expressed need to get to know a midwife, the irony was that in order to have the unsatisfactory 'familiar face' during labour, they had to relinquish their need for relationships during their pregnancies:

> *You see the problem is, if you see a different one every time you get to know them all, which is what you want, cos you don't know who's going to be at the birth – so you do want that – but you don't because you're not seeing the same person every time.*

> *There's quite a strong feeling in me that I would like it if when I went for my next appointment that it was [midwife] again. So in many ways, in practice, I'm quite happy reinforcing that relationship and yet obviously if there are six, I don't want to end up giving birth with somebody I haven't met before, so I do need to meet the others.*

It often felt as though the priority was on meeting midwives rather than meeting the woman's needs. As one woman remarked:

> *I'd rather have had some support than just a series of ladies rushing in to sort of present themselves to me and go out again, having ticked themselves off the list.*

Sometimes women called midwives during labour, but were unsure from her name over the phone which 'familiar face' would arrive. The main advantage of meeting midwives briefly on one or two occasions cited by the women was that they could check that none of the midwives were 'very unpleasant' and that there was not going to be a 'personality clash'. In these circumstances the only recourse open to women was to refuse to be attended by individual midwives. Ironically, the lack of continuity made this all the more difficult as it meant:

> *Basing my assessment of people on little comments because you know, I saw that woman at the clinic for fifteen minutes. I've no idea what she's like at all.*

They felt especially unwilling and unable to do this during pregnancy:

> *I don't know if it's because you are more vulnerable when you're pregnant and let people boss you about more. And then you think, why did I let her say that or do that to me just because I*

was pregnant. But I'd give her another chance, just for her feelings really. I didn't want to be horrible.

In the rare circumstances when a woman informed a senior midwife that she did not wish to be attended by an individual midwife, 'they actually just ignored what my stated request was'.[21] In any event, this could not address the fundamental issue of getting to know midwives.

Women knew that they needed to engage with midwives at a deeper level but could see that maternity services were not designed to make this possible. They attributed many of the difficulties they experienced to the system of care in operation rather than to individual midwives. They frequently talked about midwives as 'well-intentioned', 'friendly', 'nice people', but at the same time, 'strangers': 'I mean, the midwives are lovely, but they're still, you know, it's quite a lot of strangers'. So while midwives could be experienced as friendly and supportive, they got to know little about the woman and her life context.[22] Inevitably, given the obstetric context of community care, some women experienced midwives as unsupportive, but still felt that had they been able to get to know one midwife during their pregnancies, they could have 'engaged more' and ironed out some of the difficulties. This is confirmed in the second quotation below where the woman talks about a friend's experience:

> *My criteria for what that person would ideally be like could be much broader and much more malleable if I could get to know somebody. I could get round the little quirks or whatever.*

> *I think it's six [midwives in the team]. It's far too much. You can't really build up a rapport with your midwife which I think is the important thing really because you're in such an emotionally vulnerable phase in your life. It should be one midwife or two. Like my friend for example – that's the friend who did the one-to-one scheme. She said initially she wasn't that keen on her midwife. But in the end she just thought she was absolutely fantastic and wonderful and she said she really got to know her.*

The impossibility of getting to know midwives

Maternity services appeared to be as inflexible for midwives as they were for women. Even when women and midwives got on well, or when a midwife had attended a woman during her previous birth and wanted to attend her during her next pregnancy and birth, there seemed to be no way of facilitating this. And even when women felt strongly about getting to know a midwife and a degree of continuity was arranged, this did not work out in practice:

> *I had an appointment with the community midwifery manager because I had strong feelings about the fact that I would like to get to know, and I would want the person delivering the baby to get to know me prior to the birth so that we could be fairly clear about my needs and opinions on various forms of intervention and drug use. She agreed that three midwives would be allocated to my case. She couldn't guarantee who would be at the birth, but she could guarantee that one of three midwives would be at the birth and that I could get to know the three over the forthcoming months. This arrangement broke down almost immediately. So it seems clear that they are unable to accommodate me, but they're even unable to accommodate the compromise that they suggested to try and make me feel more comfortable.*

Midwives did what they could. Sometimes they asked women in late pregnancy if there was a midwife they would like to see again, or visited a woman in early labour to introduce themselves if they had not met before. One midwife accepted as many shifts as she could during the week of a woman's expected date of birth, but the baby arrived the following week. On-call rotas were sometimes given out, so that the woman had some idea about who would attend her. Women also did what they could. Some women called midwives early in labour or delayed calling in order to have a midwife they had met and liked. One woman took homeopathic remedies in order to have her baby when her preferred midwife was on call (in one area, rotas stopped being given to women when it became known that they were taking homeopathic remedies to induce labour when midwives who were supportive of home birth were on call). The general feeling was that there was little choice but to resign themselves to the lack of continuity, despite the inadequacies of this and the anxiety it caused:

> *I suppose I feel a kind of acceptance that that's the way it works. And yet I'm not happy with it.*

It does unnerve me that I have not got one person who I'm going to get to know quite well over the period of time.

One woman found the rhetoric of continuity and the reality of discontinuity so unacceptable that she booked with an independent midwife:

I was only going to be seeing them twice for fifteen minutes if I was lucky. That was me getting to know them. And not only that, but that was called getting to know them. That was sold as a lovely, cosy alternative, and I just thought, this is quite dishonest. I'm not going to collude. I can't collude with you and pretend that that's acceptable. I won't know these women at all.

Many women were unable to change their bookings for a variety of reasons: there were few independent midwives, they found the cost prohibitive, they were committed ideologically to the NHS, they felt that should be able to assert themselves, or they unravelled the mysteries of calling an obstetric service 'woman-centred' only late in pregnancy or after birth. On realizing that they would be unable to develop a relationship with one or two midwives during pregnancy, some women abandoned the ideal of forming trusting relationships. They focused instead on the midwives' attitudes to home birth, knowing full well that continuity of care cannot be provided by a collection of individuals, working in a controversial area:

I would rather have a midwife. Or two midwives even would be fine. Does it matter to me that I know them very well? It almost doesn't. What matters to me is that I know their views on home birth – their ideology I suppose, on how happy they are with home birth, how confident they are, if they're experienced and what procedures that they are likely to follow.

Further discontinuities

In addition to the lack of continuity within the community midwifery services, as I mentioned earlier, women were told that because of obstetric policies about risk, their midwives would attend them at home only if they gave birth between thirty-eight and forty-two weeks of their pregnancies. Otherwise they were expected to give birth in hospital attended by hospital staff. This added element of uncertainty further disrupted meaningful engagement between women and midwives because some women were reticent about engaging with their midwives until their home birth was likely to go ahead:

> *I think I asked most questions when they were here the last time, cos obviously that was when I felt things were sort of definitely happening. That I was really having it at home. So I suppose up until the thirty-eight weeks I thought I was to go into hospital anyway if the baby came before then, cos it was too early.*

Jillian Creasy's (1994) qualitative research on the experiences of women who transferred from community to hospital care during late pregnancy or labour suggested that being accompanied by a known carer made for a more positive experience.[23] While all but one of the women (who felt that her community midwives were unable to support her beliefs and needs) agreed that this was the case, the hierarchical bias towards hospital staff makes it more difficult for community midwives to practise in hospital.[24] And because maternity services de-emphasize relationships, community midwives are often excluded from transferring with women into hospital because of their workloads, rotas and shift patterns. Thus women who transferred to hospital care often felt abandoned by their community midwives. For example, the community midwives withdrew care from the following woman when she was thought to have reached over forty-two weeks in her pregnancy:

> *I just felt really like they'd completely abandoned me and I just thought, well it would be really nice because now when I'm so anxious, why don't they give me a ring and give me a bit of emotional support. And I thought this is where this whole system just falls apart and I was really, really disillusioned by it, I must say. I just thought this is the time I really need to speak to them. I don't need to see them. I don't want hours of their time. Just give me a phone call. I felt like I'd already been given over to the hospital almost. That's how I felt. It was really awful. I could have really done with just the odd phone call. I mean I didn't want that much, just how are you getting on, you know.*

Transferring to hospital was all the more difficult because of the added disjunction between the home and the hospital environment.

The transition from one to the other was described as moving from 'one world to the other' with 'different rules for both'. There was a sense of these two worlds not 'working together' and of the woman being dropped from the community services like a 'hot potato' with little understanding about the stress this causes women:

> *When I had to go into hospital the midwives weren't with me. None of my community midwives were with me . . . So the first time we went in we saw four sisters, three consultants, good-ness knows how many nurses [midwives] all in the space of one day on different shifts, all having different opinions. I was hav-ing to relate our story and they were coming up with different feelings about it. So I just felt that the whole thing didn't fit together that well. And then when I had to go back in, my mid-wife came in for about an hour with me, which was really nice of her. But she was very tired. She'd done the whole night long. But none of the other domino midwives that I'd been with would follow that on. And I kind of felt that I would have preferred for at least one of them to have been there, who knew me and could work with me. So I was left to a new nurse [midwife] to start up a new relationship. And when you're in pain, and you want to ask questions, and you have to explain the whole thing over again and you're confused, you know. The continuity wasn't there.*

Given that women transferring into hospital are moving into a differ-ent environment that is likely to have a different approach to the one they had chosen, continuity of care from a trusted midwife seems all the more important. As the quotations from the two women below demonstrate, being accompanied by their midwives gives women some protection and enables them to continue to focus on their labours rather than on negotiations with new people. Midwives can contribute to maintaining a feeling of security despite difficult changes in circumstances. In some cases, the midwife's acknowledged disap-pointment enabled the woman to express hers, so that she felt more positive about her experience than she might otherwise have done:

> *Nadine: How do you feel about having the same midwife with you, did that make a difference?*

> *Oh massively yeh, yeh, yeh totally. I mean I trusted them with it and they were very supportive and actually they were very*

disappointed that I never managed to deliver it and they were very disappointed for me, which was very touching. Yeh it was nice that they saw me through the whole thing and they remembered all the things which I'd said. Yes, it was nice that they were the ones that stayed. They were there right to the very last possible moment. I think that made a lot of difference. I think if I had been sent in and handed over to complete strangers, cos they were also able to negotiate with the doctor then as well on my behalf which was good, cos they had seen what had happened so far, because the hospital didn't actually have a birth plan or anything for me.

My midwife was great, because she didn't have to stay. So it was really good, at least I got my midwife.

Nadine: Do you think that made a difference?

It did, definitely, definitely, especially with it being [midwife] and she knew my partner really well, and she knew exactly what we wanted, and she was really good about, even though I was in hospital, you know. I was a wee bit worried about going in, but I didn't have to go through the rigmarole of signing in and you know, admissions and everything because it was [midwife] that was with me. I didn't see any other staff. I mean, it was completely quiet. She said, right, just get on with it, do what you want basically. So I think that helped as well, because I think it's the whole idea of all these strange nurses [midwives]. The first thing they want to do is give you an internal, and because [midwife] knew that I didn't want any of that – I mean, the only time she gave me an internal was when she thought he was just about coming and so I think that helped. I think if I'd had to go in and be signed over to the hospital staff, I would have hated that. It would have been people I didn't know and, as I say, I would have had to go through the whole routine. She was so good honestly. Just the fact that I didn't have to go through the hospital routine and it was [midwife] that was with me you know.

All in all, the difficulties women experienced by not being able to get to know a midwife, and the difference it made to those who did, suggests that the current controversy in the research on continuity symbolizes a dissonance between social definitions of birth that focus on the transition to motherhood where relationships are crucial, and medical definitions that focus on technical care that can be given by any competent practitioner. For women these definitions mean the difference between being treated as an autonomous subject, or a passive object of maternity services. In the same way that risk management cannot address women's safety needs, continuity of care (rather than carer) cannot address their needs for engaged relationship. Building discontinuity and lack of time into maternity services profoundly impacts on the level of interaction between women and midwives. It prevents trust developing between them, because trust develops in the context of relationships, and relationships need time to develop.

The constraints of lack of time and continuity

Communicating

A more mechanistic view of the body and bodily processes relies on clock time rather than women's time during pregnancy as well as labour. For example, the time allocated for antenatal appointments enabled midwives to carry out the physical checks but left little time for anything but superficial discussion. There was no time to form relationships that could foster 'real talk'.[25] As one woman pointed out:

> *There is so much procedure and so many stock tests to be gotten through that there is no slack in the appointments procedure for any vague chatting – as they would see it.*

Some felt that to:

> *Bring up more emotional complex issues would feel quite wrong, like you'd crossed the boundary.*

And yet time to talk was exactly what women needed:

> *I offered one of them to have a look at my bedroom and stuff, and she just seemed to want to get on to her next visit. Just somehow a distance to not really engage with you and really enter into your experience of what was going on. It's just, right, blood pressure, urine and now, any problems? You know, I didn't exactly have problems but just things to kind of think over and talk through a bit maybe . . . time.*

Again women understood that this was a structural problem that put their midwives under considerable time pressure. They did not want to add to this pressure:

> *I'm always aware that these people [midwives] are pushed for time and I don't want to blether. I feel I need to get on and out of their hair sort of thing.*

The visibility of time pressure in busy clinic waiting rooms made women:

> *Very aware of the amount of time you're spending with [a midwife] and I do think you do try to hurry along.*

This could lead to a negative spiral:

> *There was no urgency on their part to really get to know you. It's basically what the doctor would have done. So disappointing really. It's not developed a relationship.*

Exchanges could feel officious:

> *I said I'm going to have a pool and they would say, oh well, our policy is that you don't actually deliver in the water. It's been that sort of exchange.*

Overall, when women felt distanced through lack of engagement and there was so little time, it could feel too difficult to attempt to talk about their hopes and concerns about birth:

> *It [talking about birth] never seemed appropriate. They always flew in. You offered them a cup of tea to try and make a little chat. Tried to communicate. But you know, sometimes it was me as much as them. I wanted them out of the house just as quickly as they wanted to get out of the house.*

Yet within these constraints, informality and openness on the part of the midwife could encourage the devalued 'chatting' in which 'small truths' are exchanged.[26] As one woman explained, she had felt unable to talk to one midwife who asked only closed questions about physical aspects of her pregnancy:

Whereas the other one who I met just once, when she came round we found ourselves chatting. She asked us questions that encouraged us to talk, cos often I don't think of problems and worries, whereas she encouraged me to think about things slightly differently.

Another woman described how she would 'pick and choose' which midwives to talk to about her concerns on the basis of their ability to 'chat to you'. She explained that midwives who do not encourage informal chat about women's lives learn little about their pregnancies and concerns.

The assumption that communication can occur outwith relationships ignores individual communication styles and abilities. For example, one woman recognized that her midwife was the type of person:

That's actually quite nervous. So I just started to talk to her normally, and in the course of the conversation I actually realized she was quite competent, and was going to listen to me and care about me and so I got on fine with her.

Most of us relate more easily as we get to know each other and find areas of common interest. Women and midwives are no different:

The midwife who I've seen most often, I think I found it most difficult to start speaking to her. But having met her several times, I think she's probably just like me. I'm quite hard to speak to when you first meet me as well and I think over time I've definitely built up to being able to speak with her.

There's one [midwife] that I thought I wasn't going to like, and then I found out she was a runner, and I run, so that was something to talk about. It's sometimes just finding a hook.

All of the above constraints impacted on information gathering. Women often found that they had to find information on their own and because there was so little time when talking to midwives they tended to focus on getting to know 'what the procedures were'.

Getting information

The combination of lack of continuity and time and the need to control information led to innumerable comments about lack of information.[27]

There was a general consensus among the women that information (especially about home birth) was 'not handed on a plate', and depended on the women seeking it out from other women, childbirth organizations, non-NHS antenatal classes and books. They also observed that the information that was made available could seem formulaic and didactic, based on predetermined notions about what women need to know. Mary Belenky and colleagues (1986) found that women's concerns were often dismissed or controlled by experts, 'either by assaulting them with information or by withholding information'.[28] Some of the women in this book reported similar experiences of being 'bombarded with things you don't want and not getting the things you do want':

> *They [midwives] were very helpful, but one thing I would say about both of them, which does seem rather churlish, is that they seem to have been trained how to treat people and the sorts of problems people have and the sorts of anxieties people have. And when they're faced with you, which is 'a' person rather than 'the' person. You know, you're an individual, and you might ask questions in a different order, or you might ask questions you shouldn't really be asking until week 38 and that seemed to throw them and I didn't sometimes think that I was being heard. I think they had lots of answers, but some of them were to questions I hadn't posed and, do you know, I didn't feel there was a dialogue. I felt a little bit invisible. It was a bit smiley and a bit formulaic. And what about caesareans, you know, how often does that happen? I had all these questions and they tended to say things like, you don't need to worry about things like that at the moment. And I was like, is that going to stop me wanting to know? I don't think so. So in the end I just switched off and thought, I'll go and get a book.*

The women I talked to observed that obstetric knowledge and the structure of maternity services can reduce the meaning of communication to that of conveying limited information that ensures conformity: informed consent rather than informed dissent.[29] The short time for questions following the antenatal 'checks' is a gesture towards woman-centred care that cannot easily destabilize obstetric priorities. More detailed or complex information that might lead to women challenging midwives' policies was particularly difficult to obtain. For example, a number of women's babies were breech during part of their pregnancies. None of them felt that this should automatically necessitate a hospital birth but they were unable to engage midwives in discussions about this. They were told that breech babies usually turn or are born in hospital:

> *They [midwives] proclaimed the baby breech and then insisted the baby would turn and they wouldn't talk about what the implications were and they wouldn't say what their procedures were or what hospital policy was if the baby stayed that way. And I wanted to say, and what if the baby doesn't turn? Let's talk about that so that I can be prepared and make an informed decision. I need to make an informed decision. I don't want to be caught out at the last minute and for them to say to me, oh well, it's hospital policy, you have to go in, that's it.*

Because dominant values and practices are so culturally embedded they become difficult to see, discuss and resist.[30] Midwives working within dominant values are less able to see the implications of their practice,[31] and may not understand that gaps in knowledge are as constructed as knowledge itself. So while practitioners have a responsibility to enable women to make decisions, they may not be aware about the limitations of the information that they provide.[32] The onus is thus on the woman to identify, research and make decisions about complex issues. This was particularly important, but even more difficult, when women were unable to get to know their midwives. As one woman commented:

> *It all stayed vague [and] it does leave you with a lot of gaps. It means you're going in blind. I could find out a lot about the physiology of birth without asking a professional, but I can't find out about their procedures without asking them.*

Inevitably, some practices remained invisible and women were able to say only after birth that had they known that midwives might want to do a vaginal examination in order to decide when to call a second midwife, or use a hands-on technique for assisting with the birth of the baby's head, for example, they would not have agreed to these:

> *It is difficult because there's so many layers of medical expertise that you've got to get through. You've got to tell them that you don't want syntometrine or whatever. And you've got to know all these things that they're going to do just as a matter of routine. Because if I would have guessed that she was going to*

> *hold the baby's head as it was coming out, I would have put that in my birth plan, to say no, I don't want that.*

With little time to discuss these issues, the birth plan became the inadequate communication tool for the complex negotiations between women's decisions and midwives' usual practices. Women wanted to use them to convey their concerns, but discovered that birth plans are often used to steer women through difficult issues. Women's decisions were expected to be made from an acceptable menu,[33] and expressed as preferences in order to give practitioners ultimate control. If women attempted to assert 'off the menu' choices, midwives would sometimes suggest a 'wait and see' approach. This sometimes meant that they hoped to be able to help her change her mind. For example, one woman said she had decided to have a physiological (natural) third stage, but said that she had encountered 'more opposition to that than having the home birth'. She was given verbal and written information about the dangers of a physiological third stage. In later pregnancy, she said that she had been persuaded to change her mind and accept that it would be 'silly' to have a home birth and then have to go into hospital for a retained placenta. Her (reluctant) decision was documented in her birth plan. Towards the end of her pregnancy she acquired further information, and decided to go back to her original plan to have a physiological third stage. The final irony was that she was given syntometrine for the birth of her placenta because this was still in her birth plan. It was to avoid this potential inflexibility that some women did not write birth plans. The few women who had one-to-one care from a trusted midwife felt that they did not need a birth plan, but that it could be useful as an additional stimulus for discussion.

The kind of limited, impersonal and didactic information giving that women experienced did not lead to the kind of exchanges of knowledge that they needed to be able to make the best decisions they could for themselves and their babies. But as one woman commented, without getting to know midwives and spending more time with them, 'there's no way into that really'.

Communicating across ideologies

As I showed in Chapter 4, the coexistence of a dominant obstetric model of birth with muted social approaches and the midwife's conflicting role of both offering and restricting choice was confusing for women. One woman pointed out:

One minute you're a child being told to shut up and not raise difficult issues and the next minute, you're an adult, you decide what you want. But it's unclear which attitude applies to which issue.

Other women had to decipher what midwives really thought. The scene on page 147 of the woman being strongly advised to transfer to hospital, and then being told that she could stay at home, is a good example of this. Women frequently commented on the uncertainties they and their midwives faced when midwives were expected to reconcile restrictive policies with support for women:

I suppose it's that feeling of the midwives actually being very by the book and not sort of free to make their own minds up about things. I don't know what the leeway is in their criteria for doing certain things. Although I must admit, most of them did seem quite relaxed and they're in it because they want to be community midwives and they want to see home births, so I imagine they're going to be doing the best they can for you. I'm sure if I can stay at home they'll make sure I do. But on the other hand, I just hear so many people planning home births and going in [to hospital] for what seem like very small reasons and I wonder how can you sort of get round that.

This 'splitting' caused by different beliefs about birth could be unknowingly internalized by the midwife herself,[34] as one woman observed when she spoke to a senior midwife. The midwife assured her that she would be in control and that her choices would be respected, but then said 'at this point we would send a woman into hospital:

She was saying one thing and then undermining it and her language seemed to indicate a set of attitudes at odds with the message she was trying to get across.

Yet, despite the difficulties identified by women, ideological boundaries could sometimes be crossed. When women and midwives make time, away from hospital premises, they are freer to connect, communicate and question obstetric norms.[35] As women noticed, home visits over a cup of tea were more relaxed, and when:

You're more relaxed, you can ask about things. And there's things that I maybe wouldn't have asked about if I had been at the clinic.

During one of my interviews, a woman told me that she was finding it difficult to engage midwives in meaningful discussion during her pregnancy. By coincidence, a midwife arrived to see the woman partway through this interview. I left, and we resumed the interview after the midwife's visit. The woman explained to me how she and her midwife had moved from the usual, quick didactic information-giving to more thoughtful dialogue. Her description of the encounter demonstrated the commitment and skills that the woman and her midwife needed to move beyond the usual superficial talk, and why this is essential. She described how she initially negotiated ten to fifteen minutes of her midwife's time, but remarked that even this would have been too short 'to get to know somebody'. She then used some of the issues she had talked about with me to initiate a conversation about midwifery support during labour and the circumstances in which transfer to hospital would be advised. Her midwife was able to talk about how she supports women in different ways depending on the needs of the woman and that 'some women want tactile support, some women want to be spoken to, some women need reassurance, other women want somebody to be quiet, and we try and respond to what's going on at the time'. This thoughtful, more personal answer gave the woman confidence in herself and her midwives. The woman commented that this midwife and most of her colleagues talk 'very fast', and are 'purposeful and businesslike' and that her favourite midwife and another midwife 'stand out' because they 'use less words and speak more slowly'. Having more time and engaging on a more personal basis meant that this midwife was able to show her:

> *Listening side – and you know, when she said, 'So what are your questions about that?' Or when she said, 'How does that feel?' I could see that there was a sensitive side as well.*

This was extremely reassuring for the woman because she went on to explain that the fastness and efficiency used by many midwives:

> *Makes me shut down. I think that's probably the point where if I were to think about the emotional or the spiritual parts of the birth it almost feel as if they're too tender and too soft to be talked about in that fast way and so I think that that sort of thing does narrow down what we would talk about.*

The contrast in communication when women and midwives shared similar ideologies and formed close relationships highlighted the difficulties I have just described. One women who moved her booking from a team of community midwives to one-to-one care from an independent midwife explained the difference. Prior to booking with her independent midwife, the woman had felt compelled to ask a question, no matter how irrelevant to her, in the 'two minutes allotted at the end of the session' in order not to feel 'at the bottom of the class' or to 'fill a gap', whereas with her own midwife:

> *I'm now asking questions that I really want the answers to instead of filling a slot.*

She went on to say that she initially wanted to appear intelligent and capable and ask 'good questions' and that it took some time:

> *To stop doing that and just make a cup of tea and have a chat to her. I think she helped me to become more in touch with what I really needed to know or what I really needed to do in the time that we spent together – which wasn't always ask questions.*

The woman described a more informal relationship where she and her midwife could chat. This resulted in her realizing:

> *That I was enjoying the times that I spent with her and that I was feeling more and more confident, even when I hadn't cleared up any specific issue.*

As she felt more confident and comfortable with her midwife, she found that she could ask about complex issues about her autonomy, as well as specific questions about interventions. Learning about herself, her pregnancy and her midwife became:

> *Seamless, and I knew that [midwife] would respect my feelings. So it was more of a discussion. We would have discussions about things that would come up. There would be a programme on TV about birth, so we'd discuss it a bit. So we found out how each other felt that way rather than having a question and answer sort of dialogue.*

This level of communication resulted in the relationship being able to reach a point of resolution from which the woman could approach her birth calmly and confidently:

There was a kind of silence in the relationship, a stillness which was very important. And we'd done all the talking in the build up. So the talking was done. I felt confident that she [midwife] knew where I was coming from and vice versa. It was like we'd done all our dress rehearsal – what if . . . what if. And on the day there was nothing left to say really. So it just felt very calm, and I think that was the most important thing.

This personalized care that developed from the relationship was in stark contrast to the impersonalized care women described when midwives were perceived to be 'professional' but distant.

Professionalization

Does professionalization lead to impersonalization?

I explained in the introduction at the beginning of this book that in planning a home birth, women hoped that their care would be more personal and individualized than it would otherwise have been. But the structure of care that I discussed in Chapter 3 (and have just described above) frustrated women's and midwives' best efforts to personalize an essentially impersonal service. While professionalization need not lead to impersonalization,[36] the deep-rooted ideology that has shaped it inevitably has a profound impact on how midwives behave.[37] They tend to wear professionalism differently in different contexts. For example, when they are unable to develop relationships with women, have little time, and are expected to conform to obstetrically based policies, professionalism distances them from women. Women planned home births hoping that:

The care would be more personal and more concerned with me.

At home you're more likely to be attended by people that have greater respect for your personality, your individuality.

However, some felt that this was not the case because there:

Were different ones coming round all the time and there's no way of knowing when you meet any particular one that they're going to be the one that will be with you at the birth and they don't know that either.

Some women felt this to be:

> *Institutionalized in as far as I've not got to know them [midwives]*
> *and that's the same with institutions isn't it?*

They associated this kind of professionalism with the hierarchies, orders and discipline described by Mary Cronk (2000) – 'uniforms', 'black bags', 'efficiency', 'officiousness', and 'just a job':[38]

> *I just feel like it's their job. It does feel quite impersonal. I suppose*
> *I've got a certain amount of confidence in them because they've*
> *done it for quite a long time and they probably do know what*
> *they're doing. It's just the impersonal type of NHS feeling. I*
> *wouldn't say there was any common ground. There was nothing*
> *bonding between me and my midwife.*

> *Any of the ones [midwives] I've seen all look like they'd not be*
> *willing to make a huge amount of judgement on their own.*
> *They'd probably stick very much to the rule book. But that's just*
> *a feeling and I'm not saying I blame them for that.*

Woman understood that institutionalization fosters disengagement because of the sheer numbers of women and babies that midwives see on a day-to-day basis. They could see the difficulty of 'bringing that newness with them' when

> *You've been doing it for years with little respite. It's a bit like if*
> *you go for an interview. It's your one interview but the inter-*
> *viewer is – you're tense and they're a bit jaded and do you know,*
> *it's that division between you. And I don't know whether it can*
> *be crossed really'.*

But professionalization does not erase personalities and personal qualities. Thus the expectation that continuity of care can provide 'seamless' care, because midwives are interchangeable, contradicts the women's experiences of midwives' uniqueness and individuality. As women pointed out 'they're definitely all very different people'. Some were experienced as 'very formal', others as 'very friendly':

> *It's sort of quite a range. And some were much more open and*
> *friendly people. Some disclosed a lot more about their own*

experience as well which was nice. And others didn't tell you anything so it really depended on the individual.

As Carolyn Weiner and colleagues (1997) showed, personal bio-graphies contribute to how professionals do their work. Women also brought their own biographies, and suggested that the 'fit' between them was as important as their individual qualities. Attempting to neutralize biographies is not only impossible, but also undesirable. Being unable to find the person behind the professional distances women and midwives from each other, their experiences, knowledges, views about birth, family situations, and the contexts in which they practise and give birth.[39] This decreases the knowledge store from which midwives and women can draw – knowledge that contributes to safe birth, as I explained in Chapter 4.

What is lost to professionalization?

As I discussed in Chapter 3, the process of professionalization usually means accepting only objective scientific knowledge and rejecting other knowledge.[40] Women could see that this is exactly what has happened. As one commented:

The intuition side has been sort of overridden with technology – a bit of a loss of information really.

The wealth of lost knowledge reduces autonomy, as I have explained, and midwifery practice can be reduced to 'midwifery by numbers'. The midwife becomes disconnected from her knowledge and acts as a trans-mitter of evidence-based care that may or may not turn out to be bene-ficial for women and babies. For example, a woman told me recently that she was strongly advised by her midwives to comply with a policy that they said may change in the very near future, on the basis of new evidence. Midwifery is more than scientific evidence,[41] and women rec-ognized midwives as a source of evidence-based and experiential knowl-edge. They appreciated when midwives were able to help them weigh up evidence in more holistic ways, by engaging but not dictating. One woman, who knew and trusted her midwife, commented:

Her [midwife's] opinions were always given subtly and I never felt dictated to in any way, but she would if I pressed her. She would understand that I needed to know what she thought.

If professionalism means 'sticking to rules' midwives are unable to engage with women's decisions that challenge these rules. This can make women feel that midwives are 'covering their backs' rather than supporting them and 'inspiring confidence'. It ultimately decreases the woman's ability to follow her own ethical concerns. In talking about decision-making and responsibility, some women identified a cavernous gap between the active support based on skill and confidence they needed from midwives and the reluctant or apparently neutral support they experienced. This is a very important issue because women recognized that decisions are made in the context of relationships with midwives. They assumed responsibility for their decisions but at the same time needed their midwives to be with them on these decisions. One woman explained that 'it had to be you that had to take the onus' and that this was:

> *Fair enough. To a certain extent that's okay, that's acceptable. I should take the onus, but they could at least sort of encourage you a bit more.*

This issue of support for decisions is a very fraught issue because on the one hand those midwives who provide active support to women are often most likely to be accused of ignoring local policies and practising unsafely. On the other hand, it is those very midwives who from the women's point of view are most likely to provide them with safe care on their terms that they can trust.

But this kind of 'being with', honesty, empathy and respect is also undermined by the emphasis on 'efficiency' and competency demanded by institutions.[42] As I explained in Chapter 3 the mechanization and industrialization of the life world, the lack of emphasis on the emotional and spiritual aspects of life,[43] and capitalist definitions of production that have led to a live baby being the only measurable outcome of birth, often lead to midwives being judged only on their technical proficiency. Many women concluded that to expect more than technical proficiency was to expect too much, and that safe care is provided by technical competency alone. So while one woman described a midwife as 'intimidating', 'very bossy', 'abrupt' and a 'bit of a monster really', and said that her partner was 'terrified' of her, she described her as:

> *Very professional – she's obviously a good midwife and very highly trained, but not able to speak to you.*

This may reflect findings that suggest that:

> To gain a consistent overall impression people would try to avoid mixing positive and negative central traits. For example, people find it hard to imagine that a 'good nurse' could also be a 'cruel' person.[44]

This section on professionalization confirms the feminist view that a society marked by mechanization and industrialization fails to acknowledge the existence of caring work and the emotional demands posed on those who do it. Women realized this and frequently commented on midwives' exhaustion, stress and overwork. This could lead to midwives giving superficial or blanket reassurances. As one woman explained, midwives were sometimes:

> *Quick to say, oh it'll be fine – which doesn't work in dispelling people's anxieties. And I really don't like that. I find that very minimizing of my fear. But it's like any helping profession isn't it. In order to really listen to somebody in a painful, emotional state, you've got to feel it a bit yourself haven't you, and I suppose they don't want to be doing that ten nights a week while they're on shift or whatever. But I think that's the only way you're really effective.*

Quick reassurances were sometimes experiences as pseudo-mothering when:

> *What you want is a mother probably, to be mothered when you're just becoming a mother yourself.*

This type of mothering increases self-esteem, empowers and facilitates the woman to nurture her baby – 'mothering the mother to mother her baby.[45]

Engaged professionalism: the professional friend

The exceptional midwives were those who women felt crossed the boundary from professional detachment to professional engagement. They showed enthusiasm for their work and an expectation that all would go well. They were more autonomous, allowing policies and professional allegiances to recede as they moved closer to the woman. They were more able to listen to and trust the woman's knowledge.

One woman greatly appreciated her midwife's support, when there had been doubt over the likelihood of her having a home birth because her baby's head remained high in late pregnancy and early labour. When the woman felt that the baby's head was beginning to move down, her midwife acknowledged this and encouraged her to continue:

> *I just felt that she did really trust. She seemed to say, you'll know, and I did know.*

The comment from other midwives on the team, that this midwife:

> *Does her own thing made me think that that was a really, really good thing that she did do her own thing. I feel that there is a possibility that some of the other midwives might have said, no we're not happy with this.*

Where women formed relationships with one or two midwives the professional/personal divide was consistently less visible and divisive. One woman who got to know her midwife well explained the value of this and the dance between closeness (that enabled her to feel engaged and comfortable), and distance (that prevented her midwife's issues from encroaching on her own) that Sigridur Halldorsdottir (1996) describes. The woman suggested that without needing to know 'each other inside out', they had developed enough closeness to know that 'we broadly suit each other'. She also commented on the midwife's ability to be 'warm and friendly' and maintain an appropriate level of privacy without being closed – 'she has a kind of demarcation and I like that'. The woman describes the professional friend relationship:

> *The funny thing is, you build up a relationship that has a lot of trust – implicit trust in it. But at the same time you both know that it's built around a professional thing – and it is. It is built up quite quickly. So that in a way, I'm asking her to behave like a very close friend on one level and she isn't. And I know that, and she knows that and that's okay, but do you see what I mean?*

How midwives wear professionalization impacts on the level of mutual support or shared powerlessness that women and midwives experience. Whether it is used restrictively or as a way of supporting women's autonomy makes all the difference in the world. For example, one woman reported that her midwives had not attended a water birth before, but were keen to find out as much as they could. They borrowed her water birth video and showed themselves to:

> *Be very game, so I'm very grateful that they've come this far with me.*

Another woman was told: 'This is going too far, absolutely no way. None of us in the team have experience of water birth delivery, this is the most ridiculous thing I've ever heard'. This midwife refused to take a book on water birth offered to her by the woman. As Ruth Wilkins (2000) suggested, without moving outside the accepted paradigm of professionalism, women and midwives cannot move far together, challenge obstetric hegemony or develop transformatory knowledge, yet when midwives become professional friends, women are their strongest supporters, as the campaigns to support women-centred midwives demonstrate.

As far as these women were concerned, the point of developing relationships was to develop trust. Being 'friendly', 'good hearted' and 'lovely' was inadequate if they remained 'strangers'. The main quality within the relationship that women prioritized was trustworthiness. They were well aware of obstetric authority and their own vulnerability during pregnancy, birth and new motherhood and needed to be able to trust midwives to support their deep-rooted ethical concerns.

Trust

Perhaps one of the most important aspects of this research is that the women showed the intimate connection between trust and safety to be profoundly and irrefutably tenacious. Thus the current climate of facelessness and expert knowledge,[46] which promotes disengagement between women and midwives and makes it dangerous for midwives to support women,[47] is the very climate that creates danger for women and babies. There is an inherent paradox in obstetric ideology focusing on safety and at the same time decreasing safety by placing obstacles in the way of trust developing between women and midwives, as the following quotation plainly tells us:

> *I don't trust her not to panic and send me off to hospital just because things are bit slow or something. And if there was a good reason for me going into hospital I still wouldn't trust that it was a good reason, because I wouldn't know that she wasn't*

just panicking or plotting to get me away. And I don't think they trust me at all. I think [midwife] is very frightened that I'll stand there saying, 'I'm not going into hospital, I'm staying here', and put her in a really difficult situation.

The women I talked to wanted to be able to trust their midwives to meet their needs in the way that women trusted their midwives in other studies.[48] As well as entrusting midwives with their emotional and spiritual concerns, women wanted midwives to trust in the birth process and their abilities to give birth in their own ways. Women agreed with Maggie Banks' (2000) comment that 'the most essential component of [the midwife's] kit . . . is her trust and knowingness in women's ability to give birth':[49]

I get the sense that she [midwife] trusts. There's no reason for anything to go wrong. And I feel she would be there saying, 'You're going to be fine'. I think it's that that makes a midwife. Somebody who has a lot of trust in the thing of birth and is able to go with the rhythms and understand it and link in with it.

In Chapter 4, I discussed that developing confidence was one of the ingredients women identified in their definition of safety. Their confidence or lack of confidence was increased by the confidence or lack of confidence of their midwives. Many women had their own anxieties and any lack of trust and confidence on the part of the midwife influenced how the woman felt. Their observations confirmed the importance of midwives' trust and confidence in the process of birth. One woman explained that even though she had chosen a home birth:

You're not a 100 per cent sure that it's the right thing to do and that it's going to be safe and everything will be okay. But you know getting such a positive attitude off the midwife is such a big help in keeping you to your decision.

During a difficult but uncomplicated labour, another woman commented that her midwife:

Stayed as cool as a cucumber, which if she hadn't – if she'd at any point suggested that I wasn't going to make it then that would have had a huge influence on me.

A different woman experiencing a similar labour, noticed that:

Because they [midwives] were anxious, it completely changed the way I was looking at the situation. Up till then I was coping and then suddenly I was like, no. They didn't put a lot of pressure on me, only that I knew they were anxious about it.

But a patriarchal culture provides little fertile ground from which midwives can develop trust in themselves, women's bodies, and birth. Women wanted to trust midwives' abilities to recognize safety and danger but often felt they could not. They wanted:

Someone [who] does know what is risky, who I can trust, who'll reassure me if everything's fine and say, 'This is okay, don't be worried' but at the same time someone who knows when There's something wrong and we should be doing something – and I'd trust them. The problem is I don't.

To feel sure about whether or not they could trust a midwife, they needed to know her but often found that 'it's really hard to say because I just don't know them well enough'. Unusually, one woman, who knew and trusted her NHS community midwife, trusted her midwife to tell her if all was well, rather than fearing being transferred to hospital unnecessarily:

I really trust her and I trust her judgement and, I know when I go into labour and she'll come and she'll check everything and if she says everything's okay I'll believe her. I'll trust her that it is okay.

This bears no relation to the kind of blind trust that women talked about. 'Hoping for the best' or 'fingers crossed' were sometimes their only realistic options, but this kind of hope has nothing to do with trust or safety. It reflects a last resort to maintain some semblance of autonomy in the face of powerlessness. Occasionally, real trust was established in labour by a midwife unambiguously supporting a woman's decisions. One woman explained that she felt very strongly about not having a vaginal examination (VE) during labour, and had told her midwives about this, but as soon as a midwife arrived during her labour:

It was straight away into a VE. Like I just want to give you a VE, okay? I felt, oh God, this is happening straight away. I felt, the power's being taken and they were going to start taking control.

But I was really relieved when [main midwife] said, 'No, we've already discussed it and she's not going to have one'. That kind of came at the very beginning when they arrived and it really mattered then to know that I could trust her with something like that. I felt I could trust her further, because she was taking my side above her colleague's really.

It was very unusual for women to have developed complete trust in their midwives before they went into labour, in the way the quotation on page 146–7 describes when the woman's baby passed meconium and her midwife supported her to remain at home. This kind of trust can happen more easily and openly only when midwives are free to support women's autonomy, knowing that they will be protected rather than victimized if they do this. Rather than increase risk, as some fear it might, respecting women's autonomy is likely to increase safety by increasing the level of trust between women and midwives. The greater the trust, the more likely it is that women and midwives will work together towards safe decisions.

Limited trust or trusting in retrospect

Given the dissonance between midwives' policies and women's concerns, women often remained uncertain about whether or not their integrity would be respected and protected during the vulnerable period of birth. Some women were unsure about whether they would be able to focus on the challenge of giving birth, or whether they would need to 'watch out' and be ready to assert their decisions. They wondered about how possible this would be from a position of vulnerability:

I don't want decisions to be made on my behalf. You know, I got this worrying feeling that even if I said beforehand that I didn't want it [syntometrine and vitamin K], that at a vulnerable moment they [midwives] might try to persuade me. And I've heard that this actually happened to some people. You know, that even though they'd said something beforehand, people have tried to manipulate them with clever arguments at vulnerable times. And I didn't want to have to deal with that. I wanted my opinions to be respected.

Some women felt that the irresolvable gap between their ideologies and their midwives' practices and the lack of any mechanism for addressing this left them little choice but to distance themselves from the possibility of trusting midwives:

> *Nadine: How far would you say you have been able to develop a trusting relationship with your midwives?*
>
> *A trusting relationship? Well, no, I don't think that really enters into it. No, I don't think I would put any trust, and I think that maybe I tried to do that when [daughter] was born, and actually that is not the right place to repose your trust. I mean, you really have to trust in your knowledge of your body and yourself and the lasting relationships that you have with 'non-professional' people.*

(I mention the problem of women having to gain support from others, rather than midwives, in the section on support on page 197.)

A typically realistic assessment was that community midwives could be trusted to support women as far as they could without deviating too far from their policies and would not suggest transferring to hospital for 'flippant' reasons, or the 'smallest excuse' and that they would 'talk and discuss it beforehand'. In other words, many women came to the conclusion that their midwives would be competent and trustworthy in relation to the model of birth in which they were practising, but that they could not necessarily trust them to move outside this model if women needed them to:

> *If the baby's in danger, then of course do anything. But I suppose, it's just that if I don't know that I'm coming from the same value basis as somebody, then I don't know if they're going to be making decisions on the same basis as I would.*

When mutual trust developed from shared views about birth in the context of a relationship, the difference this made was indescribable. It led to women approaching birth with the kind of confidence that all the women hoped to feel in relation to their midwives:

> *The difference of knowing I'd have someone more in line with my thinking – I didn't feel that I needed a birth plan any more because I trust her opinion and that way I don't have any fears. So I don't have to swot up so much and be so defensive.*

Very few women felt the level of trust described by the woman above prior to giving birth. Many found that midwives did respect their views and support them during their births, but this was often in retrospect and sometimes following a series of disagreements about birth practices. For example, one woman who believed that her midwives were very unsupportive of her plan to give birth at home found the midwives to be 'super' during her labour and also reflected on how easy it would have been for them to persuade her to go to hospital during labour. 'She could have had me in hospital like that', snapping her fingers – but instead the midwife supported her:

> *There was no argument. I think if there had been, they could have ruined it.*

Another woman described the uncertainty she felt before birth:

> *At first I didn't know – it's when something big happens, like labour and birth, I suppose, that you really see what a person's true colours are like. I didn't know if what she was saying was maybe just to keep me happy until the birth. I didn't really know that. I didn't know if she was any more to be trusted than the others. And during the labour she was very good. So before, I couldn't really have told whether or not she would be.*

Yet feeling confident and knowing beforehand that they could trust their midwives was crucial, precisely because they knew or suspected that they would not be in a position to assert themselves while simultaneously negotiating their own internal experience of birth.

Trusting in the face of vulnerability

Women need to be able to trust midwives, not only to protect the process of birth, their integrity and their babies' well-being but also to protect their individual identities. These identities are socially, physically, emotionally, spiritually and sexually reconstituted through the complex transition to motherhood. The reconstitution of identity during transitional processes (rites of passage) such as birth means that it is vulnerable to external influences and at risk of being harmed.[50] Those present are entrusted to support birthing women to reorganize their identities in keeping with their own values, rather than those of others. Because the fragmentation and power of a rite of passage is not part of the language of obstetric birth,[51] its potential benefits and harms, and women's dependency on others to effect a positive transition remain muted. Harms are often expressed in terms of lack of control resulting in emotional harm that changes the woman in some way. As one woman explained:

> *In most of my life I'm in control of what's happening and once you're like that it's very difficult to then give control to other people, especially about something as important [as birth]. I did have postnatal depression after [child]. I wasn't myself after I had her but I just felt if I was more in control of what was happening to me, then I might have been a bit better later on.*

Another woman, like many others, said that she was not afraid of obstetric procedures or technology if they were needed and was grateful that they are available, but:

> *I think what I would find really difficult to cope with afterwards would be if I had been taken into hospital, or pressured to have a birth different from the sort that I wanted, on the basis that there might be something wrong, and then to find out that there hadn't been anything wrong. That's the kind of scenario that I really feel would be very difficult to handle. The aftermath of that. Feeling very angry and cheated. Especially if I'd been resisting and saying, no, no, I think it's okay.*

It is clear that when women and midwives engage in marginalized activities (like home birth) regulated by obstetric ideology, relationships can easily become sites of muted distrust rather than mutual trust. If women felt that midwives were practising from a standpoint that was not in tune with their own and having to protect their own vulnerabilities rather than women's, they often felt it was safer to withhold information in case it jeopardized their plans to have home births. Even basic information might be withheld. One woman 'had to tell everyone I was fine', even though she was suffering from depression 'in case that was a reason for me not to be able to have home birth' and another woman was afraid that:

> *Every time I conveyed a fear, it was going to be another black mark against me being able to stay at home. So I began to develop a habit of hiding things.*

Some women concluded that 'the less you actually tell people that something is bothering you the better it is'. Ultimately, even though women wanted to engage with midwives, if they felt unable to trust them, it felt unsafe to engage other than superficially. As one woman commented:

> *To be honest with you, I think it's easier to talk about things that have nothing to do with the pregnancy or the birth and talk to them about your house or garden and whatever.*

The reasons to respect women's values and to be worthy of her trust are many and compelling as I discuss further in Chapter 6. I would now like to expand on how women talked about the support they needed from their midwives.

Holistic support or obstetric surveillance?

By support, women meant assistance to move through pregnancy, birth and early motherhood in a way that would maintain their own and their babies' well-being and honour their integrity. Not surprisingly, concepts like 'support' can have different meanings within different contexts.[52] Within an obstetric framework, the separation of birth from its social context means that support focuses on surveillance and monitoring. Women's different and additional needs are not always easy to articulate:

> *When people stay at home, it's almost as if they're saying, well I don't need any of these things. I'm going to do it on my own. But I'm trying to say, well, in fact I do need a lot but in a different way. I don't need the drugs and I don't need surgical instruments I hope. But what I really need is support.*

As I described earlier, the women reported that the main purpose of antenatal appointments was to carry out physical health checks (checking the woman's urine and blood pressure, palpating her abdomen and listening to her baby's heartbeat) and that this took up most of the appointment time. Although many women appreciated these checks, they experienced this approach to care as limited and failing to meet other needs. All the women wanted a more holistic approach to health care and some questioned the value of fragmented care from strangers who knew nothing about them. 'Checks' on their own were considered to be of limited value:

What they did was lots and lots of checks which I didn't need. I felt like I was able to gauge my own health, and that I didn't need to be measured, weighed, checked so much and I needed something else and there wasn't anything else. The medical check went under the guise of getting to know you and I just thought, actually this is all wrong – just having my tummy measured. And if that's all that was going to happen, it was ignoring so much.

This kind of checking could feel threatening and more like surveillance. It objectifies women, treating them as 'nonentities, nonparticipants, environments, or functions'.[53] One woman felt that her midwives had only a 'monitoring role – they see themselves as monitors. They're not here to support'. However, while 'checks' could be experienced as undermining in the context of fragmented care, these same 'checks' could be experienced very differently in the context of a holistic approach from a known and trusted midwife:

The difference is because I have time to get to know [midwife]. So what happens is that she comes round, we have a cup of tea, we have a chat, then we do the check. So she will do all these things, but it seems relevant. It's like somebody you know who's caring for you, checking that you're okay. So it feels different because you're not straight in the door and on the scales, or straight in the door lying on your back with your top up. You've actually engaged as an adult with somebody first.

As I explained in Chapter 2, the underlying principles of biomedical health care emphasize abnormality and illness and de-emphasize normality and health, to the extent that the body is only visible through symptoms of illness.[54] As I also explained in Chapter 3, the relentless search for abnormality has meant that physiological, emotional and spiritual skills integral to safe birth remain relatively undervalued and underdeveloped.[55] Of course midwives have skills in these areas, but sometimes women had to ask them to put aside paperwork or stop chatting so that they could put these into practice. Women were acutely aware of midwives' physical, emotional and spiritual presence or absence. As one woman commented, during her labour

There came a stage when I really wanted them to be with me. I just remember looking really hard into her eyes and she absolutely meeting that stare and giving me strength, which is exactly what I needed.

The search for abnormality not only de-emphasizes the skills to assist births that are normal but more challenging or unusual, but also leads to more births being considered abnormal and in need of obstetric intervention. As one woman commented:

I suppose it [skill] comes from experience, but it feels like they're actually not getting the experience

because normality has become so limited in meaning.

The complex physiological emotional and spiritual skills that some midwives have been able to develop and that could transform midwives' and women's experiences of safe birthing are barely audible. Even basic alternative knowledge and skills are lacking. Women commented that homeopathy, herbalism, nutrition, shiatsu, acupuncture and other approaches can contribute to well-being during pregnancy and birth, but are not used:

There's so much wisdom that they could tap into that they don't seem to be interested in – it seems bizarre.

Generally, many women felt that the home birth service could be 'greatly improved and the systems around it could be more supportive of that choice'. Some women felt that midwifery training should be expanded so that midwives could competently and confidently attend a greater variety of normal births at home, so that women who believed that they would be safer at home could rely on good midwifery care. They could see that expanding midwifery knowledge and practice is the way to increase women's autonomy and safe birth. But this is a contentious issue because it challenges the boundary between normality and abnormality on which the demarcation between subordinated midwifery and authoritative obstetric power and knowledge rests. In other words, expanding midwifery is a direct challenge to obstetric hegemony.

Support for the birth–motherhood continuum

Whether women talked about safety, well-being or integrity, they talked about it in terms of the transition to motherhood. While there were diverse views on being a mother, birth set the scene for future family well-being and was described as a journey within the motherhood journey. This brings to mind birth practices in non-industrialized cultures that focus as much on the early mothering period as on pregnancy and birth.[56] While we must be cautious about interpreting other cultures through our own eyes and values,[57] the focus on the time after birth in some cultures contrasts sharply with practices in most of the industrialized world, where postnatal care is not necessarily provided on a statutory basis (as in North America) or provided minimally (as in parts of Scandinavia) or focuses on babies' physical health (where it is provided by paediatric nurses). Even in Britain where postnatal care is still statutorily available to all women, very few women receive midwifery care for more than ten days, and report that they receive visits less frequently than they need and that these tend to focus only on physical health checks rather than the emotional support women often need.[58]

From the perspective of the birth–motherhood continuum the role of the midwife is too narrow and time limited. So in addition to discussing how current services could be improved within the existing framework (by providing greater continuity, more time, more home visits, more information and discussion, more emotional support based on women's needs and beliefs, and more integration between home and hospital services), some women questioned the framework itself. They imagined that midwives' skills could include skills to facilitate motherhood as well as birth. It was perhaps because of this that some women felt that midwives should have children themselves, though others felt that a midwife's experience of birth and mothering, if unprocessed, might interfere with her ability to empathize with other women.[59] Speculating on Christine Bewley's (2000) work on childless midwives led me to wonder if this is more of an issue in the context of lack of continuity. It might be less important when women are able to get to know and appreciate the skills and attributes of individual midwives. It might also matter less if part of the midwives' role could be to help women connect into the social network of mothers around them.

In a culture that is based on the nuclear family and devalues motherhood there are few mechanisms for connecting communities of birthing women and mothers. Some women felt that encouragement to support each other during labour could increase connections between women because it would be part of 'your friendships' and 'that way it's ongoing'. Many women stated that their partners should be their main birth supporters as they believed that this promotes family bonding, but over half the women planned to have an additional female helper with them during birth:

I think I remember saying with [baby's] birth that it's really a woman's thing. I really felt that I needed the presence of other women – particularly women who'd been through the process.

This could be complicated when women were unable to get to know and trust their midwives and were concerned about their midwives' practices. In these circumstances, they usually selected birth companions who would support their views as well as provide emotional support. This could be threatening to midwives if they felt less able to persuade woman to conform with local policies and practices and thus less able to safeguard their own positions. So while women were sometimes surprised that birth companions were not generally encouraged by midwives, midwives themselves sometimes expressed concern about birth supporters,

They asked me if there were any AIMS people coming. They were very interested in [friend]. In fact they kept on saying – 'and they'll look after the children'. And I didn't confirm that or deny it.

Of course, some midwives were welcoming of women's chosen supporters, but only the women attended by independent midwives reported that the possibility of other supporters was actively explored and that their midwives initiated meetings with those who would be present to discuss how they would work together to support the woman. This was ideal because support needs to be cohesive to be most supportive and can feel less surportive if it is so:

I think she [midwife] was completely oblivious of what I really needed. You know, just the emotional support. Although I got a lot from my friend and partner they weren't midwives. I was looking for somebody with the expert knowledge to tell me more about what was happening, or how I was doing, or what I should be doing.

Where ideological dissonances distance women and midwives, midwives are unlikely to begin the process of re-establishing the connections women need during motherhood. Yet this is exactly what Nicky Leap's (2000) work on community building achieved. By acknowledging birth as part of motherhood, acknowledging women's needs for ongoing support and the limitations of midwifery (as currently defined), her practice actively engaged with the woman's social network in order to help women gain support from their own communities. The idea that those who support women during birth will form closer attachments to her and her baby on an ongoing basis was similar to views expressed by some of the women. The midwife's role is one of facilitating relationships between the woman and her community, potentially dissolving any adversarial boundary between midwives and female helpers at birth. Meanwhile, ideological dissonances, as I have discussed, caused conflict that women and midwives found difficult to resolve.

Dealing with conflict

The support women needed for their decisions confirms the complex feminist theories I discussed in Chapter 2 – that women's behaviour is contextual and relational, but that this partly reflects their subordination.[60] The women wanted to exert their autonomy by moving through birth in their own unique ways in the context of supportive, trusting relationships with midwives. Relying on rights was not necessarily helpful (as I discuss in Chapter 6) because lack of support for decisions undermined autonomy. While women talked to me about the dissonance between them and their midwives, most, like those described by Mary Belenky and colleagues (1986), found assertiveness problematic and conflict intolerable. Most did not want to assert their rights, make 'waves', have midwives attend them under duress, or cause a 'fuss' that might alienate health practitioners. One woman described having a scan that she didn't want. Because she was so relieved that her doctor had supported her plan to have a home birth, she did not want to refuse the scan in case her doctor withdrew her support. All the women showed great strength, skills and resources, but very few felt prepared to openly assert some of their beliefs and needs. The woman who felt in control at home and said

> *If I had a really stroppy wee woman [midwife], I would just say,*
> *go away. This is your job and you're not doing it, so go away*

was very much the exception. For most, being themselves and asserting their needs was extraordinarily difficult. A more common feeling was:

> *I just felt what I always feel with medics – just wanting them to*
> *leave it alone and stop worrying at it and not really being able*
> *to say so.*

As Mary Belenky and colleagues (1986) described, when women felt unable to assert themselves, they often judged themselves negatively, feeling that, 'I let myself down. I should have been more forthright' but adding that 'it's difficult when you're relying on someone'. Some saw themselves as 'quite cowardly' or lacking in courage about asserting themselves, 'I wanted that but I didn't go for it because I wasn't assertive enough'. But they also said that they might have felt less silenced and more able to talk about some of the ideological differences between them and their midwives had they been able to form relationships. When there was so little time to talk to relative strangers they felt that to communicate these concerns they would have 'to be bluntly assertive'. As one woman explained:

> *If I'd had one midwife who I'd built a relationship with over a lot of weeks or months then maybe I would have been able to talk to her about the kind of emotional difficulties that I had around not being able to talk about the value level and things. It would have depended on what midwife I got obviously, but had it been somebody who I developed a rapport with, a lot of those difficulties could have been a lot less, just from knowing somebody and knowing where they're coming from and even just having longer to work out how it is that I can say things that otherwise would feel difficult – because that's another way round having to be bluntly assertive – working out how you say this in a way that can be heard. You know, for me it can take quite a long time of negotiating around with somebody to find out what they can hear and what they respond well to and what I wouldn't be able to say.*

A plethora of popular western literature urges us to resolve conflicts openly, but as I have described, the midwives' need not only to steer women,[61] but also to avoid conflict,[62] is overwhelming. One woman commented that she was persuaded to talk to a midwife again before deciding whether or not to have her involved in her care, but the midwife avoided her. And some observed that differences could perhaps be resolved with individual midwives, but that this is impossible in the context of teams of midwives and short antenatal appointments: 'even if you manage to reach an understanding with one of them', she may not attend the birth 'and it's quite exhausting to have to make that effort six times over'. Another pointed out:

> *You chat about the same things with each of them that comes. You never really scratch the surface. I think it would have been*

better if you'd known who you were going to get and I know that's really difficult, but at least you could have said, right, well, that's who I'm going to get. Let me try and knock her into some sort of shape before the event. Whereas you can't try and knock six of them into shape by meeting them all once each.

There was an expectation that women and midwives should resolve any difficulties between them, yet there were no apparent skills, mechanisms or support to help them to do this. There was apparently little understanding that conflicts were often about the need for women to be autonomous and the need for midwives to prevent this, if it might lead to women moving outside their policies or sphere of practice. The expectation that conflict could be resolved put pressure on women and midwives but was often unachievable. As one woman explained:

One of the midwives – we really didn't get on with. So then this woman [senior midwife] phoned up and said, 'Can I send her round to you? Part of her job is to make you feel at ease and if she's failed to do that I think she needs to sort that out with you.' And I was pretty against it really. I thought, look, we just don't get on. It's not cos she's a bad midwife it's just cos we don't get on and I said that. But she persuaded me that the adult thing to do was to meet her. We did feel at the end of it that we'd talked through a lot of the problem. But at the same time I'm glad she wasn't on and we didn't have to deal with her [during labour].

Keeping in mind even just a few of the women's considerations (their dependency on fragile relationships with midwives, their need to feel supported in their decisions, the obstetric expectation of compliancy, professional alliances, and the potentially punitive attitudes towards those who challenge obstetric beliefs), their difficulties in asserting themselves look rather more complex. Their reluctance to cause conflict seems more of a pragmatic, self-protective decision not to alienate midwives or attract punitive measures. For many women avoiding conflict was a high priority. This explains why feminist theories found that women's caring attitude could override their need to assert themselves, even when this caused them suffering,[63] and why this could be interpreted as women having to internalize conflict in a culture that prevents them asserting their autonomy safely.[64]

Can relationships transform?

The work that was done on ethics of care and relationality by feminists such as Mary Belenky and colleagues (1986), Carol Gilligan (1985), Nel Noddings (1984) and Sara Ruddick (1989), and taken further by Nancy Goldberger and colleagues (1996), Linda Nicholson (1999) and Ann Oakley (2000), is undoubtedly crucial. But what does this mean for relationships between women and midwives? Can caring relationships be transformatory without being oppressive, taken for granted, or seen as merely a symptom of patriarchal power relations? Is it possible to develop healthy relationships that are both nurturing and able to address differences?

There seemed no doubt that trusting relationships with known midwives, who shared a similar birth philosophy and had time to be with women could increase women's knowledge, self-development and autonomy.[65] But when women met different, overworked midwives, who could share their ideals only to some extent, relationships seemed more likely to coerce and oppress. Women often felt unable to say or do what they felt was right for themselves, their babies and their families. So while caring relationships may be the basis for healthy self development,[66] they become dysfunctional if caring is an expectation of women but not of men, or demands that women and midwives must be self-sacrificing. This leads to the current paradox of expecting midwives to nurture women and women to nurture babies within industrialized, impersonal, and time-deprived services that nurture no one.

Enabling relationships to develop between women and midwives forges alliances between them. This can begin to undo the divisiveness and reduce the coerciveness of dominant obstetric ideology. As Helen Stapleton's (2004) work confirms this is even more powerful when women and midwives begin to shape birth culture together, because 'the force of the paradigms that govern medical knowledge is such that *individual* dissenting voices, whether of patients or physicians, have scant hope of claiming a hearing'.[67] Perhaps this is why continuity of care is threatening. Together, women and midwives really begin to question obstetric meanings of birth and uncover their own knowledge based on their own experiences. Together they begin to reveal 'what is "not supposed to exist"'.[68] As long as women and midwives are kept apart by obstetric ideology, most women will struggle to assert their autonomy in childbirth and most midwives will uphold obstetric thinking and practices. Trusting relationships with midwives who have developed their own autonomy, that balance closeness and distance maintain safe spaces for women to develop their own knowledge and autonomy without floundering, as this next woman suggests:

> *Birth is a natural normal everyday process and it doesn't need to be made right by the medical system. There was nothing in any of my births that would have required me to be in hospital and it feels like an invasion that . . . What am I trying to say? They were all there waiting for it to go wrong, and it wasn't going to go wrong and they saw it as their place to do that whereas that's my responsibility. It's my place to do that and I know when it's necessary. Women love their babies. I would never put my baby in danger and I don't know anyone who would. The medical field is there when one needs it and one knows oneself when one needs it. I think what women need is not to be patronized and ignored. I think we need information, unbiased information, not about how to do it, but about the possibilities. What movements make some labours easier, what things women find make labour progress better, what to do when your baby's in a breech position, what to do when different things occur during a normal pregnancy and birth. Knowledge is what we need, you know, it's in women's hands, that's where it should be. That feels right because we can work out for ourselves. We're not stupid, you know. I felt I was treated as if I was stupid in some way or not able to have a baby and of course we're the ones who do it. You know, it seems that we've come a long way, but not half far enough. In some ways it's in the dark ages because we're not trusted. We're not trusted to have our babies. I think there is an enormous place for women's knowledge. I think the barriers have to be pushed in order to make that space.*

Strong, trusting relationships could lead us out of 'tick box' midwifery, where women are expected to make acceptable decisions about pregnancy and birth at designated times and then expected to adhere to these. It may be possible to imagine skilled, knowledgeable and autonomous midwives bridging the 'cultural gulf' between women's knowledge and that of dominant obstetric ideology. It may even be possible to imagine women's decisions arising over time in dialogue with midwives. In other words, forming relationships could be a way of shifting the focus from the 'immortality strategy' (managing risk to ensure a live woman and baby), to the more procedural view of safety that I discussed in Chapter 4 that would address a broader concept of safety.

This chapter has focused on the impact of coercive obstetric thinking on individual relationships between women and midwives. Chapter 6 looks at this coerciveness in more general terms. It considers the consequences to women's integrity and identity of an ethics that hampers women's attempts to journey through pregnancy and birth in their own ways, and midwives' attempts to journey with them.

Notes

1 Jenny Green 1999: 8.
2 Foucault 1980; Mackenzie and Stoljar 2000; McNay 1992; Murphy-Lawless 1998a; Shildrick 1997.
3 Belenky et al. 1986; Debold et al. 1996.
4 Davis-Floyd and Sargent 1997; Jordan 1993.
5 Cronk 2000; Edwards 1996; Robinson 1999.
6 Kirkham 1999b; Stapleton et al. 1998.
7 See, for example, Gaskin 2003; Rooks 1997; Schlenzka 1999.
8 Clarke 1995; Kirkham 1999b.
9 Freire 1972.
10 Hadikin and O'Driscoll 2000; Shallow 1999; Stapleton et al. 1998.
11 Starhawk 1990.
12 Wagner 1995.
13 Kirkham 1999b.
14 Stapleton 2004.
15 Murphy-Lawless 1991.
16 Edwards 2004a, 2004b.
17 Levy 1998, 1999b.
18 Murphy-Lawless 1998b.
19 Chesney 2004.
20 Leap 2000.
21 See also Gardner 2004.
22 Wilkins 2000.
23 See also Walker 2000.
24 Shallow 1999.
25 Belenky et al. 1986.
26 Spacks P. (1982), in Belenky et al. 1986: 116.
27 Comaroff 1977; Kirkham 1989; Stapleton et al. 1998.
28 Belenky et al. 1986: 194.
29 Goer 1999.
30 Davis-Floyd and Sargent 1997; DeVries et al. 2001; Jordan 1993; Oakley and Houd 1990.
31 Wagner 2001.
32 McLeod and Sherwin 2000: 268.
33 Mander 1993, 1997.

34 Debold et al. 1996.
35 Mercer and Skovgaard 2004; Wilkins 2000.
36 Pairman 2000; Smythe 1998; van Olphen Fehr 1999.
37 Oakley 2000.
38 Cronk 2000: 22.
39 Bewley 2000.
40 Downe 2004; Oakley 2000.
41 Downe 2004.
42 Halldorsdottir 1996; van Olphen Fehr 1999.
43 Hall and Taylor 2004; Siddiqui 1999.
44 Hadikin and O'Driscoll 2000: 50.
45 Mander 2001: 82.
46 Giddens 1991.
47 Hadikin and O'Driscoll 2000.
48 Lemay 1997; van Olphen Fehr 1999.
49 Banks 2000: 132.
50 Davis-Floyd 1992; Shildrick 1997.
51 Adams 1994; Coslett 1994; Rabuzzi 1994.
52 Treichler 1990.
53 Adams 1994: 246.
54 Leder 1990.
55 Hall and Taylor 2004.
56 Kitzinger 2000; Priya 1992.
57 Oakley 2000: 55.
58 Patricia Hamilton talked about her research on this at the Fourth International Home Birth Conference in Amsterdam in March 2000.
59 See Mander 1996.
60 Belenky et al. 1986; Debold et al. 1996; Gilligan 1985; Nicholson 1999; Ruddick 1989.
61 Comaroff 1977; Levy 1998, 1999b.
62 Kirkham 1999b.
63 Belenky et al. 1986; Gilligan 1985; Ruddick 1989.
64 Debold et al. 1996.
65 See also Belenky et al. 1986: 217; Stanton 1996.
66 Ruddick 1989; Starhawk 1990.
67 Code 2000: 192.
68 Harding 1996: 446.

6 'They think it's best'
The ethical implications of obstetrics

The real political contest, on issue after issue, is a struggle between value systems – the confident scientific rationalism of the government elites versus the deeply felt human values expressed by people who are not equipped to talk like experts and who, in fact, do not necessarily share the experts' conception of public morality . . . The public's side of the argument is described as 'emotional' whereas those who govern are said to be making 'rational' and 'responsible' choices. In the masculine culture of management, 'emotion' is assigned a position of weakness, whereas 'facts' are hard and potent. The reality, of course, is that the ability to define what is or isn't 'rational' is itself laden with political self-interest, whether the definition comes from a corporate lobbyist or from a federal agency . . . For elites, the politics of governing is seen as a continual struggle to manage public 'emotions' so that they do not overwhelm sound public policy.[1]

Chapters 4 and 5 demonstrate women's broad concerns about safety and the value they place on engaged, trusting relationships in order to achieve that safety. They show women's strengths and vulnerabilities in the face of an ideology that values neither their concerns nor relationships. This chapter expands on some of the themes of Chapters 4 and 5 by looking at the more detailed interactions between women's thinking and their experiences of maternity services. It explains why concepts such as choice and control exist mainly at a rhetorical level and why rights are problematic.[2] It explains the impact of the day-to-day coercions in maternity services on women's bodies, minds and psyches that hamper rather than enable them to develop their autonomy.

This chapter looks at the costs of challenging normative values and practices. It is about how the 'immortality strategy' has led to decades of obstetric discourse focused on risk and death,[3] to the extent that women's qualitative experiences of birth have all but been forgotten about. It is about how women engage with obstetrics from their own ethical positions and about the autonomy and freedom they feel they need to be able to focus on birth without fear. The tension between engagement and disassociation is as much a feature of this chapter as it was in Chapters 4 and 5.

Resisiting obstetric coercion

The catalyst for this chapter was first and foremost the experiences and fears that women expressed about being coerced, manipulated or forced into agreeing to practices that they believed to be inappropriate. Some women were afraid that an obstetric approach may extend into their homes or that they may be transferred to hospital and thus to the full force of obstetric ideology: in both cases being exposed to physical and emotional violations that might compromise their own and their babies' and families' well-being and integrity. By looking at how services might be otherwise, I hope to add to the compelling discussions about why we need to sensitize health care ethics to the feminist concerns of embodied diversity and vulnerability in order to change how practitioners respond to pregnant and birthing women.[4]

Meanwhile, the sheer effort and courage needed by women (and those midwives who support them) to resist obstetric practices and exert autonomy is overwhelming. The coerciveness of birth practices, the assumption of authority described by Robbie Davis-Floyd (1992) and Brigitte Jordan (1997), the treatment of women's bodies as brute matter, the inevitability of obstetric practices taking precedence and drowning out women's voices, and the failure to attend to the experience of giving birth to a new and cherished family member are clear in the extract below where a woman describes the birth of her previous baby in hospital. In this stark example, we can see how institutionalization of obstetric practices perpetuates professional behaviour that in other circumstances would be viewed as intolerable. It exemplifies the disassociations of modernity described by Carol Gilligan (in an interview with Mary Hamer 1999) and Charlene Spretnak (1999) and the disrespect for and violence towards women discussed by Jo Murphy-Lawless (1998a). It raises many of the issues I discuss in the rest of this chapter:

> I [had] my head down, and my bum up and I was rocking. And he [partner] was like asking me shall we get anybody and I said, yeh, and I wish I'd never now because he went off, and got a

nurse or a midwife. She'd taken one look at me, and gone, oh, we'll have to get you up to labour ward – can you walk? I got off the bed, made it about five steps, got hit by a contraction and – no, hang on. She said we've just got to make it to the lift, and we got into the corridor and I was having another one. I remember being against the wall and going oh no, cos I could feel it [baby] coming down inside me and there were people coming to visit [during visiting hour] and I was thinking, oh no, don't let me have it here in the corridor. Put me back in the room. And she got a damn wheelchair, and she goes, sit on that, and I went, you must be joking. She said, no. Sit down. I remember sort of trying to get on this wheelchair. I could feel it between my legs, this big lump, if I sat down, so I was trying to hold myself up on the arms of the wheelchair and not push my bum down and she whisked me off. I was whizzing about and she's got me in this lift and it was awful, because I was caught in the panic of her running, and I was going, oh my God, hang on, I'm going to fall off the chair. And we got in the lift and upstairs and it was just like, mad running about and get the dress off, get a gown on, get on the bed. In comes somebody to examine me, and I'm going to her, it's there, no need to put your hands in me, you don't have to. Oh but I will, and right enough, she didn't get in very far. She went, oh yes, so there is. Well, I told you that, didn't I. Believe you me, I can feel it. And at this point she said, she was going to put a drip in my arm, and I'm like the head is here. I am frantically trying to get on all fours and they told me to get back because I was putting the baby in distress so I turned round again, and I was sort of sitting up, and she was going on about, she had to put the drip in my arm because I had signed the consent to say that I would allow them to put a line in my wrist. It was like something out of a Carry On film. There I am trying to get away from her because I was trying to concentrate and she's trying to get me to keep my arm still. She was struggling with my arm and eventually she seems to have given up or finished. By this time I was more concerned about the midwife who was stretching my vaginal skin around the head of the baby, and it was stinging like hell. And I was saying to her **GET OFF ME, LEAVE ME ALONE**, and she was going oh no, no, no, she has to do this, and I was going, just leave me alone and screaming and shouting. And it was all over before I knew it, she's going, look, and [partner's] going to me, it's there, it's there, it's head's there. And I looked down, and he *was looking up at me all scrunched up. And that was the other thing I didn't like. She promptly then pulled the body out. I was in this relaxed – oh thank God, he's here – the vital bits were there, he was breathing and crying, he was like looking at me and she pulled him out. I wish she'd waited for me, or just for him to come with the next slither. But this anxiety to get it out. I remember thinking, don't give me that injection, I'm not having that injection, and I wanted them to leave the cord, but I hadn't said it to them, and before I knew it, I was clamped. Well, the next thing I noticed was she's got a hold of the cord, and I said, let go of my cord. I said, **LET GO OF MY CORD**, and she went like, oh, I'm just helping, I'm just seeing if it's loosened, and I was going, don't pull the cord, and she was going okay, okay, don't panic. And then they've said, could I get on all fours, could I kneel up because some fifteen minutes have gone by, and the placenta wasn't coming. And I said, oh, I've got ages yet, just leave me. She said, oh no, you have to get up, there's only twenty minutes, and I'm saying oh, no, no, no, you're not going to touch that until at least an hour has gone past. So I knelt up and I've heard someone going, oh, where's all that blood come from, looked round, and there was this pool of bright red blood round behind me, and I'm thinking, oh, what's happened. Bloody thing in the arm. No sooner had she put it in, I've put my hands behind me, because she was asking me to push my bum on the bed, when the head was being born and I was going like, I don't want to, I was trying to push my bum up off the bed and as I did it, I must have knocked the thing out of my arm, so all the time I'm like, pushing down, I'm pumping blood out of the thing. So it was like, oh, that's okay, we know where the blood's come from, cos I was thinking, oh God, don't let me be haemorrhaging. I ended up bruised from the finger tips to the elbow. You know, that was just a pointless exercise to fulfil a piece of paper really. So, yeh, the placenta came fine, and it was all okay and we thought that was it. I wasn't giving them the baby and he was quite happy. He was looking around and I mean, I don't want you to go and bath him or anything, just leave him. Oh, they had to weigh him and they wanted to do a glucose check, and like, hang on a minute, I don't like this. Like why are you doing this when the only solution seems to be to give them food. And they were saying I didn't understand anything about it. This was after they weighed him, because up until that point, I would say that everyone thought he was a perfect little baby.*

Yes, he looked small, but I'm sure in comparison to me he didn't look that small, and it was like, they put him on the scales and attitudes changed. It was like they wanted to whisk him away, they wanted the paediatricians, they wanted blood, and I was going no, no, no, hang on, hang on, the paediatrician's checked him over and he's fine. His breathing is mature, he's full term, he's okay, he's just small, he's not in a bloody trance, he's not in a hypoglycaemic state. Anyway, we're having this big, big row by now cos I'm saying, well, I'm going home and I'll feed the baby. I'll stay awake all night, I don't care, that's what I did with my last baby. I took him out the nursery, and stayed awake all night, and fed him, and let them prick him again the next morning, and they said he's stable, whatever that means. And my GP said he would come cos I'd said to him that I wanted to discharge myself immediately and he said he would come to the house to look at the baby for me, so I couldn't see the problem myself. He was born at ten to nine, and by now it was about eleven o'clock, and we're arguing and arguing and nothing's happening. I'm going like, I can't feed the baby while you're rowing with me. I'm like, just go away please. I have bottles, I have formula, I have a breast pump, I have boobs, I have milk, I'll spoon feed him, I will drip it in his mouth if necessary, I will get food into the baby. I'm not going to walk off and put him to sleep and leave him am I? And so we went out looking for the paperwork, and it was thrown on the desk in front of us and that was it – off we went. But it was great when we got back [home].

None of the above is unusual, and none of the practitioners are 'bad' people. In a rule-bound, faceless institution, as Mavis Kirkham (2004) points out, practitioners cannot easily do otherwise. Indeed, women became acutely aware that their increasing vulnerability during pregnancy and birth was likely to be exploited:

When you're pregnant, you're so vulnerable, it's not just like the me you know normally. Your emotions are running high, you feel so vulnerable and you don't know. And when they start implying that in some way you're going to be hurting your child, then I think that's a dreadful, dreadful thing to say.

And as another woman explained, vulnerabilities have to be manipulated when local policies are at odds with women's decisions, even if this means that practitioners have to breach their trust:

I was manipulated in all sorts of ways throughout the service they gave me, including the negotiations when we were talking about the pool. I think that's a strong manipulation to negotiate something and then when I'm in labour, when I'm at my most vulnerable, renegotiating. I do feel strongly about it. You know, if you're promised something, then they should come up with it. And it's that blip between what is negotiated and what happens that made me feel unsafe and unable to trust what was going on.

Manipulation can be subtle and out of awareness: offering a woman an epidural rather than suggesting the birth pool she had hoped to use, asking her if she consents to syntometrine as she is birthing her baby, not helping her off the bed when she had planned to use upright positions. The list is endless. Coercion may be less subtle and quite deliberate. The point is that women's ethical decision-making and health-care ethics are based on incompatible views about how people make important life decisions and what kind of support they need to be able to put these decisions into practice.

Asserting ethical positions

So far, I have challenged two rather different theories about how women are, how they live their lives and how they make decisions about birth and motherhood. In Chapter 2, I described the patriarchal definition of people as separate beings aspiring to rationalism. The following quotation sums up this view – that individual autonomy is:

> Broadly defined as the ideal of self-legislation – characterize[d by] an ethics of modernity in which the subject ideally acts independently of interests, bodily desire, others, prejudice or tradition.[5]

The other theory is based on the notion that women are so inherently caring, and so connected to those around them that they are unable to care for themselves if doing this causes conflict of any sort. As I quoted on page 54:

> Even when women held strongly to their own ways of doing things, they remained concerned about not hurting the feelings of their opponents by openly expressing dissent. They reported that

they were apt to hide their opinions and then suffer quietly the frustration of not standing up to others. Some women described feeling either petulant, private resentment of others or self-admonishment for being so unassertive.[6]

These are crucial debates because how we define subjectivity defines autonomy and ethics, and all of these define how we treat pregnant and birthing women. Understanding this is fundamental to women's lives because as they explained, birth 'is not a separate part of your life. It's one of the things that forms you' and 'something really major happens to you, your body, physically and emotionally which will change your life for absolutely ever'.

If empty rationalism and subservient caring are both oppressive in different ways and negate the individual woman, who she is and all she aspires to; and if they can be used to persuade her to accept birth ideology and practices that do not feel right for her and her baby, can we develop new theories? As I discussed in Chapter 2, feminists have been using postmodernism to grapple with theorizing a different sort of autonomy and ethics that acknowledges that each of us attempts to forge a life based on a diverse collection of concerns and that we are all positioned differently in relation to dominant power and knowledge. The idea that 'very few people have wholly privileged identities. Very few people have wholly subordinated identities,'[7] makes sense of the tensions feminists have uncovered between domination and resistance and gives us hope that new theories about ethics and autonomy more closely aligned with women's concerns can indeed be developed.

In order to develop these theories, feminists have had to engage with complex theories about subjectivity (how people are and develop, how they relate to themselves, their surroundings and each other, and how they live in their bodies). These theories provide useful insights into some of the ethical struggles around birth and why it is difficult but possible for women to exert autonomy.

Ethical decision-making

Can we breathe life into the empty moral subject?

The trouble is, that, as we have seen, the subject of modernity is unchanging and there is a uniformity and equality assumed between subjects that bears no relation to reality. The feminist idea that we function in a social web or network means that interrelatedness is the principle from which we develop as individuals. Thus autonomy and ethics are circumstancial processes that emerge through the interactions between people, and the embodied concerns of pregnant and birthing women are an integral aspect of rather than an impediment to autonomy.[8]

When ethics is based on a subject which endlessly and unsuccessfully attempts to empty itself of subjectivity, autonomy is twisted into a negation of women's very real concerns about birth. It is this cold emptiness of modernist thinking that facilitates the daily abuse in and on women's minds, bodies and spirits in the name of protecting babies. Yet as women frequently said, they felt that *they* were in the best position to protect their babies:

> *I don't really support the idea that pregnant women are not really fit to make decisions. I think they are perfectly fit. They're actually probably more fit to make decisions because they are completely focused on their task. They are only mothers at that point and nothing else. And to say they don't have the best interest for their children at heart – I think it's a huge insult to women, an absolute insult to women.*

Health-care discourse reduces mothers' heartfelt concerns for their children's well-being to consent to practices and treatments that it deems appropriate. It absolves itself by subscribing to two rather paradoxical beliefs: that individuals are equal and thus free to choose and exert their rights, and that we are all the same and all hold similar beliefs. The subordination and exclusion of those who are different and hold different beliefs remain conveniently invisible.[9] So while the notion of consent may seem unproblematic in health-care ethics, it is immediately problematic if we look beyond sameness and equality and acknowledge the differences and vulnerabilities of pregnant and labouring women. The assumption of equality vanishes when a body is giving birth in a system that is insensitive to women's bodies and ignores how women tend to respond to those around them. But this assumption means that obstetric practices become 'irresistible',[10] and consent turns into compliance.[11] One of the women who felt that she and her midwives held different views about birth said that they attempted to reassure her by telling her that 'of course we won't do anything without your consent'. But as she pointed out:

> *Well, what sort of consent are you going to be giving at that point [during labour] . . . and that's not ever frankly discussed.*

Having a trusting relationship with a midwife who understands the woman's beliefs and concerns seemed to be one of the best ways of transforming vulnerability and uncertainty into strength and confidence. This next quotation is from a woman who booked with an independent midwife. It is a rare example of a woman's sense of autonomy being developed during pregnancy and continuing through birth:

> *I worry a little about presuming you won't be compos mentis. I mean, I was myself. There were times when I was elsewhere but that's another matter. I wasn't another person. I had my sense of humour. I had my faculties and I had my own wishes. I was in a lot of state but I wasn't in so much of a state that I did not know what I wanted. And I don't know how many people would feel confident that that would be the case. I felt confident in advance and that was the reality – that I was capable of making decisions.*

The importance of engagement that I described in Chapters 4 and 5 become particularly clear over the issues of choice and control.

'How can you make a good choice out of five bad choices?

The current concepts of choice and control are little more than empty rhetorical responses to criticisms of obstetric paternalism. They have little to do with women's autonomy. It has been recognized that maternity services are obstetrically orientated and provide too little choice for women, as I discussed in Chapter 3. But without asking searching questions about the thinking behind obstetric policies and practices, choice is predicated onto a host of underlying constraints that serve to limit it. Yet as Joseph Raz suggests, it is only by 'having a sufficient range of acceptable options' that choice can lead to greater autonomy.[12] Women made similar comments – that they needed not only options, but also 'the means to do it', but found that even basic options were lacking:

> *How can you make a good choice out of five bad choices? And I just thought, now where would I want to give birth here. And I thought nowhere. Not on this horrible plastic chair. Not on this horrible high plastic bed. You know, none of those were in any way inviting for me to lie on or sit on or squat on. The bed was too high. You couldn't kneel on the floor. I thought, this is not a good place to have a baby.*

More fundamental choices about whether or not to engage with the maternity services, whether or not to call a midwife in labour and having some control over who would attend birth seemed to be off the choice agenda (one or two women became aware of this when they heard about a local woman who had given birth without midwives; one of them commented that, 'it just sort of opened my eyes – that you can do it on your own'). As I have already suggested, choice is limited to a predetermined obstetric menu available to some women in some circumstances,[13] leaving women and midwives with minimal or illusory choices. And when women (or midwives) question why their decision-making should be restricted to a pre-selected menu or 'shopping list',[14] they are deemed irresponsible. For example, one woman's GP was contacted to find out if she was of 'sound mind' when she asked searching questions about obstetric interventions.

Despite the rhetoric of choice, there is still an assumption that obstetrics knows best and that if women have the 'right' information, they will make the 'right' choices and if midwives explain the 'right' choices well enough, women will follow their advice. Decision-making outside the box is defined as a communication failure or an act of deviancy on the part of the woman, midwife, or both. This infantilizes woman and midwives and reduces their abilities to develop their ethical positions and exert their autonomy by putting decisions into practice. It also ignores the fact that while authoritative knowledge is powerful, it is nevertheless culturally shaped rather than correct. This is not to suggest that *all* interactions between individual women and midwives are coercive, or that choice is uniformly oppressive, but when choice is embedded in a dominant ideology it is generally oppressive. As Carolyn McLeod and Susan Sherwin (2000) comment:

> Patients' autonomy is generally reduced to the exercise of 'informed choice' in which the information provided is restricted to that deemed relevant by the health-care provider (and by the health-care system, which has determined what information is even available by pursuing certain sorts of research programs and ignoring others). Even in 'ideal' cases in which patients have strong autonomy skills and full access to all the available information, it is important to recognize the influence that oppression may have on the information base and, thereby, on the meaningful options available to patients.[15]

As I suggested in the previous chapters, women need information in order to make decisions,[16] but the information given to them by practitioners is usually based on obstetric knowledge. Access to information about other birth knowledges and the values on which obstetric knowledge is based depended on them finding this out for themselves:

> *I have to know everything about it. I can't just have the normal knowledge of a normal person to have a baby. I've got to have all the knowledge of all the nurses [midwives] and the obstetricians because they won't advise me according to what they know I want. They will advise me according to their own set of rules and what they want and that's not unbiased. They didn't give me unbiased information, and allow me to make my own decision. They specifically veered me towards their own outcome.*

They frequently talked about having to know a great deal, but felt that the onus should not be so exclusively on them to search out information:

> *You've to know your stuff and I think, that's not right. I shouldn't have to know my stuff.*

But they felt they had to 'arm' themselves in order to make decisions that felt right to them. The same kind of confusion that I described on page 147 about transferring to hospital because of meconium staining arises when women are asked to make choices about other issues that obstetrics has strong opinions about. A woman described being asked to make a choice about vitamin K, for example:

> *She only told me the good side and then said, this has got to be your choice. And I didn't understand if it was so good, why it needed to be my choice.*

Again the onus is on women 'to find the other side' and make sense of obstetric choice.

To claim that information is in any way unbiased is to fall back on the claim that rationality is free of external influences.[17] Knowledge is always sought and constructed from particular viewpoints and information giving is always influenced by a variety of interests and constraints.[18] The vacuum assumed by the rhetoric of choice is not a vacuum at all, but is filled with a complex interaction of interests that I have described and that are described in detail in the chapters of Mavis Kirkham's (2004) edited book on the subject.

But as the women pointed out, knowledge about obstetrics' limitations and knowledge about other birth practices were of no help if midwives lack knowledge and skills. Not only does this limit the range of options open to women, but gives the false impression that courses of action that they had wanted to avoid are in fact chosen by women themselves:

> *Once you go into hospital it's forget everything that you've learnt or put on your birth plan.*
>
> *Nadine: Did you feel that?*
>
> *(Sighing) I kept hoping that it wasn't the case, but it was very much the case. And eventually you get so fed up, that it's just like, oh do anything to end this pain. And so (sighs) you are then asking for whatever it is that they're going to do, when if they had been in tune with you from the beginning it might not have been necessary to do what ends up happening. If people would be much more involved with you, mobilizing you and trying to help you cope without diamorphine, then it might not get to that, okay, let's just get this over with, however it has to be done. You have no choice, you haven't really got any choice. The choice that I made was let's get this finished and over with or do what I had been doing for the past four hours, for another couple of hours. So okay, let's get this over with.*

At the same time, this illusion of choice could become a distraction from the enormous task of giving birth when women 'were having to listen to everything they were saying and thinking well, do I want that'.

All in all, women's decision-making did not correspond to the expectation that 'correct', choices should be made at designated times and adhered to. Like the women in Robin Gregg's (1995) study, their decisions were made from 'a lifetime process of developing beliefs and attitudes'.[19] Their journeys through childbearing were a time of change and growth. As they accumulated knowledge and adapted it to their own beliefs and lifestyles, they might plan home births in late pregnancy, or want to avoid routine practices that they had initially accepted as necessary. They needed midwives who could journey with them, provide them with more information as they digested earlier information, and discuss and weigh up uncertainties. Making a decision 'on the spot' with relative strangers with whom 'you never really scratch the surface' could not begin to fulfil the need for engaged dialogue that enables the continuum of decision-making.

In describing the limitations of choice, they confirmed Jo Green and her colleagues' (1998b) findings that limiting choice means that control is necessarily reduced.

'You still don't have a great deal of control'

Home birth, as I described on page 90, is often assumed to provide women with ultimate control.[20] But the women suggested that if control means asserting their own meanings of birth, then control at home is relative rather than absolute. Women expected to feel more in control at home than in hospital:

> *It's your own home. The midwife is coming into your home and they're a visitor whereas you're like a visitor in the hospital.*

They hoped to avoid the complete lack of control that some had felt in hospital, so that their expectations might end up being closer to the reality of giving birth.

> *I realized that one of the other reasons [I felt disempowered] is that whatever you think that you can do in terms of mobility, when you go into hospital, it just can't happen because the room's too small. There's lino on the floor, so it's not very comfortable to get onto the floor. The beds are hard. There's machinery about and there's no way, that even if you wanted to that you could realistically walk up and down the corridors, because they'd be wanting you back in the room. So even if everybody thinks it's a good idea to be mobile, it's just not practical in hospital. And I didn't realize that until I got into the labour ward and I really needed to concentrate, and I just thought, I can't do it here. And at that point I actually got quite frightened and wondered what was going to happen next and didn't feel at all like I was going to be in control.*

Of course control is never absolute. Even if we leave aside the more complex ideas about how we are formed through interactions with others and our environments, we live in a society that has developed systems of control in every area of our lives over thousands of years. We would be misleading ourselves and others to think that we control our lives. And when women report:

The consultant said to me, you don't need to bring a birth plan, because if you come into hospital it won't be taken into consideration.

we cannot maintain the myth that women have control. The rhetoric of choice and control tends to focus on the individual rather than on societal constraints. Yet as I mentioned earlier, social norms usually decide where, how and with whom women give birth.[21] As I also described in Chapters 2 and 3, social norms have exerted control over women's knowledge, bodies, autonomy, midwifery and birth practices. This is why this book has focused on women's experiences within a social context: 'We must . . . evaluate society and not just the individual when determining the degree to which an individual is able to act autonomously'.[22]

Women's reported experiences of being in control varied. Some women described subtle differences between hospital births where midwives tended to be 'telling me when to do things and giving advice and saying push now, or do this now, or whatever' compared to home birth where midwives more often 'sat back and let me get on with things'. Some described healing home birth experiences following hospital births where they felt they had no control. Many women felt that they had control over some issues, but not others

In terms of having who I wanted here, I could do that more freely, and just have things as I wanted them. But in terms of being assertive with the midwife, I don't think I was at all. I just felt really vulnerable physically.

In your own home people can't be telling you what to do – well they could be telling you what to do, but not quite in the same way as they can in the hospital.

Others felt controlled by obstetric ideology even in their own homes and pointed out the paradox between the rhetoric of choice and obstetrics' need to control women:

I thought it [the home birth service] was almost a form of controlling people. I don't think there's a great deal of choice about it is there? It is just a monitoring service. It doesn't allow you any opportunities to get to know a midwife, or trust a midwife. It's just about monitoring you and doing all the things they do in hospital but doing it in the community. I do feel that your knowledge is totally overridden and I don't think I appreciated that until I had a baby at home and realized that even although you're in your own home you still don't have great deal of control.

The greater the level of discordance between a woman's beliefs about birth and local birth practices, the less able she felt to exert her autonomy and make decisions she felt would be right for her and her baby These women sometimes felt their homes, their mental health, and their ability to make decisions and become mothers were scrutinized and judged. They were acutely aware of the lack of autonomy women really have:

> *I feel like I'm complying. I feel that I couldn't just go off and do it [give birth on my own] because, I've been told in the past that I'll be committed to a mental hospital. So I have in the back of my head – sort of big brother. I'm complying, you know. I'm doing what I have to do.*

Women did what many of us do when faced with a hostile system or one that they felt unable to change. They distanced themselves from what seemed like a futile struggle and as I explained on page 192, withdrew from midwives. One woman explained that she had been too concerned during her previous pregnancy to build up a relationship with midwives and take them into her confidence. She described herself this time round as:

> *Much more businesslike. My approach is just, let them get on with their side of it and I get on with my side. [In fact], if you let these people into your confidence, then really you're putting yourself in a dangerous position.*

Another felt that although she would have appreciated support she had to rely on her own resources. Although she felt enabled to be 'blunt' about her views, this was because she had disengaged – 'I don't need them!' This disengaged autonomy left women without the support that they needed, unable to create the safest circumstances for themselves and their babies, and without a sense of real autonomy.

On issues that challenged local policies exerting control was extremely difficult and required extraordinary effort. One woman described stressful and lengthy negotiations with midwives and paediatricians in the throes of labour because her baby had passed meconium and staff insisted that the baby should be suctioned and possibly resuscitated at birth. The usual practice in her local hospital was to cut the umbilical cord at birth so that the baby could be removed from the mother and suctioned and resuscitated in another room. The woman insisted that the equipment should be brought into the labour room so that her baby could be treated beside her. Bringing equipment to the women and baby, so that the physiological processes at birth can remain as undisturbed as possible, is supported by evidence[23] and is already normal practice in some British maternity units, but she was told this was impossible, so:

> *I had to make absolutely sure that they knew that they couldn't take my baby away. That was not a possibility and that they would have to take me with the baby if the baby had to go anywhere. So I felt that I was in control of my personal and my baby's safety but only because I couldn't trust them.*

This kind of situation highlighted how undermining women's autonomy creates two deeply conflicting needs – the need to 'watch out' in order to protect their integrity and the need to feel safe enough to 'let go' in order to give birth:

> *It's a confusing one, because I kind of want both ends of the spectrum. I want to be able to give up control completely and just be able to go with it. And I also want to have complete control over the space and what's happening in it, you know, who's doing what to me or the baby. And they don't feel very compatible, those two different states of being – completely surrendering to a very powerful process and also kind of going, hang on a minute, I don't like what you're doing there.*

The highly complex tensions contained within the rhetoric of choice and control are supposedly ironed out by a series of rights. It is not surprising that women found rights to be equally confusing and problematic.

The problem with rights

Rights arise from the same patriarchal thinking as choice and control. As I have suggested on a number of occasions, this thinking has no concept of relational decision-making that women usually engage in. Rights are adversarial and need to be asserted, often against the wishes of others. Yet women wanted to maintain the fragile relationships they had with their midwives and found it exceptionally difficult to assert themselves, even if this meant being attended by a midwife that, 'I had been dreading and not actually wanting to come'.

In a unique example of open conflict, one woman described the difficulties of asserting herself and how discussions with her midwife became increasingly undermining and coercive. She had been told by her midwives that she could not have a home birth and therefore put her plans in writing to them. She was then informed that she had left the decision too late and that she couldn't be accommodated because there were already two home births booked in the month her baby was due to be born. When the woman said she still intended to have a home birth:

> *She was almost aggressive. There was no smile, there was very definite eye contact, very square shoulders, very drawn up posture, very stiff. You know, that was quite frightening. But because I knew it was my right to have a home confinement I thought, no, I'm not going to let you dissuade me and I met her match for match. The more angry and adamant she got, the more adamant I got that this was my choice. But it's when you get home that you start to think, God what a big head to head I've had there, and these are the women that are supposed to be coming and giving me care and if I alienate them I won't get the best care. Or perhaps I have made a bit of a silly choice.*

The midwife visited her at home the following day, to tell her that she was not making a sensible, informed or appropriate decision and reiterated that it was too late. The woman repeated her intention to give birth at home. Her midwife then told her that 'anything could go wrong' and asked her if she wanted her child to die. When the woman was still not persuaded, she 'covered the home birth disasters' – the woman bleeding to death before help could arrive and the baby not breathing at birth.

> *It left me feeling very isolated. I would have been so much happier had she come in and said, okay we're a wee bit concerned, we'll go over a few points but at the end of the day if this is where you choose to deliver we'll give you all the support we possibly can. Whereas now I'm left with feelings of – what if something does go wrong, and am I going to get the told you so syndrome or the, what do you expect you had a home confinement? That's not a nice feeling cos you end up with self-doubt – whether you are making the right decision or*

whether you are strong enough to actually go the whole way with it.

As another woman pointed out, appealing to rights is usually a response to conflict. This reduces safety as it inevitably causes polarization. In the event of a problem arising women might find it more difficult to transfer to hospital if they need to:

> *All the way along I'd said if there's a problem I'd love to go into hospital and I think if there's an emergency I'll be very grateful for it. But then it became like a battleground. And now I feel if I go into hospital I feel like they've won and I've lost.*

Of course rights have contributed to reducing unacceptable abuses against people and to changes in maternity services.[24] They have also protected home birth in the face of obstetric opposition. But rights do not necessarily lead to change,[25] and using their rights was clearly problematic for women and a far cry from the support they desired. As Carol Gilligan noted, the idea that we are separate individuals leading separate lives with a collection of rights to use as we choose is clearly anathema to many women.[26] So even though all the women knew that they had a right to a home birth, for example, most did not want to insist on that right. Comments went along the lines of 'I found out that I had a legal right, but I didn't really want to invoke that'. Women did not want to 'make waves' or seem 'pushy'. Nor did they want to oblige midwives to attend them under duress. Rights could not guarantee support or increase confidence:

> *The most important thing to me was to feel supported. From what I could gather, a home birth wasn't going to have much benefit if I wasn't with people who I felt were supportive.*

> *I hadn't considered an independent midwife cos I didn't think I'd need one. I thought I had a positive attitude. I'd seen a successful home birth and I thought, I'll be able to give birth. I was quite unconcerned until later on – until I actually met them one to one and met my GP. And when I actually felt that trickle-down effect of losing my confidence, I thought, well, hang on a minute. Maybe I do need someone more supportive.*

As I suggested earlier, women are unlikely to make choices that are not positively supported by practitioners. And as Iris Marion Young

(1997a) pointed out, inequalities between ideologies and individuals are such that negative liberty (making a choice a legal right) needs to be replaced by positive liberty, where the choice is supported enough for it to become a reality.[27] The difference this kind of support made to women is clear:

> *I think that she [midwife] made me more and more confident to explore areas. It was important for me that I did what I wanted, and when I found that my midwife was really interested in the way that I thought, it made me feel more confident. I just felt like she was saying, yeh whatever you do, it's fine by me and I think that did help me to grow because I thought that she trusted my ideas and she found them interesting. It made me follow through instead of just wishing. I got more and more confident about getting exactly what I wanted.*

For women, refusing treatment was even more difficult than claiming their rights. The guilt and blame introduced by obstetric morality, combined with women's concerns about their babies, are not conducive to claiming rights, but are even less conducive to refusing treatments:

> *Looking back on it, it might have been better to fight for it a wee bit more [home birth]. Cos I hadn't really wanted to do that [be induced] and I suppose looking back on it, I think, I should have just said, no, I'm not doing that, I'm just going to let it happen itself, cos it had started. It was just not quick enough.*

As women discussed their needs during birth, it became clear that choice, control and rights were imposed concepts that were somewhat alien to women's main priorities.

What does control mean?

Control usually means 'power over' – the kind of power that is 'linked to control and domination' and is ultimately 'backed by force'.[28] Women experienced this as they struggled to hold onto their priorities. Those women who were least prepared to relinquish their autonomy, were most likely to feel this pressure. For example,

> *They [midwives] would try and get me to assure them that if something was going wrong, that I would go into hospital, that I wouldn't be saying, no. I have to be at home.*

But these women, like others,[29] wanted to avoid being controlled without controlling or 'dictating' to others. They wanted to feel safe.

> *I mean, control isn't something that I would necessarily put lots of emphasis on. It's not that I want to be able to necessarily dictate so much what goes on. More that I don't want strong influence on me because I know that if I have that influence I bend to it and in the long run that's no good for me. It's much better if I'm doing what actually feels natural, I think. But also I suppose it comes down to knowing. Knowing what's going on. Knowing who's going to be there. I mean, the idea of having students, having a midwife popping in and out, and perhaps a doctor popping in and out feels very unstabilizing to me. I suppose it's more dissipating control. There's not so much of an issue of who is in control, when it's at home, because it's not my wish to be pushy but more that there's no one in control. That things can just flow.*

When women talked about control, this usually related to whether or not the woman felt a passive recipient of care – an object being done to – or felt that she was central to her own experience. Passivity was often associated with hospital rather than home:

> *In hospital all you do is go there and they seem to do everything for you. You don't really* think *very much for yourself any more.*

Though with the encouragement of a midwife, a woman who transferred into hospital described regaining her centrality during the birth of her baby:

> *Everything was happening to me and people talking and talking at me. It just felt like I wasn't there. I was frightened [during the first stage of labour]. All these things happening to me and not with me. But in second stage I felt I was really part of it. It was my experience. I felt I'd reclaimed it, and these other people were just helping me to have my experience. Whereas the first half was like taken away.*

Women described diverse needs for control in their lives, but control during birth seemed to be missing the point: an inadequate substitute for stability, safety, and freedom to be themselves. Ideally control could be abandoned and women could instead plan familiar, predictable and 'low load' birthing environments,[30] so that external distractions would be reduced to a minimum ('it seemed to be all about removing obstacles') and they could focus on the task of giving birth. As two women explained:

> *It requires a certain amount of quiet round about you, and trust and respect, and when that isn't given, it's easy to doubt yourself or not to be able to hear what's going on [in your body].*

> *I think I would have not been able to just be inside myself, so much. I think I would have been much more aware of the things that were going on around me and aware of my surroundings in a way that I didn't need to be here, cos I knew what was around me.*

While women wanted to avoid being controlled, they wanted their midwives to be strong, empowered and inspiring in order to give them the confidence and strength they needed to birth their babies. They wanted to see 'more power given back to the midwives' to 'make them a lot better at their jobs'. Those midwives who stood by women were highly valued and appreciated by women. The midwife on page 189, who supported the woman's decision to avoid vaginal examinations, continued to support her during a long third stage, despite pressure from the local hospital to transfer her to hospital: 'they had insisted that she bring me in, and she said she didn't think it was necessary, that I was healthy and everything was fine'. The woman went on to explain that:

> *I was really glad that [midwife] was there. Afterwards I was crying when I thought of what could have happened if we had had another midwife. I just kept saying thanks be to God, thanks be to God, cos I would have been in hospital. I felt just so relieved that we had a midwife that respected me and [partner] and our relationship and just knew that we could do it ourselves. It could have been so different.*

Of course, the modernist view that individuals are self-contained and impermeable means that health-care ethics cannot easily take into account the effects of one person on another. This makes it difficult for practitioners to understand the difference between 'power with' (or being with) and 'power over'.[31] This view of the individual mutes the potentially beneficial or harmful impacts of relationships between practitioners and women, even though these are keenly felt by women.[32] 'Power with' results in parents feeling that 'we did it ourselves'.[33] But if we do not understand that this comes from the practitioner actively engaging, facilitating, protecting, and being with, the pull towards 'power over', even in partnership models of care, is strong.[34]

Starhawk (1990) suggests that practising 'power with' leads to women developing 'power-from-within'.[25] By this she means that the woman develops a positive sense of herself, that she is aware of and nurtures connections with others and her environment and that she is able to challenge those who exert 'power over'. This is similar to the kind of relational autonomy that I have been describing and the kind of stance that women attempted to work towards as they negotiated the move from control (obstetrics' ways and time) to freedom (women's ways and time).

Moving from control to freedom

Understanding that power-from-within is about the move from control to freedom gives authority to a word that is used frequently by women, but largely discounted by obstetric thinking – 'relaxed'. So while obstetrics is based on a complex system of controlling women's (disconnected) birthing bodies, this is completely at odds with how these women described the need to feel completely free of any sort of control in order to focus and really listen to their (connected) birthing bodies. There was a general consensus that the process of birth cannot and should not be controlled, 'because it happens at its own pace' and 'because you get so taken over don't you?' Comments such as 'how can you manage an involuntary process?'[36] and 'when will we be released from this obsession to control [labour]?',[37] were echoed by those of the women:

> No don't push, and then push, and then don't push, and then push. And I'm going hang on, hang on. That's like you telling me when to poo. I mean, it's impossible isn't it. I'm constipated and you're trying to manage it. Like it doesn't work.

Yet women sometimes felt that the natural birth rhetoric (from the 1950s) is where the woman expected to exert control over her birthing body still informs recent thinking and assumes that women will be in control, especially at home:

It does seem that is what is expected from the midwives' point of view – or in this situation anyway. Because they see you as staying at home, they basically assume that you're going to be in control. That you'll be able to tell them what to do all the time.

But being relaxed meant being released from control and being free to open their minds, bodies and spirits to the power of birth within them. Because of the cultural constraints on women that I discussed in Chapter 2, finding their own power often depended on how empowered their midwives were. Yet, as we know, often midwives feel fearful or trapped by obstetric policies and practices. Often they can support women only to 'beat the system', rather than protect a space for them to give birth in their own time and way. It was in this context that midwives might exhort women to push their babies out, even if they had no urge to push, in an effort to 'get this baby out before the doctor comes back'. I once witnessed an experienced midwife becoming increasingly directive towards a woman in labour as she tried to balance the woman's desire to stay at home with local policies on the appropriate length of labour. The woman birthed her baby at home, but not in her own time and way, and not in a way that enabled her to feel the power of birth within. For women and midwives finding their 'power-from-within' requires the kind of trust between them that I discussed in Chapter 5. But as women pointed out, if lack of continuity made it difficult for them to trust and feel at ease with midwives, it was no less difficult for midwives to trust and feel at ease with them:

Lack of continuity is really a problem, also for midwives, because to be fair, to give them a chance to get to know women a bit and to feel comfortable in her home. You know, those things take time.

Midwives need relationships as much as women if they are to help them feel relaxed enough to give birth.

Stabilizing the environment

The ability to 'relax' was seen by the women as crucial, but not one that is necessarily easy to achieve. They understood that in a culture increasingly fixated on control, where women's bodies are particularly constrained,[38] their bodies may not easily 'let go'. Whatever their views on control, one of the reasons they planned home births was to create a level of certainty for an uncertain process, and free themselves from a whole set of temporal, spatial and behavioral constraints likely to feature in hospital. In hospital, birthing bodies are expected to comply with hospital culture.[39] As some women commented, they were often 'hooked up to goodness knows what. I couldn't move. I couldn't get off the bed'. They were aware that being at home would free their bodies in ways that would not be easy in hospital, so that they might be able to relinquish control of the process of birth, knowing that the environment would remain familiar and stable. Women's homes could be organized around their bodies:

> I know which bits of furniture are the right height, the right shape, to be useful. I'm also looking forward to the fact that there'll be soft stuff on the floor and that I can maybe put something like a sleeping bag underneath the plastic sheeting and I can really use the floor. In hospital, on a lino, you can be uncomfortable to go on all fours or on your knees. I mean, that's almost like the first thing that I think about when I think about having the baby at home – how I can manoeuvre myself comfortably. I know that that'll happen [losing control] and when that happens, what will I do? So that I can have worked it out beforehand cos in hospital you don't get any chance to do that at all. And that's what I found very much last time – that you had no idea what you were going into. In a hospital birth there's absolutely no control over your environment. I mean, for people like myself who are totally used to controlling their environment it's really scary and unnerving and that relates to both feeling disempowered and also feeling like you're out of control.

Unlike David Machin and Mandy Scamell's (1997) findings, the women I talked to saw being at home as a way of minimizing the disjunction that usually occurs between home and hospital. They attempted to weave certainty into the uncertain process of birth wherever they could in order to prepare themselves for this challenging rite of passage:

> If you're in hospital and sometime in the past you've thought, this is what I'd really like to do, it just goes completely out of the window once you're actually in hospital being told what to do by staff, because they think it's best. So it's only after a couple of months when you've been home, that you think, it was like a different world when you said, or wrote down, I wanted to do that. It bears no relation to what actually goes on. So, I

see, and I don't know how this is going to work, but I see being at home as a way of joining up what you thought when you were pregnant and what you wanted when you were pregnant, and what actually happens in the labour.

It is possible that in the absence of trusting relationships, the environment took on greater importance than it might otherwise have done. One woman who booked with an independent midwife noticed that 'because we felt so happy with [midwife] and there were so few variables it didn't matter that one of them was rather major [moving house at the end of pregnancy]'. But there was a limit to how far women's homes could minimize differences in ideology. Walls do not necessarily provide a barrier to obstetric thinking and practices if these are brought by midwives. Nor do they necessarily protect the woman from seeing herself through others' eyes:

The midwives sat, one on each sofa and watched me all the time. They didn't leave me in peace at all. I was moving around – well I was moving my hips with a contraction and that was fine. But I really felt that I couldn't do that in front of them. Most of the time I spent going out of the room. I'd go into the bathroom for a contraction or I would just go out into the hallway. But I really didn't feel like labouring in front of them. I just felt uncomfortable in their presence basically.

Even when women found midwives very supportive, the disadvantages of discontinuity meant that some women felt 'most at ease when they weren't there at all', and were either on their own or with those they knew well. Without knowing women, it is difficult to know how midwives could be more in tune with or responsive to women's diverse needs. In the next two quotations, for example, one woman felt her midwife should have left her alone at times and the other was distressed when her midwife suggested doing this:

Perhaps if the midwives had on occasion been able to just take themselves out, that would have been a good idea, just for focus and to be able to concentrate and to be able to talk very openly with my husband about what I felt. Because there were things that I could say to him that he would know what I meant. I would be able to share some of my real fears and anxieties, which I felt I couldn't share in front of the midwives because they might take them more seriously than they were actually meant. Like the time when I said I'm going to die. And they said, no you're not, no you're not – when I just wanted to be able to express some of this. I didn't want anyone to do anything about it, but I sometimes wanted just to express things that I felt a bit inhibited to do.

In retrospect I was a little annoyed with what happened with the midwife. About the possibility of her going away. It placed a burden of decision on me at a time when I felt she should be here for me. The only time I didn't feel in control was when she said she might leave for a couple of hours.

Helping women feel relaxed is not as easy as it sounds. But as they talked more about moving from control to freedom, they explained more about what this means and what they need to achieve this.

'Letting go': but not 'losing the plot'

Women talked about simultaneously 'letting go' and 'concentrating', not unlike Carol Macmillan's description of passivity and agency,[40] and Nel Noddings' description of active passivity:

> I let the object act upon me, seize me, direct my floating thoughts . . . My decision to do this is mine, it requires an effort in preparation, but it also requires a letting go of my attempts to control. This sort of passivity . . . is not a mindless, vegetable like passivity. It is a controlled state that abstains from controlling the situation.[41]

They talked about losing control in different ways, and as I have suggested saw this as an essential, or integral part of giving birth:

Cos it's like trying not to go to the toilet when you need to go. You know you better lose control otherwise you're going to be in trouble.

It would be like the way that you open up to have an orgasm. Like if you strain, then it doesn't happen. Whereas if something melts inside then it does.

As they pointed out, 'you have to feel safe enough to be able to do that' and when it happened it could feel 'exhilarating' or 'freeing'. The focusing and concentration, where the smallest distraction could defocus the woman, was almost palpable in some of the interviews:

> *I don't know – control – it's a funny word. I was kind of going with my labour and at times I was thinking of losing control. For me losing control would be like either just losing the plot completely and not being aware of what's going on any more or letting myself go and I mean all the time I was breathing, I was focusing on breathing so much that I was actually wondering while I was breathing, how women had time to scream cos I was doing such deep breaths in and then blowing out. So I was really focusing on it so much I was really wondering, when do they scream? If I'd found time to scream I would have done it, but I didn't. I just thought, God, cos it's such a distraction if you scream you'd be lost – you've lost the rhythm of breathing as far as I could see.*

Each woman planned her own way of focusing and steadying herself, but often felt she could best do this on their own, or with those she knew well, as midwives might bring a certain level of distraction:

> *I think probably, the longer I can be on my own and come to terms with – you see this is what I want to do. I panicked when I first got in labour with [first baby] and of course the more I panicked, the worse it got and the more I got myself into a state. Whereas this time I really want to have a clear head I really want to – relaxation techniques, breathing techniques. I really want to get myself on a wavelength where I'm completely in control myself. And I want to get on that before I have anybody [midwives] coming in. I really feel as if I want to get myself sort of steady before anybody comes in and starts listening to the baby's heartbeat and you know, doing all this carry on.*

While 'letting go', 'surrendering' and 'going with the flow' were described positively by most women, there seemed to be a fine line between this and 'losing the plot'. The involuntary 'losing the plot' was experienced negatively by one or two women who had long, painful labours and who felt that they had coped less well than they expected:

> *I felt I'd failed. Not failed, but just I should have done it better. I was expecting to be able to cope throughout the labour. I did have this quite high ideal that I constantly wasn't living up to.*

This is perhaps Tess Cosslett's (1994) point, that natural birth has its own norms and costs. Interestingly, two women who knew and trusted their midwives found their difficult experiences of birth were 'humbling' but still 'empowering', whereas a third woman who was attended by supportive and caring midwives she did not know, talked about her experience as 'humiliating' and later became postnatally depressed. While some feminists and others criticize the natural birth discourse for setting women up to fail, it might be more useful to look more closely at how maternity services fail them.

Women who transferred to hospital were particularly able to see the paradox between their need to be free to focus and obstetrics' need to monitor and control. Their experiences highlighted the paucity of language to articulate this paradox, as well as the strength women needed to be able to resist 'losing it' in difficult circumstances. This quotation comes from a woman who was accompanied to hospital by a midwife she knew well and trusted:

Nadine: Did you feel in control would you say?

I did unless I was strapped onto the monitor and then it really changed me. So no, I didn't feel very much in control then. But when I was doing all my different positions I was completely in control.

Nadine: Would you be able to describe how it feels to be in control or not?

I think when I did feel in control I wasn't even really aware that I was in hospital. I was very aware of thinking positive, and I was very aware of every time I felt a pain. I was very aware of thinking, right this is bringing your baby closer and closer and it did make me feel much more in control. I think I fairly much switched off when I felt in control, and I wasn't really aware of my surroundings and then I was in myself. I was aware of what I was feeling, I was aware of my baby coming closer and closer, but I wasn't actually aware of anything around me. God, it's hard to explain, actually.

Nadine: So when you felt out of control how did that feel?

Well, just the opposite really. I was really aware of, oh God, I'm in this hospital, I'm sitting on this hospital bed. I'm stuck to this hospital monitor and you even smell the hospital. Then you start losing it a wee bit and everything seems much more clinical. But

I was very aware of not wanting to feel like that. So if I did start feeling like that, I was trying to get myself out of it and thinking – I read this somewhere in a book – I was thinking myself just like a flower, and like opening a petal at a time and I was thinking of myself dilating. So I think every time I felt like I was losing it, I was trying to bring myself back by thinking – right, you've got a contraction coming, it's going to be painful, but it's going to bring your baby a wee bit nearer to you. So I was trying not to be out of control. I was very aware of trying not to lose it because when I did lose it, I really felt like that last contraction was just so painful – you panic, and when you panic and you're not in control it really is a hundred times worse. So I really tried, and I think I did really well.

Other women described feeling alienated from their own resources in hospital when monitored:

You can't move and so you get completely cut off from any of my own resources.

They described routine obstetric practices interfering with their need to focus and those who transferred to hospital talked of restrictions in hospital gradually reducing their abilities to respond freely to their labours:

The bit at home I was in control of definitely and I felt much more relaxed. Even if it was painful, I do remember being in control of the pain. Whereas being at hospital, I don't remember being in control of the pain. I remember feeling it had completely taken me over. I couldn't stop it and I couldn't get my head round it and I couldn't go with it. And I think that happened quite gradually. But I do think a lot of the things like putting the belt on me, trying to get me back onto the bed when I was walking around and all that sort of gradually ebbed away at my ability to cope with it all.

Distractions of any sort were experienced as obstacles to giving birth. And as women planned for birth, it became clearer to them that pharmaceutical pain relief could also be distracting.[42] It could prevent them from tuning into their bodies, and undermine their abilities to focus on and work with their labours, because 'you can't feel where you are', and 'once I had that gas and air, it felt like I was there but not present', and:

> *I would want to be in control of myself because I'm the only one that knows, that can feel what's going on. I'm the only that can look into my own body so hopefully, even if I can explain what I'm feeling or what I think I should be doing then they can suggest – maybe you should change position, or maybe you should breathe like this. But hopefully I will be fully aware. That's why I don't want to take any drugs to make me disorientated or unsure.*

Managing unruly bodies

Possessing women's bodies

Women's complex discussions about the vulnerability, sensitivity and power of birth and their bodies, and their experiences of obstetric control support the feminists' views in Chapter 2 that bodies are neither unfeeling or disassociated from the person,[43] and that power is dramatically played out in and on bodies .[44] But as I suggested, their constant cycles of 'leakiness',[45] and their ability to be more than one, are particularly disconcerting to the view of the individual as self-contained or bounded.[46] As we can see, health-care practices need to possess, process, and constrain them. The detached thinking behind these practices make their violence and abuse seem normal and acceptable to practitioners in hospitals where this detachment is reflected.[47] But for some women, 'it's like going to jail or something', because their bodies becomes almost like inanimate third parties that can be possessed by the practitioner. For example:

> *Suddenly I'm there with my boobs out, and I've got one woman [midwife] squeezing this nipple, and another woman [midwife] trying to get the baby on here. And they're all playing with my nipples like it's some sort of third party, and I'm sitting there going, my God, what's happening.*

> *I asked about stitches and if they did them in the subcuticular way. Because I realized that it made a difference to swelling and I wanted to know. I thought I don't want to be faced with it happening and then not be able to say, what are you going to do? And when I asked these sorts of questions, I didn't think*

that they thought that was appropriate for me to ask. It would be like asking a mechanic how he was fixing my car.

This kind of detached, rationalist thinking has led to mechanistic birth practices that assume control of women's bodies.[48] It begins antenatally. One woman described antenatal care in hospital as 'loads of waiting' interspersed with weight, height and blood pressure checks, 'like you're on a car assembly line getting a little bit done at a time'. Another described how she found the herding in hospital antenatal clinics abhorrent:

> *At your twelve weeks appointment in hospital people are taken in fours, and so you might have to give a urine sample in fours, and get weighed in fours and it's just like a sheep pen, and it was horrible. It was really dehumanizing.*

Others felt that even in the community, there was a degree of inflexibility that undermined their ability to take responsibility:

> *They had this reel in motion, and I would get in the way of that every now and again.*
>
> *Nadine: How would you get in the way of it?*
>
> *Just by being too assertive or asking them lots of questions or not doing things in the right order or my concerns weren't fitting into the plan. And also you don't seem to be allowed to participate in the system in any sort of piecemeal fashion. You go for it or you don't. Like you have to get all the tests done, all the weighing and the protein test which you can easily do at home. You don't need anyone to do them. I had to take the whole package if I wanted anything at all and I found that very frustrating.*

This kind of thinking and appropriation extends through birth to the 'product' of birth – the baby.[49] Women frequently expressed distress about babies being taken from or not given to them at birth, or being weighed, measured, cleaned and dressed sooner than they wished, or against their wishes. This assumption of ownership was highlighted when a father wanted to receive his baby as it was being born, and the midwife assumed this to be illegal:

She said she'd have to ring her supervisor about it but she really thought it was illegal. That midwives had to deliver the baby.

As I explained in Chapter 2, the disembodied discourse of health and ethics hides how bodies are appropriated and violated. It also hides practitioners' needs to distance themselves from women's bodies. Alice Adams (1994) provides an insight into this in her analysis of 'A Night in June'. A doctor attempts to extract a baby by reaching into the woman's womb and rationalizes the sexual violence by depersonalizing the woman.[50] Literature on abuse has not tended to cover birth, but when it has, there are similarities between women's experiences of abuse and those of traumatic birth experiences.[51] The implications for women and practitioners are profound. Over half of the women in this book described incidences in hospital or at home that they found distressing and violating. Others described incidences that they did not describe as overtly violating, but which were nonetheless carried out against their previous stated wishes, or in the face of resistance at the time. While supporting a friend who had planned a home birth but transferred to hospital, one woman described how impersonal services, where practitioners focus on obstetric procedures, are insensitive to women:

Here's my friend just lying there naked sort of thing. And it's just like she hardly existed, it was quite difficult for her voice to be heard. So I think the whole thing was pretty horrible for her.

As I suggested on page 59, even seemingly innocuous gestures can exert power over bodies. More invasive practices during labour such as vaginal examinations were particularly problematic for some women. Monitoring the baby's heartbeat could also be experienced as invasive by some.

Checking and monitoring women's birthing bodies

Of course women had different views about monitoring during labour (just as they did during pregnancy, as I discussed in Chapter 5). While some women found it reassuring, some found it invasive. The practice of monitoring babies and women during birth is integral to obstetric safety and thus midwifery care. But while research has considered different methods of monitoring babies' heartbeats,[52] and the accuracy of vaginal assessments,[53] no research has been done to determine whether or not these practices are beneficial. With notable exceptions, few have questioned these or considered how women feel about them.[54] Without exception, all the women in this study wanted monitoring to be kept to a minimum, with few or no vaginal examinations. Some women began to question the necessity of any routine practices. They reasoned that if continuous monitoring of the baby's heartbeat is potentially disadvantageous, does it need to be monitored at all if the woman feels all is well? And if intermittent monitoring is beneficial, how can we know how often it needs to be done? In other words, if women's knowledge and birth can be trusted so far – can it be trusted further? These questions cannot easily be asked or answered within an obstetric framework.

Women asked these questions because, as I explained above, they needed to be completely free of distractions. Some felt that they knew that their labours were progressing well and that their babies were safe and could see no reason to interfere with the all-consuming challenge of coping with their contractions. A number of women felt that monitoring and examinations not only interfered with the birth process, but also undermined their confidence and instincts. Some felt that vaginal examinations might make them 'close up'. Some considered using a pool in order to avoid interference and were dismayed to learn that midwives could bring sonicaids that could be used in water:

> *My heart sunk, and I thought, oh, they're going to chase me in the pool.*

Some felt that monitoring the baby's heartbeat introduced anxiety and control and necessitated a midwife's presence every fifteen minutes, when they would have preferred to be alone with their partners:

> *I was assured that they would only do them [vaginal examinations] out of necessity, but I still don't understand why they're necessary. Somehow I have the feeling that they can't observe women and feel that things are all right without having to use physical monitors all the time. That is what I find slows me down, interferes with me. And then I was looking for reassurance after every time I was checked, to make sure I was all right, when in actual fact, I didn't ever think it was necessary or helpful. It comes back to confidence again. I think that they are the trained individuals and I am not, and yet I feel they could use their powers of observation better, just to watch a woman and see. Somehow, just to experience the woman, I suppose, a whole experience rather than breaking it down all the time by*

measuring and calculating and feeling that you're controlling something you're not controlling. It's something that moves completely on its own. And it's actually only hindered, I think, by the interference.

Like it was a bit, stop we have to control something that kind of a way, but it did remove me from how I was feeling a little bit and started me thinking, how is the baby? And then I was relieved that the baby was fine. I don't know if it's really completely necessary. I really can't imagine how you would not know if the baby wasn't okay yourself and that little bit of control that they had was a small bit irritating. Like I said, when I did hear the heart beat was fine it was a relief. But I wouldn't have had to feel relieved if I didn't think that they were worried it mightn't have been okay.

Obstetric practices control the natural rhythms of women's birthing bodies by using invasive and painful practices that remain unacknowledged by disembodied ethics. But are deeply felt by women's sensitive, feeling, knowing bodies that carry the memories of the violence inflicted on them. In fact memory plays no part in defining health care ethics despite evidence that birth has temporal influences on women:

> The activity of remembering an event in my life by representing it to myself not only preserves my knowledge of the event but also rekindles the emotions associated with that event, leaving me to some extent in a similar condition as the one I was in when I experienced the event.[55]

While this may be self-evident to women, it plays little part in obstetric thinking.

Hurting women's bodies

Some women commented on the pain caused by some interventions. While the pain of contractions was often seen as acceptable pain – pain 'as it should be' – some women were distressed by unexpected, unwanted, or unnecessary pain. One woman commented that she was unaware that her primary midwife would want to do a vaginal examination in order to decide when to call the second midwife. She reluctantly agreed:

I just thought, oh, right, that's what we have to do. Whereas afterwards you think, well, did we need to do that?

During the examination, the midwife told her that she was going to keep her hand inside her during a contraction:

Well, what can you say about that when it's actually going on? It seemed a bit unnecessary. I did find it a horrible part of it – and painful, and not really part of the process of getting [baby] out necessarily. I don't think I really trusted the midwife after that.

Another woman very reluctantly accepted an induction using oxytocin that she had been very keen to avoid because of the overwhelming pain she experienced from this during her previous labour. She was unsure about whether she was strongly advised to agree to this because it was necessary or because the midwife:

Was getting snash from the consultant. I mean, to be fair, I didn't know this woman. I had no relationship with her, so I couldn't tell whether she was reacting to an outside force that was saying, get this woman on a drip now. Just tell her anything.

In hindsight, she felt she should have refused because her labour had already started and the induction caused her a great deal of distress both during and after her baby's birth.

It is difficult to know whether or not birth practices are experienced as more invasive when carried out by relative strangers. Do trusting relationships, where women are the focus of attention, reduce their experiences of pain and violation? There are suggestions that the context in which invasive practices are carried out may be as important as the invasiveness of the practices themselves.[56] Knowing what we now know about women's embodied experiences, it is not surprising that unless complications developed, women felt most empowered and least harmed when invasive practices were avoided or kept to a minimum.

The trouble is that as feminist theorists from a wide variety of disciplines have concluded, disembodied modernist thinking alienates women from their bodies making the violence of obstetrics possible and difficult to resist.[57] Both women and midwives are part of the same oppressive culture and are subject to the same violating experiences,[58] but few midwives have examined their personal or professional experience of violation.[59] Few have considered their own embodied experiences.[60] Forgetting bodies unwittingly continues a long tradition of silencing about the harm done to women in the name of science. It alienates women and midwives from themselves, their bodies, each other, and ultimately, their worlds. As I explained above, it prevents midwives from understanding the 'midwife effect',[61] their embodied influences on birth and that nobody (no body) can have no effect. It also hampers the efforts of those women who seek to reclaim the power of birth and their bodies. In other words, attempting to erase the body and its ability to feel, childbirth is not only sanitized of the everyday oppressive practices carried out on women's bodies, it also mutes the power, desire, sensuality and spirituality as potential experiences of childbearing.

The pleasurable potential of bodies

I suggested in Chapter 2 that feminist theorists have expanded on Michel Foucault's theories about power and argued that his views about disciplinary power and how it creates disciplined and disciplining embodied subjects are too narrow. They suggest that there is space for embodied *productive* power where bodies can resist attempts to control and constrain them.[62] Of course, given the expectation of selfless nurturing coupled with patriarchal definitions of sexuality that reduce women to passive objects of desire, it is not surprising that the power and sensuality of birth are 'barely audible'.[63]

But women's discussions supported feminist notions of embodied resistance as well as oppression. They talked about bodily pleasure as well as pain and power as well as vulnerability – though they found it difficult to talk about the powerful and sensual nature of birth given the clinical language of obstetrics and its disempowering birth practices. However, these women's experiences resonated with the small amount of literature that acknowledges the pleasure and power of women's bodies and birth.[64]

For many women, pregnancy and birth held spiritual and sensual qualities and for many was clearly part of their woman-ness and sexuality. These were often mentioned when women talked about why they were planning home births. (Where women felt 'asexual', this was usually in terms of dominant definitions of sexuality. That is, that they did not want to have sex with their partners and felt unattractive because of their size and shape.) Starhawk (1990) comments that the erasure of spirituality and the erotic are the bedrock of patriarchal oppression and that controlling women's sexuality undermines women's sense of worth and 'is the cornerstone of the structure of domination'.[65] The women's views on sexuality and spirituality suggested that this is indeed the case. They saw medicalization as a threat to the fragile continuum of sensuality and spirituality through birth and motherhood:

> *As a pregnant woman your sexuality is huge, and profound, but it's quite fragile. And I don't find my sexuality is very robust. So I can feel very sexy, but if somebody makes me feel insecure, I'm crushed. And I think I would say that a hospital experience would end up making me feel really bad about my sexuality. I think every bit of spirituality just gets left by the by, if you were in hospital. It certainly would for me. How can I have space to have these feelings. But the issue of sexuality would go the other way. It would probably make you feel less so. In a medical environment you're much more of a slab of meat and I don't want to feel like a slab of meat. Because you are big and you are different and you're not sexy in a way that a skinny available woman is sexy. It's a different thing and as soon as you're laid out on a couch, that's enough to switch it and you become a sow. And if you're at home with candlelight and privacy you can be big and beautiful. But put you under a strip light and you're not, and it's that fast.*

The diversity of women's views on sensuality and spirituality is reminiscent of Luce Irigaray's (1985) metaphor of women's sexuality – 'this sex which is not one'. For example, some women felt the power and sensuality of birth:

> *I do remember what a sexualizing experience it was and how animal and sexy it was to give birth. I was really sore, but I still felt really quite animal, and that was very powerful. That was very, very helpful to give birth.*

Others found that giving birth was a spiritual experience that they may not have been able to experience in an institutionalized environment. At home 'it wasn't being clashed by a sterile, clinical environment'. For others, giving birth was both sensual and spiritual:

> *I felt more the spiritual side at the beginning and then when [partner] got up after my waters broke and was massaging my back for me, I remember we said afterwards, it was like we fell in love all over again kind of. It wasn't the sexual aspect of it so*

much as just a real closeness that kind of developed as labour went on for me. It was just very relaxing and kind of passionate. And I remember just looking at him sometimes and really seeing him in a way I had never seen him before. Kind of knowing that we were making this amazing thing happen. So it was lovely to be able to have those feelings and to be able to express them. I did find great relief actually in kissing his neck for some reason – actual pain relief. And when I was leaning over, he was sitting on the bed I think and I was kneeling on the ground in front of him with my arms round his neck and just looking into his eyes and being able to kiss him. And again because we were here [at home], we were able to express that. So yeh, it was very fulfilling the whole thing, in a spiritual way and in a physical way.

One woman had been called 'weird' by members of her family when she mentioned the possibility of birth and sexuality. Some women were hesitant about expressing feelings of sexuality around birth, as this was not something that they had heard about from other women or read in books. Yet one woman said:

I found the whole pregnancy – this will maybe sound strange – but it is quite sexual. Oh God, how do you explain it.

Some women found that although birth was painful, there was something orgasmic about it too:

Suddenly I had all this energy and I just felt great and you know, I was really quite – I suppose I was really quite turned on would be the word to use. I mean it was absolute agony, but there's something there that is like when you're having great sex, when you feel this great sort of emotion overwhelming you, and you do feel quite turned on. Well, it was a similar sort of feeling and then you suddenly just feel this woosh, and out the baby comes and it's just like – I don't know, I mean, you just glow suddenly. I don't know (sighs) it's hard to explain. Well, with me, I feel it when the shoulders come out and the baby sort of wooshes out with all the water. It's like, I just suddenly thought, I'm a mummy, I mean it just made me feel so emotional. I was so proud of myself as well. It was just like, a great big smile on my face. It was like I did it. And all these emotions just suddenly sweep over you.

A number of women found that birthing their placentas was a sensual experience because 'it's all squishy and soft' and 'lovely and warm', giving a feeling of 'relief' and 'satisfaction'. One woman described it as similar to:

> '*A first kiss with your favourite boyfriend. That mmm in your belly feeling. That's how it was for me – like ping, big electric thing, then I just felt it slide out. It was like, wow, like perfect and it felt lovely. I remember it felt really good on the cervix.*

The politicizing power of birth

Following their experiences of planning and having home births, these women, wanted others to know that they could have their babies at home and that birth can be empowering and pleasurable. They also deplored the muting of this knowledge:

> *That's the one thing that really angers me as well is that information isn't there. All right, it is there, but it's not being distributed as widely as information about hospital births and all the technical side of everything. When you fall pregnant it seems like you just have to go and do your own research, and it's like you've to struggle really to get what you want. If you want a home birth it's like you're going against the norm. And it just really makes me cross that it's expected for one to go to hospital.*

> *Afterwards I couldn't get over how emotional I felt about other women's experiences – how much I felt, God I wish everyone could know that they can do it – know that it's the powers in them, rather than outside. And along with tears of joy, you have this conflicting feeling of, it can be like this for everybody and why isn't it? I hate the idea that the power isn't seen to be the woman's but it's just like you're a patient and the baby has to be taken out of you rather than your body can work wonders. I really feel that doctors don't see that at all. They really have no respect for the power the woman has, even female doctors. I mean, it's just like not taken into account.*

Just as the woman in Kirsi Viisainen's study observed that we have such powers inside if only we knew how to use them, so that we would dare to go against the direction given by society and do what we feel is right.[66]

Like women in other studies,[67] women also made links between birth and other areas of their lives. All described themselves as having been more politicized by planning home births in a culture that marginalizes this. This brought both benefits and costs. It could act as a catalyst for enhancing our abilities to challenge lack of information, injustices and oppressions and counteract passivity, but it could also be uncomfortable as those contrasting comments show:

> *The political effect has continued and I think it's made me just feel more on-the-ball. I think there's something kind of washed out and passive about people when they've had this really managed, probably awful experience that they want to put in a cupboard. These things just chip away at them, and they become a bit pallid. And I think it's kept it a vibrant issue. Do you know what I mean?*

> *It's like once you start you can't stop. You have to keep questioning and it's not always easy. It creates conflict. In my family and [partner's] family there's a lot of trust put in doctors and I've always had that trust as well really. And it's difficult for us to try and go against that now. I suppose we had the strength of the home delivery behind us. That gives us confidence. But it's still difficult. You had to go out and seek out the information. You're not going to be told by the people that are supposed to know about health care.*

As woman questioned accepted meanings of birth, they thought more about their ethical responsibilities towards themselves, their babies and others. In doing this they could see that both health-care ethics and ethics of care are coercive and cannot necessarily help them to safeguard their babies and themselves while at the same time maintaining connections with those around them.

What birthing ethics means for women

Much of the discussion in this chapter is about bringing women back into the picture and looking at their priorities. This challenges obstetric knowledge and technologies and the adversarial woman/baby division (a division that prioritizes the baby's health and has led to a growing concern with fetal and paternal rights). It examines the curiously simultaneous disappearance and management of women's bodies in obstetrics. A disappearance and reappearance that in between times removes the woman from her body and mutes the close relationship between mother and baby.[68] I come back to Jo Murphy-Lawless' (1998a) observation that the 'ongoing experience of being a mother' holds more meaning than the obstetric 'immortality strategy',[69] and also to the quotation on page 122 that supports this view:

> *My responsibility is to form a relationship. It's almost like that the birth is a rite of passage, and by the end of it you've been through it together and you're in relationship to the baby. The baby is what comes at the end of the process of giving birth, and I think the more connected I am with the birth, the more connected I am with the baby. And maybe my responsibility is to be open to having that connection with the baby.*

Any sense of relationship between mother and baby in obstetric ethics means the woman being selfless and complying with obstetrics' focus on the baby. Yet for these women, birthing ethics was about protecting and nurturing their babies *and* themselves. It was in this sense that they challenged disconnected obstetric ethics and ethics of care by suggesting that nurturing is an important aspect of birth but it need not be selfless or exclude multiple responsibilities or women's autonomy. In other words, nurturing their babies, themselves, and relationships was seen as mutually inclusive rather than exclusive. Focusing on protection and well-being rather than selflessness and sacrifice seems a healthier starting point for women and their families.[70]

The costs of autonomy

'A heap of guilt'

Sandra Bartky (1997) observed that liberatory politics bring both gains and losses to women.[71] Why else she asks, isn't every woman a feminist? As I described in this and the previous chapters, becoming politicized and challenging deeply held patriarchal values can have empowering gains but also devastating costs. Reclaiming the self from selfishness is no easy matter when being selfless is valorized, and attempting to reclaim birth is deemed to be selfish. By using the relationship between the woman and her baby coercively rather than positively, a spectre of so-called selfishness embeds itself in women's psyches potentially causing unbearable blame and guilt:

The line that they tend to use seems to be – no matter what your wishes are concerning the birth and where you'd feel more comfortable, surely you should consider the baby. And how would you feel if something happened to the baby. So I feel like, if something did go wrong and something happened to the baby I would have a heap of guilt, mainly from what they've said. Because they've put it on me, that I'm making an irresponsible choice that they're going along with. And if anything happens, it's my fault.

One of the women who transferred to hospital for what she felt were dubious reasons and had a technological birth there, explained how women are trapped by the rhetoric of selfishness and yet suffer its consequences deeply and personally. Before the birth of her baby she expressed the view that while one could argue that having an easier birth and calmer atmosphere might be better for the baby, it is 'probably quite a selfish thing for the mother'. The extreme distress she experienced at the end of her pregnancy and during her baby's birth made her feel very differently about this:

I mean it [birth] was just taken totally away from you in every sense. I was always a bit wary about the whole thing about empowerment. But I mean it's just so true. I just lost every will to fight and confidence in my own body. Everything. It was just gone. I mean I do feel incredibly robbed after the experience of childbirth. I find that really quite difficult to cope with [crying].

Feeling 'other'

Given the high costs of challenging a culture's authoritative knowledge, it is easy to see why women here and elsewhere are pulled towards complying with the dominant values of our culture. As women in Kirsi Viisainen's and my study commented:

It is easier to do what everybody else does, people do not want to step out from line, especially not Finns. They want to be like everybody else so that no one can say that they are different.[72]

I was just trying to be good and do everything as it was meant to be done. You know, according to the system. That's why I went to all these [parentcraft] classes in hospital. Just trying to be a good parent, you know. Following all the rules.

While feminists have strived to represent women as other than 'other', home birth is firmly located in the margins of our society. As I said earlier, women frequently rejected labels of 'radical', 'different', or 'making a fuss', but were nonetheless described as 'other' in a variety of ways, to the extent that some women started to label themselves. For example, one woman initially did not see herself as 'unusual' but came to see herself as 'rebellious'. Another woman made what she felt was a sensible decision to birth her placenta physiologically and came to see this as 'silly'.

Stereotypical views of women who plan home births seemed to be held, even by some of the midwives who attended them. One woman was asked if she could have chocolate biscuits in, 'because we find that a lot of our home birth ladies are nuts and berries ladies'. Of course midwives should have their needs for sustenance met and many of the women spontaneously talked about looking after their midwives. One or two had 'midwives' biscuits' or a 'midwives' tin'. But the woman experienced this particular comment as 'being put into that – you must be weird' category. Some women who plan home births may well share similar views and lifestyles, but stereotyping them merely erases the individual women and her concerns, increases her sense of 'otherness' and decreases her feeling of self-worth and confidence.

Some women felt alienated from other women in their own social networks. Their experience of planning a marginalized activity could lead them to feel marginalized themselves:

> *You've had your baby at home and everybody else has had theirs in hospital. Because they have an experience, they talk about it, and you're the odd one out. But you know, I tend to be that sort of person I think. I tend to do things differently or be the odd one out.*

The experience of 'otherness' can be doubly silencing and distancing in relation to other women in the community: on the one hand, women who have home births are labelled 'other', but on the other hand, their experiences go unnoticed:

> *I'm sure that they see it as something of an oddity, you know, me having had [baby] at home. But I don't think they really think about it very much. I think for them there's this paradigm. So it's almost as if I'd had [baby] in hospital as far as they're*

*concerned, because they never noticed that I had her at home,
you know.*

Thus, as I suggested earlier, far from developing closer bonds within a
community of birthing women, some women felt unable to share their
experiences and felt obliged to hide their sense of empowerment and
achievement. While 'I wished I could share it a bit more' this was difficult because 'anything I say seems like a judgement when so many
women have bad experience'. Some also resented the assumption that
a home birth must be an easy birth:

*The assumption is always, if you stayed at home it must have
been really easy. And I suppose I would sometimes like a bit of
credit for taking control and for doing something difficult.*

Women experienced this enforced 'otherness' and the subsequent muting and distance from midwives, family and friends as painful and
undermining. Although they understood that this was to do with societal pressures, the oppression they felt could be frustrating and
divisive:

*Women just have this weakness imposed on them. They
accept it and I find that I've become angry about that. I don't
feel very proud of it because you know, it isn't very generous
of me. But I just think they're colluding. And they need to
take action you know. It is possible. We have had a women's
movement in this country for many years now. When are they
going to just say: 'Right. That's enough.' And I just think it's
time for people to take action and not just be sorry and sad
afterwards – sad as that is. It amazes me that, since I've been
pregnant I have not had one story of a women who's had a
reasonable birth experience and I must have heard about fifteen. And I think that's very sad. But then I also think if
everybody feels like this how come it's still going on. What
are all these women playing at. Why don't they do something.
So it's a funny one cos how can you be angry with a woman
who's had a horrible birth experience. I think that's what happens – your heart goes out to them in one way. But then in
another – how can you say to that woman – well I hope for
the next time you're going to kick that GP's arse and say
you're not putting me in there again mate, it was crap. But*

they don't. They just go, huh. Put it to bed, get on with their lives'

Women were keenly aware that obstetric ideology was at odds with their own beliefs and that many of their difficulties stemmed from this. Nonetheless, when they were unable to forge their own meanings of birth, they often perceived this as a personal failing. They blamed themselves for not having informed themselves well enough, not communicating better, not being assertive enough, or having let themselves and their babies down in some way. As one woman said sadly and quietly: 'maybe I hadn't really managed to communicate with them. You know, I'm not such a great communicator'. And yet, how can women speak out in dangerous territory? As I suggested in Chapter 5 on page 200, we need to 'play safe' to protect ourselves. I have often remained silent, talked tentatively, dumbed down what I wanted to say, or attempted to package my views in the language of others. We cease to be ourselves in a myriad ways,[73] and frequently work under cover,[74] attempting to do 'good by stealth', to use midwife Mary Cronk's phrase. The cost is high whether we speak out or not.

The difficulties of going against the norms of our culture cannot be underestimated. While the potential exists for women to resist obstetric definitions of birth, protect themselves from potential abuse, create their own support network and develop a stronger sense of agency, power, and confidence in their abilities to make appropriate decisions, there is also the potential for these to be overridden and for them to have traumatic and undermining experiences. Indeed, it may seem dangerous to have expectations of autonomy, but *all* the women were glad that they had planned home births, and even those who transferred to hospital said that they would plan them again in a subsequent pregnancy.

Why is it important to develop integrated ethics?

Being at home attenuated obstetric thinking and practices but did not affect its core values. It penetrated women's homes, so that being at home could offer only a buffer to its 'coercive contract'. Uneasy attempts to mesh obstetric ideology with women's concerns through the rhetoric of 'choice' fails to facilitate women's ethical decision-making.[75] The notion of choice in obstetrics implies that it is almost external to actors, whereas Catriona Mackenzie (2000) suggests that autonomy is negotiated 'among three related elements of the person:

her point of view; her self-conception; and her values, ideals, commitments, and cares, in short, what matters to her'. She goes on to suggest that 'we cannot simply choose to abandon our cares or give up what matters to us. Or rather, we cannot do so without forfeit or loss'.[76] Decision-making is thus deeply implicated with personhood and autonomy. In other words, undermining decision-making potentially undermines the person, their sense of themselves and their self-esteem.[77]

If obstetrics does not rethink and expand its ethical code, it cannot stop treating women inhumanely. Its values decrease women's autonomy, ignore their feelings and knowledges, and harm their bodies, minds and spirits. By fending off other birth knowledges and practices it also continues to inhibit the possibilities and potential of birth. The abuse of childbearing women stems not from abusive individuals (though this can be the case), but from dominant structures that promote collective indifference through which abuses are carried out on women day in and day out under the auspices of what is right, necessary and ethical. An integrated ethics, sensitive to birthing women would have to develop definitions of autonomy that incorporate specifically located, embodied, potentially vulnerable and changing subjects.[78] It would have to acknowledge relational autonomy, where increased self-knowledge and ethical decision-making develop through dialogue with engaged others.[79]

Otherwise the midwife has to negotiate an (un)ethical climate, where her need to avoid risk to herself is pitted against the woman's integrity. For example, a woman's ethical decision not to have her baby's heartbeat monitored could expose the midwife to stressful enquiries, in which her license and livelihood could be at risk. However, enforcing practices on women is unlawful, untenable and unethical and can stop women from engaging with midwives. Forcing women to choose between having midwives who may not protect their integrity or having their babies without midwives is hardly an ethical solution.

The sense of empowerment or disempowerment and its ongoing effects is evident in the women's account. While some women were devastated by their perceived inability to exert their autonomy and resist obstetric ideology and practices, others described personal change and growth that led to them feeling more powerful as agents of their own and their children's lives when they had been able to define their own meanings of birth:

It's left me with a feeling that I didn't handle the situation very well. I should have really handled the situation better. I should have been stronger. I should have held out. I should not have given in. I should have been strong and said, no I don't want to be induced. But the pressures I was under at the time – I was left feeling, why didn't you just say no?

If I have a crisis of confidence, I think back to the birth and it's a very good anchor for me. You know it makes me believe in my ability to make good choices and I think it's made a tremendous impact on how I can make decisions. It just feels pivotal – a pivotal part of my politics really. It's almost like it drew together lots of sides that I had already and made them a more cohesive part of my life.

Notes

1　William Grieder 1992, quoted in Spretnak 1999: 109–110.
2　See also Kirkham and Stapleton 2004; Simpson 2004; Stapleton 2004.
3　Murphy-Lawless 1998a: 47.
4　Bartky 1997; Bordo 1997; Shildrick 1997; Thompson 2004; Young 1990a, 1990b.
5　Colebrook 1997: 21.
6　Belenky et al. 1986: 84.
7　Meyer 2000: 160.
8　Cornell 1995; Griffiths 1995; Shildrick 1997.
9　Reiger 2000; Young 1997a.
10　Machin and Scamell 1997.
11　See also Kirkham 2004.
12　Joseph Raz, quoted in Brison 2000: 285.
13　Kirkham 2004; Kirkham and Stapleton 2001; Mander 1993, 1997.
14　Stapleton 1997.
15　McLeod and Sherwin 2000: 267.
16　Green et al. 1998b: 178.
17　Colebrook 1997.
18　Weiner et al. 1997.
19　Gregg 1995: 125.
20　Campbell 1997: 4; Green et al. 1998b: 19; Martin 1987: 143; Murphy-Lawless 1998a: 245.
21　Trevathan 1997: 80.
22　McLeod and Sherwin 2000: 259.
23　Mercer and Skovgaard 2004.
24　Reiger 2000.
25　Kaufmann 2004.
26　Carol Gilligan, in Hamer 1999.
27　Gregg 1995: 10–11.

28 Starhawk 1990: 9.
29 Green et al. 1998b; Kitzinger 1990.
30 Hodnett 1989; Lemay 1997.
31 Starhawk 1990.
32 Robinson 1999.
33 See also Leap 2000.
34 Fleming 1994, 1998; Guilliland and Pairman 1995; Pairman 2000.
35 Starhawk 1990: 10.
36 Odent 1999: 31.
37 Walsh 2003: 656.
38 Bartky 1997; Stewart 2004b; Young 1990a.
39 Gatens 1996.
40 Carol Macmillan, in Belenky et al. 1986: 117.
41 Noddings 1984: 163.
42 Leap and Anderson 2004.
43 Diprose 1994; Pateman 1989; Young 1990b, 1997a.
44 McNay 1992.
45 Shildrick 1997.
46 Adams 1994; Douglas 1966; Marshall 1996; Rabuzzi 1994; Shildrick 1997; Young 1990b.
47 Foucault 1977; Starhawk 1990: 95.
48 Murphy-Lawless 1998a.
49 Duden 1993; Davis-Floyd 1992: 57.
50 Adams 1994: 40–41.
51 Kitzinger S. 1992.
52 Goddard 2001.
53 Crowther et al. 2000; Robson 1992.
54 Bergstrom et al. 1992; Central Sheffield University Hospitals 1998; McKay and Barrow 1991; Warren 1999a, 1999b.
55 Mackenzie 2000: 130.
56 Green et al. 1998b: 205.
57 Belenky et al. 1986; Brodkey and Fine 1992; Debold et al. 1996; Fine and MacPherson 1992; Hamer 1999; Pizzini 1992; Starhawk 1990; Young 1990b.
58 Rouf 1999; Thomas 1994.
59 Tilley 2000.
60 Kirkham 1999a.
61 Robinson 1999, 2004c.
62 See, for example, Bartky 1997; Diprose 1994; Griffiths 1995; Grosz 1993; McNay 1992.
63 Fine and Gordon 1992: 45.
64 See, for example, Adams 1994; Chester 1997; Gaskin 1990, 2003; Irigaray 1985; Kitzinger 2000; Lorde 1997; Rabuzzi 1994; van Olphen Fehr 1999.
65 Starhawk 1990: 25.
66 Viisainen 2001: 114.
67 Davis-Floyd 1992: 293.
68 Davis-Floyd 1992: 57; Duden 1993; Gregg 1995: 80; Jordan 1997; Murphy-Lawless 1998a; Shildrick 1997.
69 Murphy-Lawless 1998a: 47–48.
70 Downe and McCourt 2004.

71 Bartky 1997: 143.
72 Viisainen 2000b: 808.
73 Belenky et al. 1986; Debold et al. 1996.
74 Hutchinson 1990; Levy 1998.
75 Kirkham 2004.
76 Mackenzie 2000: 133, 135.
77 Shildrick 1997; Smythe 1998.
78 Colebrook 1997; Cornell 1995; Shildrick 1997.
79 Colebrook 1997; Diprose 1994.

7 Where now?

Birth is not only about making babies. Birth is also about making mothers – strong, competent, capable mothers who trust themselves and know their inner strength.[1]

I would like to conclude this book by suggesting that shifting the focus from the dominant mainstream meanings of birth to the diverse concerns of women, not only addresses specific issues about birth, but also the difficult dilemmas that we face nowadays. The difficulties women described between them and their midwives exemplify struggles between competing ideologies that are currently being played out locally and globally. These struggles impact on how and where maternity services are provided, and on women's agency (their ability to determine their own lives), whether they are childbearing women, midwives or both. They also impact on global trends towards increasing the power and material wealth (through largely unsustainable technologies) of the powerful and decreasing the (largely) sustainable material and spiritual wealth of the disempowered. In other words, the women's thoughts and experiences in this book contribute to the lesser heard stories that tell us about how and where dissenting voices meet the concrete blockages of oppressive ideologies. They also tell us about the remarkable abilities of marginalized groups (in this case women planning home births and community and independent midwives) to develop and act on their own ethical beliefs, despite the debilitating constraints of dominant beliefs and practices. For example, obstetric beliefs and practices prevent women and midwives from developing their own knowledges and skills. They prevent them from forming trusting relationships that promote safe birth. They oblige them to compromise in ways that are often detrimental to the well-being of women, babies, midwives and ultimately society.

What can we learn from these women?

Barbara Rothman observed that, 'Birth is not only about making babies. Birth is also about making mothers – strong, competent, capable mothers who trust themselves and know their inner strength'.[2] These women explained that being encouraged to become strong, competent, capable mothers helps them to protect their babies and keep them safe, before, during and after birth. Their abilities to do this depends on being encouraged to develop their autonomy skills, by being listened to, trusted, respected and treated as capable individuals. This enables them to make good decisions.[3] To focus on choice is missing the point because, as I explained in Chapter 6, choice comes from the misleading assumptions of modernity about how people relate to each other and how they make decisions. Women negotiate safety for themselves and their babies and families through ethical decision-making that unfolds best in the context of trusting relationships with those who can engage with them and focus on what really matters to them. Enabling autonomy through the facelessness and technocratization of our maternity services is impossible.[4] The exodus of midwives from midwifery seems not so surprising when we understand that they are expected to make the impossible, possible without the knowledge and skills they need.[5] All too often, women and midwives end up improving their skills of compromise rather than developing those they need to be more autonomous.[6]

As I explained at the end of Chapter 6, decision-making is a manifestation of a person's beliefs and lifestyle. It is a statement about who they are and what they care about. It is this connection between personhood and autonomy,[7] that brings birth practices to the very heart of feminist theorizing. This connection also explains why a book about a small group of women planning home births has profound implications for women and midwives in hospital situations. If women who are assumed to be well informed and assertive find it difficult to put their deeply held ethical beliefs into practice with midwives who are a little more accessible and removed from the hospital setting, it is infinitely more difficult for women and midwives in institutionalized settings. They have no knowledge about each other or how far each has been deprived of opportunities to develop and act on their beliefs and values. Yet women's integrity depends on being able to fulfil their own meanings of birth to the best of their abilities. They need the support of midwives, because without that support they are less able to make decisions and assume responsibility in the way they need to.

Can the midwife seamstress weave safety from autonomy?

Of course, we must acknowledge that women's experiences of birth are adversely affected by poverty, abuse and other oppressive factors that midwives can do little about:

> Health care by itself cannot, of course, correct all the evils of oppression. It cannot even cure all of the health-related effects of oppression. If health-care providers are to respond effectively to the problems, however, they must understand the impact of oppression on relational autonomy and make what efforts they can to increase the autonomy of their patients and clients.[8]

It is no coincidence that the chapter on relationships between women and midwives falls between those on safety and autonomy. As is clear from Chapter 5, the experienced midwife seamstress knows that safety and autonomy are woven together through her personal skill and integrity, the integrity of her relationship with the woman and the level of integrity between community and hospital services. But for midwives to enhance women's autonomy, much needs to be done to enhance autonomy within midwifery itself. For example, self-awareness must be developed, because 'to lack self-awareness is to lack autonomy'.[9] This means exposing midwives to critical feminist (and other) analyses of society so that they understand how midwives have been co-opted by obstetric ideology and socialized into practices that reduce rather than increase their and women's autonomy. It means creating a midwifery culture from education to management that develops midwives' autonomy capacities, because the impact of midwifery culture on autonomy has been clearly demonstrated.[10]

In essence, women need strong, competent, courageous midwives who can be trusted and are able to support their decisions and thereby protect their and their babies' physical, emotional and spiritual safety. For women to be more autonomous, they must be attended by autonomous midwives.[11]

Is lack of skill the greatest barrier to safety and autonomy?

None of the above cuts any ice without a broad knowledge and skill base to support it. As I observed earlier, and as is particularly clear in Chapter 4, one of the repeated and most significant explanations that women gave for midwives' lack of autonomy was the lack of low-tech, physiological, emotional and perhaps spiritual midwifery skills. These skills are needed to facilitate normal birth, keep it normal, and respond safely to as many complications as possible that would otherwise necessitate obstetric interventions. What midwifery means and what it can do is as hotly contested an issue as place of birth because the two are very much related. For midwifery to move beyond its present limited scope, it would need support from the culture as a whole and from the bodies that support and regulate midwives. Not surprisingly, while the Nursing and Midwifery Council (NMC 2002) is supporting midwifery to the best of its abilities, it is not entirely clear whether or not its guidelines can uphold autonomous skilled practice that supports women's autonomy, or whether these guidelines are still hemmed in by obstetric ideology – because this is not entirely clear within law or the wider culture. This is not to diminish the crucial efforts of many who work for change: their work is never insignificant. And because this book focussed on women's experiences, it cannot begin to do justice to those skilled and courageous midwife seamstresses who advocate and support women to make their own decisions day in and day out, often at their own personal cost. Neither does the book properly address the important midwifery innovations that continually emerge. But achievements (particularly within the NHS) are against the odds. They often falter when they meet the oppositional forces of obstetric ideology and gender-blind norms, that fail to support midwives as women. Potentially transformatory moves to create midwifery birth centres are often 'dumbed down',[12] though freestanding birth centres are emerging.[13] Autonomous experiences occur almost by chance, rather than by design. Sustainable change depends on enough women and midwives supporting the idea that a broad skill base for midwives together with structures that promote trusting relationships between women and midwives and between midwives themselves will assist midwives to engage with women in ways that increase the likelihood of childbearing being a positive force in their lives (a contribution that maternity care purports to make).

How do we create values from postmodernism?

Feminist readings of postmodernism have posed searching questions about how we could formulate any coherent approach to the development of birth practices that are inclusive of women's beliefs and needs and that avoid unhelpful polarities,[14] one of which is the home/hospital dichotomy. If we want to move beyond stereotyping women and midwives, cosmetic changes in hospital, and assumptions that only home birth can be paradigmatically different, analysis needs to focus inclusively on women, practitioners, beliefs, and places of birth. Clearly, the current libertarian solution of more accurate and unbiased information along with the right to choose is inadequate for numbers of reasons already described. And as I explained in Chapters 1, 2 and 3 knowledge is socially constructed, intimately connected with societal norms, and thus never without value.

If we look at research findings, we know that women and babies attended by skilled midwives in out of hospital settings receive fewer interventions and sustain less injuries. We know that whatever women's views on technological or natural birth prior to birth, satisfaction rates are higher among those women who have fewest interventions.[15] We know that some of the most positive accounts come from women who had home births, and/or had one or two trusted midwives throughout the childbearing period.[16] We know that where midwives provide more holistic support, and where place of birth is more flexible, more women plan to give birth at home later in pregnancy or during labour.[17] The women in this book suggest that having normal births at home often provided benefits beyond their expectations. But, as I have discussed, none of this necessarily leads us out of the polarities that feminists have criticized.[18] As Rosalyn Diprose (1994) contends, attributing technology to patriarchy is unhelpful to women and risks replacing one set of oppressive values with another. In other words, we can all too easily 'reduce "plurality" to variations on the Same'.[19]

There are complex issues here about how women's values and beliefs interact with a technocratoic society and how they might prioritize different, even competing needs and meet these priorities in ways that maintain the integrity of who they are. In a complex society women need help to negotiate their own values and needs with what is now possible and available:

> *I didn't want anything injected while the baby was in me, and gas and air seemed the safest option. Epidurals – it's tempting. A cousin of mine had what she called a mobile epidural and she could still push but felt no pain at all. I thought, oh gosh, that's the way to go isn't it really? I mean, why do I put myself through this?*
>
> *Nadine: And how did you answer that question?*

How did I answer? I don't know. I mean actually my husband said, 'You know, you should consider it'. I said, but then it means going into hospital, and he said, 'Well if you're really apprehensive about the pain, maybe that's the way to do it'. But I want the baby at home so much that I'll forgo anything which means I'll be hooked up to something. When you are hooked up, even with a so-called mobile epidural, I can't imagine that you can sort of wander around too much. The whole point is that you're anaesthetized from the waist down. You can't walk around if you're anaesthetized. You can't stand up. So, I mean, it would just in a sense betray everything that I was hoping for and wanted.

Is the way forward socializing birth, so that technology can be used to support women and babies, and midwifery practices when necessary, instead of further technocratizing it and using social practices to humanize it? This means developing technologies of the body that are sensitive to women's and babies' bodies and birth and that increase rather than decrease women's autonomy. Currently, these two agendas of socializing birth and developing appropriate technologies often maintain a distance from each other. Women, midwives and researchers need to contribute to both agendas to be most effective. Safety will never be realized through conflict, thus we need to resolve the problem of different values through attention to diversity and the particularities of women's lives rather than thoughtlessly applying the currently popular notion of standardization.

In conclusion

Midwifery offers the possibility of providing engaged, individualized, holistic care from a dedicated practitioner with in-depth knowledge and experience to any and all childbearing women. There is a great deal of merit in the idea of fostering and enabling this role rather than continuing to limit it by adhering to obstetric ideology, or fragmenting it by introducing subsidiary roles that might further undermine it.[20] There is a great deal of merit in making midwives more visible and providing bases for them in women's communities, so that they and women can develop their meanings of birth together. The role of midwifery and midwives in women's lives is powerfully exemplified by the quotation below, from a woman who had a distressing experience of birth followed by a positive one assisted by known and trusted midwives. In a few words, she brings together the substantive themes in this book – that women and birth are simultaneously powerful and vulnerable, that birth is a potentially empowering or disempowering rite of passage that requires skilled and attentive support, that it affects the woman's sense of herself profoundly and that the midwife is one of the main bridges between vulnerability and empowerment, through her ability to 'be with':

> My daughter's birth was a true healing for me; both my body and my spirit were healed and put back together again. With the help of my midwives, I discovered the strength to reclaim my body and my baby.[21]

And as one of the women in this study thoughtfully commented, when talking about her decision to engage an independent midwife

> *I think at the time, when I did it I thought it was a luxury and that the community midwives would be okay as well, but that this would be better. But now I don't think that at all because I realized what I needed was not a home birth but a need for a midwife. I probably needed that more than I needed a home birth. But getting to know [midwife] and having her there and having the same care afterwards with the same person that you'd got to know was the main thing that I needed.*

Notes

1 Thompson 2004: 137.
2 Barbara Rothman, quoted in Thompson 2004: 137.
3 A collection of essays edited by Catriona Mackenzie and Natalie Stoljar (2000) provide a detailed analysis about self-knowledge (Meyer 2000), self-definition (Mackenzie 2000; Meyer 2000), self-trust (McLeod and Sherwin 2000), self-esteem (Benson 2000; Mackenzie 2000) and self-reflection (Stoljar 2000). These demonstrate how decisions are made in relationship with others who are able to listen, trust and respect (McLeod and Sherwin 2000: 262). Thus women need a sense of their own 'worthiness' in order to make their own decisions (Mackenzie 2000: 133), but can be undermined and alienated from their own self-reasoning by others (Benson 2000: 76). In other words, 'being assertive or confident to express your own opinions and feelings has a lot to do with trusting your own judgement about their accuracy and relevance in discussion with others' (McLeod and Sherwin 2000: 273). So, exchanges with others are influential: 'other's speech to and about us and ours to and about them are crucially important in the development and endurance of our autonomous selves' (Brison 2000: 287). And even though self-worth is complex, and (fortunately) women are resilient, 'one assailant can undo

a lifetime of self-esteem' (Brison 2000: 141), as birth accounts sometimes demonstrate.

4 Kirkham 2004.
5 Clarke 1995; Kirkham 1999b.
6 Kirkham 1999b, 2004; Kirkham and Stapleton 2001; Levy 1998, 1999b.
7 Griffiths 1995; Mackenzie and Stoljar 2000; Meyer 2000.
8 McLeod and Sherwin 2000: 276.
9 Meyer 2000: 157.
10 Kirkham 1999b, 2004; Kirkham and Stapleton 2001.
11 Edwards 2000: 80.
12 Shallow 2003.
13 Anderson 2000b; Rosser and Anderson 2000; Leatherbarrow et al 2004.
14 Fielder et al. 2004.
15 Green et al. 1998b: 173–175.
16 Lemay 1997; McCourt and Page 1997; Noble 2001; O'Connor 1992;
Ogden et al. 1997a, 1997c; van Olphen Fehr 1999; Sandall et al. 2001b.
17 Leyshon 2004; Sandall 2001b; Smethurst 1997.
18 Annandale and Clark 1996; Cosslett 1994; Diprose 1994; Fielder et al.
2004.
19 Code 2000: 198.
20 Mander 2001: 168–169.
21 Noble 2001: 113.

References

Ackermann-Liebrich, U., Voegeli, T., Gunter-Witt, K., Kunzi, I., Zullig, M., Schindler, C., Maurer, M., and Zurich Study Team (1996) 'Home versus hospital deliveries: follow up study of matched pairs for procedure and outcome', *British Medical Journal*, 313: 1313–1318.

Adam, Barbara (1992) 'Time and health implicated: a conceptual critique', in Ronald Frankenberg (ed.) *Time, Health and Medicine*, pp. 153–164, London: Sage.

Adam, Barbara (2000) 'Interview: Barbara Adam', *Network: Newsletter of the British Sociological Association*, 77: 1–4.

Adams, Alice E. (1994) *Reproducing the Womb: Images of Childbirth in Science, Feminist Theory, and Literature*, Ithaca, NY: Cornell University Press.

Alexander, Heidi (1987) *Home Birth in Lothian*: Edinburgh Health Council, Torphichen Street, Edinburgh.

Alldred, Pam (1998) 'Ethnography and discourse analysis: dilemmas in representing the voices of children', in Jane Ribbens and Rosalind Edwards (eds) *Feminist Dilemmas in Qualitative Research*, pp. 147–170, London: Sage.

Allison, Julia (1996) *Delivered at Home*, London: Chapman and Hall.

Alment, E.A.J., Barr, A., Reid, M., and Reid, J.J.A. (1967) 'Normal confinement: a domiciliary and hospital study', *British Medical Journal*, 27: 530–534.

Anderson, Joan M. (1991) 'The phenomenological perspective', in Janice M. Morse (ed.) *Qualitative Nursing Research*, pp. 25–38, Newbury Park, CA: Sage.

Anderson, R. and Murphy, P.A. (1995) 'Outcomes of 11788 planned home births: attended by certified nurse-midwives: a retrospective descriptive study', *Journal of Nurse-Midwifery*, 40: 483–492.

Anderson, Tricia (2000a) 'Feeling safe enough to let go: the relationship between a woman and her midwife during the second stage of labour', in Mavis Kirkham (ed.) *The Midwife–Mother Relationship*, pp. 92–119, London: Macmillan.

Anderson, Tricia (2000b) 'Have we lost the plot?', *The Practising Midwife*, 3(1): 4–5.

Anderson, Tricia (2004) 'The misleading myth of choice: the continuing oppression of women in childbirth', in Mavis Kirkham (ed.) *Informed Choice in Maternity Care*, pp. 257–264, Basingstoke: Palgrave Macmillan.

Andrews, Alison (2004a) 'Home birth experience 1: decision and expectation', *British Journal of Midwifery*, 12(8): 518–523

Andrews, Alison (2004b) 'Home birth experience 2: births/postnatal reflections', *British Journal of Midwifery*, 12(9): 552–557.

Ann and Heidi (2001) 'Mother as midwife', *AIMS Journal*, 13(1): 12–14.

Annandale, Ellen, and Clark, Judith (1996) 'What is gender? Feminist theory and the sociology of human reproduction', *Sociology of Health and Illness*, 18(1): 17–44.

Annandale, Ellen, and Clark, Judith (1997) 'A reply to Rona Campbell and Sam Porter', *Sociology of Health and Illness*, 19(4): 521–532.

Armstrong, David (1987) 'Bodies of knowledge: Foucault and the problem of human anatomy', in Graham Scambler (ed.) *Sociological Theory and Medical Sociology*, pp. 59–76, London: Tavistock.

Arney, W.R. (1982) *Power and the Profession of Obstetrics*, Chicago: University of Chicago Press.

Aspinall, Kate, Nelson, Barbara, Patterson, Trisha, and Sims, Anita (1997) *An Extraordinary Ordinary Woman*, Sheffield: Ann's Trust Fund, 43 Sydney Rd, Sheffield S6 3GG.

Assiter, Alison (1996) *Enlightened Women*, London and New York: Routledge.

Banks, Maggie (2000) *Home Birth Bound: Mending the Broken Weave*, Hamilton, New Zealand: Birthspirit Books.

Baird, D. (1950, 1969) *Combined Textbook of Obstetrics and Gynaecology* 5th and 8th edns. Edinburgh: E&S Livingstone.

Barbour, Rosaline S. (1990) 'Fathers: the emergence of a new consumer group', in Jo Garcia, Robert Kilpatrick and Martin Richards (eds) *The Politics of Maternity Care: Services for Childbearing Women in Twentieth-Century Britain*, pp. 202–216, Oxford: Clarendon Press.

Barkley, Margaret (1998) 'Childbirth and embodiment: reflections on subjectivity and language', paper presented at Annual Conference of the British Sociological Association, Edinburgh University, April.

Bar On, Bat-Ami (1993) 'Marginality and epistemic privilege', in Linda Alcoff and Elizabeth Potter (eds) *Feminism/Postmodernism*, New York and London: Routledge.

Barrett, Michele (1992) 'Words and things: materialism and method in contemporary feminist analysis', in Michele Barrett and Anne Phillips (eds) *Destabilizing Theory: Contemporary Feminist Debates*, pp. 201–219, Cambridge: Polity Press.

Bartky, Sandra Lee (1997) 'Foucault, feminity, and the modernization of patriarchal power', in Katie Conboy, Nadia Medina, and Sarah Stanbury (eds) *Writing on the Body: Female Embodiment and Feminist Theory*, New York: Columbia University Press.

Bastian, Hilda (1993a) 'Personal beliefs and alternative childbirth choices: a survey of 552 women who planned to give birth at home', *Birth*, 20(4): 186–192.

Bastian, Hilda (1993b) 'Who gives birth at home and why? A survey of 552 women who planned to give birth at home', *Home Birth Australia Newsletter*, 33(February): 19–23.

Beard, R. (1977) 'Changes in Obstetrics: an interview with Richard Beard, *British Medical Journal*, 23 July, p. 251.

Beck, Ulrich (1992) *Risk Society: Towards a New Modernity*, London: Sage.

Bedford, Helen, and Elliman, David (2000) 'Concerns about immunisation', *British Medical Journal*, 320: 240–243.

Beech, Beverley A. Lawrence (1990) *The History of AIMS – 1960–1990* AIMS. Available from AIMS, 5 Ann's Court, Grove Road, Surbiton, Surrey KT6 4BE.

Beech, Beverley A. Lawrence (1991) *Who's Having your Baby: A Health Rights Handbook for Maternity Care*, London: Bedford Square Press.

Beech, Beverley A. Lawrence (2001) 'UKCC's failure to protect mothers and babies', *AIMS Journal*, 13(1): 10–11.

Beech, Beverley (2003) *Am I Allowed?* Available from AIMS, 5 Ann's Court, Grove Road, Surbiton, Surrey KT6 4BE.

Belenky, Mary F., Clinchy, Blythe M., Goldberger, Nancy R., and Tarule, Jill M. (1986) *Women's Ways of Knowing: The Development of Self, Voice and Mind*, New York: Basic Books.

Bell, Diane, and Klein, Renate (eds) (1996) *Radically Speaking: Feminism Reclaimed*, London: Zed Books.

Benhabib, Selya (1995) 'Feminism and postmodernism', in Judith Butler, Selya Benhabib, Drucilla Cornell and Nancy Fraser (eds) *Feminist Contentions: A Philosophical Exchange*, New York and London: Routledge.

Benhabib, Selya, Butler, Judith, Cornell, Drucilla, and Fraser, Nancy (1995) *Feminist Contentions: A Philosophical Exchange*, New York and London: Routledge.

Benoit, Cecilia, Davis-Floyd, Robbie, Van Teijlingen, Edwin R., Sandall, Jane, and Miller, Janneli F. (2001) 'Designing midwives: a comparison of educational models', in Cecilia Benoit, Raymond DeVries, Edwin R. van Teijlingen and Sirpa Wrede (eds) *Birth by Design: Pregnancy, Maternity Care, and Midwifery in North America and Europe*, pp. 139–165, New York and London: Routledge.

Benson, Paul (2000) 'Feeling crazy: self-worth and the social character of responsibility', in Catriona Mackenzie and Natalie Stoljar (eds) *Relational Autonomy: Feminist Perspectives on Autonomy, Agency, and the Social Self*, pp. 72–93, New York and Oxford: Oxford University Press.

Bergstrom, L., Roberts, J., Skillman, L., and Seidel, J. (1992) '"You'll feel me touching you sweetie": vaginal examinations during the second stage of labor', *Birth*, 19(1): 10–18.

Bergum, Vangie (1989) *Woman to Mother: A Transformation*, Granby, MA: Bergin & Garvey.

Bewley, Christine (2000) 'Midwives' personal experiences and the relationships with women: midwives without children', in Mavis Kirkham (ed.) *The Midwife–Mother Relationship*, pp. 169–192, London: Macmillan.

Biesele, Megan (1997) 'An ideal of unassisted birth: hunting, healing and transformation among the Kalahari Ju/'hoansi', in Robbie E. Davis-Floyd and Carolyn G. Sargent (eds) *Childbirth and Authoritative Knowledge: Cross-Cultural Perspectives*, pp. 474–492, Berkeley, CA: University of California Press.

Bluff, Rosalind, Holloway, Immy (1994) '"They know best" women's perceptions of midwifery care during labour and childbirth, *Midwifery*, 10: 157–164.

Bordo, Susan (1997) 'The body and the reproduction of femininity', in Katie Conboy, Nadia Medina and Sarah Stanbury (eds) *Writing on the Body: Female Embodiment and Feminist Theory*, pp. 90–110, New York: Columbia University Press.

Bortin, Sylvia, Alzugaray, Marina, Dowd, Judy, and Kalman, Janice (1994) 'A feminist perspective on the study of home birth: application of a midwifery care framework', *Journal of Nurse-Midwifery*, 39(3): 142–149.

Bourgeault, Ivy Lynn, Declercq, Eugene, and Sandall, Jane (2001) 'Changing birth: interest groups and maternity care policy', in Raymond DeVries, Cecelia Benoit, Edwin R. van Teijlingen and Sirpa Wrede (eds) *Birth by Design: Pregnancy, Maternity Care and Midwifery in North America and Europe*, pp. 51–69, New York and London: Routledge.

Bourgeault, Ivy Lynn, Benoit, Cecilia, and Davis-Floyd, Robbie (eds) (2004) *Reconceiving Midwifery*, Montreal: McGill-Queen's University Press.

Braidotti, Rosi (1997) 'Mothers, monsters and machines', in Katie Conboy, Nadia Medina and Sarah Stanbury (eds) *Writing on the Body: Female Embodiment and Feminist Theory*, pp. 59–79, New York: Columbia University Press.

Brison, Susan J. (2000) 'Relational autonomy and freedom of expression', in Catriona Mackenzie and Natalie Stoljar (eds) *Relational Autonomy: Feminist Perspectives on Autonomy, Agency, and the Social Self*, pp. 280–299, New York and Oxford: Oxford University Press.

Brodkey, Linda, and Fine, Michelle (1992) 'Presence of mind in the absence of the body', in Michelle Fine (ed.) *Disruptive Voices: The Possibilities of Feminist Research*, pp. 77–95, Ann Arbor, MI: University of Michigan Press.

Brodribb, Somer (1992) *Nothing Mat(t)ers: A Feminist Critique of Post-Modernism*, New York: New York University Press.

Brown, Stephanie, Lumley, Judith, Small, Rhonda, and Astbury, Jill (1994) *Missing Voices: The Experience of Motherhood*, Oxford: Oxford University Press.

Browner, Carole H., and Press, Nancy (1997) 'The production of authoritative knowledge in American prenatal care', in Robbie E. Davis-Floyd and Carolyn

F. Sargent (eds) *Childbirth and Authoritative Knowledge: Cross-Cultural Perspectives*, pp. 113–131, Berkeley, CA: University of California Press.

Burnett, C.A., Jones, J.A., Rooks, J., Chen, C.H., Tyler, C.W., and Miller, A. (1980) 'Home delivery and neonatal morbidity in North Carolina', *Journal of the American Medical Association*, 244(24): 2741–2745.

Burt, Sandra, and Code, Lorraine (eds) (1995) *Changing Methods: Feminists Transforming Practice*, Peterborough, UK: Broadview Press.

Butler, Judith (1995) 'Contingent foundations', in Selya Benhabib, Judith Butler, Drucilla Cornell and Nancy Fraser (eds) *Feminist Contentions: A Philosophical Exchange*, pp. 35–57, New York and London: Routledge.

Butter, I., and Lapré, R. (1986) 'Obstetric care in the Netherlands: manpower distribution and differential costs', *International Journal of Health Planning Management*, 1: 89–110.

Campbell, Rona (1997) 'Place of birth reconsidered', in Jo Alexander, Valerie Levy and Carolyn Roth (eds) *Midwifery Practice Core Topics 2*, pp. 1–22, London: Macmillan.

Campbell, Rona, and Macfarlane, Alison (1994) *Where to be Born? The Debate and the Evidence*, 2nd edn, Oxford: National Perinatal Epidemiology Unit.

Campbell, Rona, and Porter, Sam (1997) 'Feminist theory and the sociology of childbirth: a response to Ellen Annandale and Judith Clark', *Sociology of Health and Illness*, 19(3): 348–358.

Caplan, M., and Madeley, R.J. (1985) 'Home deliveries in Nottingham 1980–81', *The Society of Community Medicine*, 99: 307–313.

Cartwright, Elizabeth, and Thomas, Jan (2001) 'Constructing risk', in Raymond DeVries, Cecilia Benoit, Edwin R. van Teijlingen and Sirpa Wrede (eds) *Birth by Design: Pregnancy, Maternity Care, and Midwifery in North America and Europe*, pp. 218–228, New York and London: Routledge.

Central Sheffield University Hospitals (1998) *The Central Sheffield University Hospitals Evidence-Based Guidelines for Midwifery-led Care in Labour*, Sheffield: Central Sheffield University Hospitals.

Chalmers, Iain, and Haynes, Brian (1994) 'Reporting, updating, and correcting systematic reviews of the effects of health care', *British Medical Journal*, 309: 862–865.

Chamberlain, David (1998) *The Mind of your Newborn Baby*, Berkeley, CA: North Atlantic Books.

Chamberlain, Geoffrey, Wraight, Ann, and Crowley, Patricia (1997) *Home Births: The Report of the 1994 Confidential Enquiry by the National Birthday Trust Fund*, New York and London: Parthenon.

Charles, Nickie, and Hughes-Freeland, Felicia (eds) (1996) *Practising Feminism: Identity, Difference, Power*, London and New York: Routledge.

Chesney, Margaret (2004) 'Birth for some women in Pakistan: defining and defiling'. PhD thesis, University of Sheffield.

Chester, Penfield (1997) *Sisters on a Journey: Portraits of North American Midwives*, New Brunswick, NJ: Rutgers University Press.

Clair, Robin Patric (1997) 'Organizing silence: silence as voice and voice as silence in the narrative exploration of the treaty of new echota', *Western Journal of Communication*, 61(3): 315–337.

Clarke, Rachel A. (1995) 'Midwives, their employers and the UKCC: an eternally unethical triangle', *Nursing Ethics*, 2(3): 247–253.

Clarke, M.J. and Stewart, L.A (1994) 'Obtaining data from randomised control trials: how much do we need for reliable and informative meta-analyses', *British Medical Journal*, 309: 1007–1010.

Clifford, James, and Marcus, George E. (eds) (1986) *Writing Culture: The Poetics and Politics of Ethnography*, Berkeley, CA: University of California Press.

Code, Lorraine (1993) 'Taking subjectivity into account', in Linda Alcoff and Elizabeth Potter (eds) *Feminist Epistemologies*, pp. 15–48, New York and London: Routledge.

Code, Lorraine (1998) 'Voice and voicelessness: a modest proposal?' in Janet A. Kourany (ed.) *Philosophy in a Feminist Voice: Critiques and Reconstructions*, pp. 204–230, Princeton, NJ: Princeton University Press.

Code, Lorraine (2000) 'The perversion of autonomy and the subjection of women: discourses of social advocacy at century's end', in Catriona Mackenzie and Natalie Stoljar (eds) *Relational Autonomy: Feminist Perspectives on Autonomy, Agency, and the Social Self*, pp. 181–209, New York and Oxford: Oxford University Press.

Colebrook, Claire (1997) 'Feminism and autonomy: the crisis of the self-authoring subject', *Body and Society*, 3(2): 21–41.

Comaroff, Jean (1977) 'Conflicting paradigms of pregnancy: managing ambiguity in antenatal encounters', in A. Davis and G. Horobin (eds) *Medical Encounters: The Experience of Illness*, pp. 115–134, London: Croom Helm.

Confidential Enquiry into Maternal and Child Health (2004) *Why Mothers Die 2000–2002: The Sixth Report on the Confidential Enquiries into Maternal Deaths in the United Kingdom*, London: Royal College of Obstetricians and Gynaecologists.

Cooper, Yvette (2000) Letter to Nicholas Winterton MP 19th June 2000 – in response to letter from Beverley Beech, chair, AIMS to Nicholas Winterton.

Cornell, Drucilla (1995) 'What is ethical feminism?', in Selya Benhabib, Judith Butler, Drucilla Cornell and Nancy Fraser (eds) *Feminist Contentions: A Philosophical Exchange*, pp. 75–106, New York and London: Routledge.

Cosslett, Tess (1991) 'Questioning the definition of "literature": fictional and non-fictional accounts of childbirth', in Jane Aaron and Sylvia Walby (eds) *Out of the margins: Women's Studies in the Nineties*, pp. 220–231, London: Falmer Press.

Cosslett, Tess (1994) *Women Writing Childbirth: Modern Discourses on Motherhood*. Manchester and New York: Manchester University Press.

Cowan, Jane K. (1996) 'Being a feminist in contemporary Greece: similarity and difference reconsidered', in Nickie Charles and Felicia Hughes-Freeland (eds) *Practising Feminism: Identity, Difference, Power*, pp. 61–85, London and New York: Routledge.

CRAG/SCOTMEG Working Group on Maternity Services (1993) Roadshows February–May 1993, London: HMSO.

CRAG/SCOTMEG Working Group on Maternity Services (1994a) 'Innovations in Practice: Abstract of Presentations March 1994', London: HMSO.

CRAG/SCOTMEG Working Group on Maternity Services (1994b) 'Innovations in Practice: Abstract of Presentations October 1993', London: HMSO.

CRAG/SCOTMEG Working Group on Maternity Services (1994c) 'Innovations in Practice: Summary of Submissions October 1993–March 1994', London: HMSO.

CRAG/SCOTMEG Working Group on Maternity Services (1994d) 'Report on Obstetric and Neonatal Flying Squads', London: HMSO.

Creasy, Jillian Margaret (1994) 'Women's experience of transfer from community-based to consultant care in late pregnancy or labour', unpublished MPhil thesis, University of Sheffield.

Cronk, Mary (1992) 'A doubly difficult birth', *Nursing Time*, 88(47): 54–56.

Cronk, Mary (1998a) 'Hands off the breech', *The Practising Midwife*, 1(6): 13–15.

Cronk, Mary (1998b) 'Midwives and breech birth', *The Practising Midwife*, 1(7/8): 44–45.

Cronk, Mary (2000) 'The midwife: a professional servant?', in Mavis Kirkham (ed.) *The Midwife–Mother Relationship*, pp. 19–27, London: Macmillan.

Crotty, M., Ramsay, A.T., Smart, R., and Chan, A. (1990) 'Planned home births in Australia 1976–1987', *Medical Journal of Australia*, 153: 664–671.

Crowther, Caroline, Enkin, Murray, and Keirse, Marc J.N.C. (2000) 'Monitoring the progress of labour', in Murray Enkin, Marc J.N.C. Keirse, James Neilson, Caroline Crowther, Lelia Duley, Ellen Hodnett and Justus Hofmeyr (eds) *A Guide to Effective Care in Pregnancy and Childbirth*, pp. 281–288, Oxford: Oxford University Press.

Cumberlege, G. (1948) *Maternity in Great Britain: A Survey of Social and Economic Aspects of Pregnancy and Childbirth, Undertaken by a Joint Committee of the Royal College of Obstetrics and Gynaecology and the Population Investigations Committee*, London: Oxford University Press.

Dalmiya, Vrinda, and Alcoff, Linda (1993) 'Are "Old Wives' Tales" justified?', in Linda Alcoff and Elizabeth Potter (eds) *Feminist Epistemologies*, pp. 217–244, New York and London: Routledge.

Damstra-Wijmenga, Sonja M.I. (1984) 'Home confinement: the positive results in Holland', *Journal of the Royal College of General Practitioners* 34 (August): 425–430.

Davies, Charlotte Aull (1996) 'Nationalism: discourse and practice', in Nicky Charles and Felicia Hughes-Freeland (eds) *Practising Feminism: Identity Difference Power*, pp. 156–179, London and New York: Routledge.

Davies, Jean (2000) 'Being with women who are economically without', in Mavis Kirkham (ed.) *The Midwife–Mother Relationship*, pp. 120–142, London: Macmillan.

Davies, J., Hey, E., Reid, W., and Young, G. (1996) 'Prospective regional study of planned home births', *British Medical Journal*, 313: 1302–1306.

Davies, Lorna (2004) 'Feminist approach to midwifery education', in Mary Stewart (ed.) *Pregnancy, Birth and Maternity Care: Feminist Perspectives*, pp. 143–56, Edinburgh: Books for Midwives.

Davis, Margaret Llewelyn (ed.) (1978) *Maternity: Letters from Working Women*, London: Virago.

Davis-Floyd, Robbie E. (1992) *Birth as an American Rite of Passage*, Berkeley, CA: University of California Press.

Davis-Floyd, Robbie E. (2002) 'The technocratic, humanistic, and holistic paradigms of childbirth', *MIDIRS Midwifery Digest*, 12(4): 500–506.

Davis-Floyd, Robbie E., and Davis, Elizabeth (1997) 'Intuition as authoritative knowledge in midwifery and home birth', in Robbie E. Davis-Floyd and Carolyn F. Sargent (eds) *Childbirth and Authoritative Knowledge: Cross-Cultural Perspectives*, pp. 315–349, Berkeley, CSA University of California Press.

Davis-Floyd, Robbie E., and Dumit, Joseph (eds) (1997) *Cyborg Babies: From Techno-Sex to Techno-Tots*, New York: Routledge.

Davis-Floyd, Robbie E., and St John, Gloria (eds) (1998) *From Doctor to Healer: The Transformative Journey*, New Brunswick, NJ: Rutgers University Press.

Davis-Floyd, Robbie E., and Sargent, Carolyn F. (eds) (1997) *Childbirth and Authoritative Knowledge: Cross-Cultural Perspectives*, Berkeley, CA: University of California Press.

Daviss, Betty-Anne (1997) 'Heeding warnings from the canary, the whale, and the Inuit: a framework for analyzing competing types of knowledge about childbirth', in Robbie Davis-Floyd and Carolyn F. Sargent (eds) *Childbirth and Authoritative Knowledge: Cross-Cultural Perspectives*, pp. 441–473, Berkeley, CA: University of California Press.

Daviss, Betty-Anne (1999) 'From social movement to professional project: are we throwing the baby out with the bath water?', Philippines Proceedings, paper presented at the International Confederation of Midwives, Philippines.

Daviss, Betty-Anne (2001) 'Reforming birth and (re)making midwifery in North America', in Raymond DeVries, Cecilia Benoit, Edwin R. van Teijlingen and Sirpa Wrede (eds) *Birth by Design: Pregnancy, Maternity Care, and Midwifery in North America and Europe*, pp. 70–86, New York and London: Routledge.

Debold, Elizabeth, Tolman, Deborah, and Brown, Lyn Mikel (1996) 'Embodying knowledge, knowing desire: authority and split subjectivities in girls' epistemological development', in Nancy Goldberger, Jill Tarule, Blythe Clinchy and Mary Belenky (eds) *Knowledge, Difference, and Power: Essays Inspired by Women's Ways of Knowing*, pp. 85–125, New York: Basic Books.

Declercq, Eugene R. (1994) 'A cross-national analysis of midwifery politics: six lessons for midwives', *Midwifery*, 10: 232–237.

Declercq, Eugene, DeVries, Raymond, Viisainen, Kirsi, Salvesen, Helga B., and Wrede, Sirpa (2001) 'Where to give birth? Politics and the place of birth', in Raymond DeVries, Cecilia Benoit, Edwin R. van Teijlingen and Sirpa Wrede (eds) *Birth by Design: Pregnancy, Maternity Care and Midwifery in North America and Europe*, pp. 7–27, New York and London: Routledge.

Delphy, Christine (1996) '"French feminism": an imperialist invention', in Diane Bell and Renate Klein (eds) *Radically Speaking: Feminism Reclaimed*, pp. 383–392, London: Zed Books.

Denzin, Norman K., and Lincoln, Yvonna S. (eds) (1994) *Handbook of Qualitative Research*. Thousand Oaks, CA: Sage.

Department of Health (DoH) (1993) *Changing Childbirth: Report of the Expert Maternity Group Part 1*, London: HMSO.

DeVault, Marjorie (1990) 'Talking and listening from women's standpoint: feminist strategies for interviewing and analysis', *Social Problems*, 37(1): 96–116.

DeVault, Marjorie (1994) 'Speaking up, carefully', *Writing Sociology*, 2(2): 1–3.

DeVries, Raymond G. (1989) 'Caregivers in pregnancy and childbirth', in Iain Chalmers, Murray Enkin and Marc J.N.C. Keirse (eds) *Effective Care in Pregnancy and Birth*, pp. 143–161, Oxford: Oxford University Press.

DeVries, Raymond, Benoit, Cecilia, van Teijlingen, Edwin R., and Wrede, Sirpa (eds) (2001) *Birth by Design: Pregnancy, Maternity Care, and Midwifery in North America and Europe*, New York and London: Routledge.

Dickens, Charles (1844/1998) *Martin Chuzzlewit*, Oxford: Oxford University Press.

Dickersin, Kay, Scherer, Roberta, and Lefebure, Carol (1994) 'Identifying relevant studies for systematic reviews', *British Medical Journal*, 309: 1286–1291.

Diprose, Rosalyn (1994) *The Bodies of Women: Ethics, Embodiment and Sexual Difference*, London and New York: Routledge.

Di Stefano, Christine (1990) 'Dilemmas of difference: feminism, modernity, and postmodernism', in Linda Nicholson (ed.) *Feminism/Postmodernism*, pp. 63–82, New York and London: Routledge.

Dolan, Bridget, and Parker, Camilla (1997) 'Caesarean section: a treatment for mental disorder?', *British Medical Journal*, 314: 1183–1187.

Donnison, Jean (1988) *Midwives and Medical Men: A History of the Struggle for the Control of Childbirth*, 2nd edn, New Barnet, UK: Historical Publications.

Doran, C. (1989) 'Jumping frames: reflexivity and recursion in the sociology of science', in *Social Studies of Science*, pp. 515–531, London: Sage.

Douglas, Mary (1966) *Purity and Danger: An Analysis of the Concepts of Pollution and Taboo*, London: Routledge and Kegan Paul.

Douglas, Mary (1992) *Risk and Blame*, New York: Routledge.

Downe, Soo (2004) *Normal Childbirth: Evidence and Debate*. Edinburgh: Churchill Livingstone.

Downe, Soo, and McCourt, Christine (2004) 'From being to becoming: reconstructing childbirth knowledges', in Soo Downe (ed.) *Normal Childbirth: Evidence and Debate*, pp. 3–24, Edinburgh: Churchill Livingstone.

Downe, Soo, McCormick, Carol, and Beech, Beverley Lawrence (2001) 'Labour interventions associated with normal birth', *British Journal of Midwifery*, 9(10): 602–606.

Duden, Barbara (1993) *Disembodying Women: Perspectives on Pregnancy and the Unborn*, Cambridge, MA: Harvard University Press.

Durrand, A.M. (1992) 'The safety of home birth: the Farm study', *American Journal of Public Health*, 82: 450–453.

Durward, Lyn, and Evans, Ruth (1990) 'Pressure groups and maternity care', in Jo Garcia, Robert Kilpatrick and Martin Richards (eds) *The Politics of Maternity Care: Services for Childbearing Women in Twentieth-Century Britain*, pp. 256–273, Oxford: Clarendon Press.

Edwards, Nadine (1994) 'Policies for homebirth in Scotland', *AIMS Journal*, 6(3): 13.

Edwards, Nadine (1996) 'Women's decision-making around home birth', *AIMS Journal*, 8(4): 8–10.

Edwards, Nadine (1998) 'Getting to know midwives', *MIDIRS Midwifery Digest*, 8(2): 160–163.

Edwards, Nadine Pilley (2000) 'Women planning home births: their own views on their relationships with midwives', in Mavis Kirkham (ed.) *The Midwife–Mother Relationship*, pp. 55–91, London: Macmillan.

Edwards, Nadine Pilley (2001) 'Women's experiences of planning home births in Scotland: birthing autonomy', unpublished PhD thesis, University of Sheffield.

Edwards, Nadine (2004a) 'Protection – regulations and standards: enabling or disabling?' Part 1 *Midwives*, 7(3): 116–119.

Edwards, Nadine (2004b) 'Protection – regulations and standards: enabling or disabling?' Part 2 *Midwives*, 7(4): 160–163.

Edwards, Nadine Pilley (2004c) 'Why can't women just say no? And does it really matter?', in Mavis Kirkam (ed.) *Informed Choice in Maternity Care*, pp. 1–29, Basingstoke: Palgrave Macmillan.

Ehrenreich, Barbara, and English, Deirdre (1973) *Witches, Midwives and Nurses: A History of Women Healers*, London: Writers and Readers Publishing Cooperative.

Ehrlich, Susan (1995) 'Critical linguistics in feminist methodology', in Sandra Burt and Lorraine Code (eds) *Changing Methods: Feminists Transforming Practice*, pp. 45–73, Peterborough, UK: Broadview Press.

Eichler, Margrit (1988) *Nonsexist Research Methods: A Practical Guide*, London: Allen & Unwin.

Eisenstein, Zillah (1989) *The Female Body and the Law*, Berkeley: University of California Press.

England, Pam, and Horowitz, Rob (1998) *Birthing from Within*, Albuquerque, NM: Partera Press.

English National Board for Nursing, Midwifery and Health Visiting (ENB) (1999) *Midwifery Practice: Identifying the Developments and the Difference. An Outlook Report Arising from the Audit of Maternity Services and Practice Visits Undertaken by Midwifery Officers of the Board*, English National Board.

Enkin, Murray (1994) 'Risk in pregnancy: the reality, the perception and the concept', *Birth*, 21(3): 131–134.

Enkin, Murray, Keirse, Marc. J.N.C., and Chalmers, Iain (1989) *A Guide to Effective Care in Pregnancy and Childbirth*, Oxford: Oxford University Press.

Eskes, Martine, and van Alten, Dirk (1994) 'Review and assessment of maternity services in the Netherlands', in Geoffrey Chamberlain and Naren Patel (eds) *The Future of Maternity Services*, pp. 36–46, London: RCOG Press.

Evans, Frances (1985) 'Managers and labourers: women's attitudes to reproductive technology', in Wendy Faulkner and Erik Arnold (eds) *Smothered by Invention: Technology in Women's Lives*, pp. 109–127, London: Pluto Press.

Evans, F. (1987) *The Newcastle Community Midwifery Care Project: An Evaluation Report*, Newcastle upon Tyne: Newcastle Health Authority.

Evenden, Doreen (1993) 'Mothers and their midwives in seventeenth-century London', in Hilary Marland (ed.) *The Art of Midwifery*, pp. 9–26, London and New York: Routledge.

Expert Working Group on Acute Maternity Services (2003) *Implementing a Framework for Maternity Services in Scotland: Report of the Expert Group on Acute Maternity Services*, Edinburgh: NHS Scotland.

Featherstone, Mike, Hepworth, Mike, and Turner, Bryan S. (eds) (1991) *The Body: Social Process and Cultural Theory*, London: Sage.

Field, Peggy Ann, Marck, Patricia Beryl, Anderson, Gwen, and McGreary, Karen (1994) 'Introduction', In Peggy Ann Field and Patricia Beryl Marck (eds) *Uncertain Motherhood: Negotiating the Risks of the Childbearing Years*, pp. 10–15, Thousand Oaks, CA: Sage.

Fielder, Anna, Kirkham, Mavis, Baker, Kirsten, and Sherridan, Angela (2004) 'Trapped by thinking in opposites', *Midwifery Matters*, 102: 6–9.

Filippini, Nadia Maria (1993) 'The Church, the state and childbirth: the midwife in Italy during the eighteenth century', in Hilary Marland (ed.) *The Art of Midwifery*, pp. 152–175, London and New York: Routledge.

Finch, Janet (1984) 'It's great to have someone to talk to: the ethics and politics of interviewing women', in Colin Bell and Helen Roberts (eds) *Social Researching: Politics, Problems, Practice*, pp. 70–87, London, Boston, Melbourne Henley: Routledge.

Fine, Michelle (ed.) (1992) *Disruptive Voices: The Possibilities of Feminist Research*, Ann Arbor, MI: University of Michigan Press.

Fine, Michelle, and Gordon, Susan Merle (1992) 'Feminist transformations of/despite psychology', in Michelle Fine (ed.) *Disruptive Voices: The Possibilities of Feminist Research*, pp. 1–25, Ann Arbor, MI: University of Michigan Press.

Fine, Michelle, and Macpherson, Pat (1992) 'Over dinner: feminism and adolescent female bodies', in Michelle Fine (ed.) *Disruptive Voices: The Possibilities of Feminist Research*, pp. 175–203, Ann Arbor, MI: University of Michigan Press.

Flax, Jane (1990) 'Postmodernism and gender relations in feminist theory', in Linda J. Nicholson (ed.) *Feminism/Postmodernism*, pp. 39–62, New York and London: Routledge.

Fleissig, A. and Kroll, D. (1997) 'Achieving continuity of care and carers', *Modern Midwives*, 7(8): 15–19.

Fleming, Valerie E.M. (1994) 'Partnership, power and politics: feminist perceptions of midwifery practice', unpublished PhD thesis, Massey University, New Zealand.

Fleming, Valerie E.M. (1996) 'Midwifery in New Zealand: responding to changing times', *Health Care for Women International*, 17: 343–359.

Fleming, Valerie E.M. (1998) 'Women-with-midwives-with-women: a model of interdependence', *Midwifery*, 14: 137–143.

Flint, Caroline (1991) 'Continuity of care provided by a team of midwives: the Know Your Midwife Scheme', in Sarah Robinson and Ann M. Thomson (eds) *Midwives, Research and Childbirth vol. 2*, pp. 72–103, London: Chapman and Hall.

Ford, C., Iliffe, S., and Owen, F. (1991) 'Outcome of planned homebirths in an inner city practice', *British Medical Journal*, 303: 1517–1519.

Foucault, Michel (1972) *The Archaeology of Knowledge*, trans. A. Sheridan, London: Tavistock.

Foucault, Michel (1977) *Discipline and Punish: The Birth of the Prison*, New York: Pantheon and London: Allen Lane.

Foucault, Michel (1980) *Power/Knowledge: Selected Interviews and Other Writings 1972–1977*, ed. Colin Gordon, Brighton: Harvester Press.

Frankenberg, Ronald (1992) '"Your time or mine": temporal contradictions of biomedical practice', in Ronald Frankenberg (ed.) *Time, Health and Medicine*, pp. 1–30, London: Sage.

Fraser, Nancy (1992a) 'Introduction', in Nancy Fraser and Sandra Lee Bartky (eds) *Revaluing French Feminism: Critical Essays on Difference, Agency, and Culture*, pp. 1–24, Bloomington, IN: Indiana University Press.

Fraser, Nancy (1992b) 'The uses and abuses of French discourse theories for feminist politics', in Sandra Lee Bartky and Nancy Fraser (eds) *Revaluing French Feminism: Critical Essays on Difference, Agency, and Culture*, pp. 177–194, Bloomington, IN: Indiana University Press.

Fraser, Nancy (1995) 'False antitheses: a response to Seyla Benhabib and Judith Butler', in Selya Benhabib, Judith Butler, Drucilla Cornell and Nancy Fraser (eds) *Feminist Contentions: A Philosophical Exchange*, pp. 59–74, New York and London: Routledge.

Fraser, Nancy, and Nicholson, Linda (1990) 'Social criticism without philosophy: an encounter between feminism and postmodernism', in Linda Nicholson (ed.) *Feminism/Postmodernism*, pp. 19–38, New York and London: Routledge.

Freire, Paulo (1972) *The Pedagogy of the Oppressed*, Harmondsworth: Penguin.

Friedman, Marilyn (2000) 'Autonomy, social disruption, and women', in Catriona Mackenzie and Natalie Stoljar (eds) *Relational Autonomy: Feminist Perspectives on Autonomy, Agency, and the Social Self*, pp. 35–51, New York and Oxford: Oxford University Press.

Furedi, Frank (1997) *Culture of Fear: Risk-taking and the Morality of Low Expectations*, London: Cassell.

Gardner, Jenny (2004) 'Jenny's story', *Birth and Beyond*, 21: 2–3, 40 Leamington Terrace, Edinburgh, EH10 4JL.

Gaskin, Ina May (1990) *Spiritual Midwifery*, Summertown, TN: Book Publishing Company.

Gaskin, Ina May (2003) *Ina May's Guide to Childbirth*, New York: Random House.

Gatens, Moira (1996) *Imaginary Bodies: Ethics Power and Corporeality*, London and New York: Routledge.

Gelbart, Nina (1993) 'Midwife to a nation: Mme Coudray serves France', in Hilary Marland (ed.) *The Art of Midwifery*, pp. 131–151, London and New York: Routledge.

Giddens, Anthony (1991). *The Consequences of Modernity*, Cambride: Polity Press.

Gilligan, Carol (1985) *In a Different Voice: Psychological Theory and Women's Development*, Cambridge, MA: Harvard University Press.

Glucksmann, Miriam (1994) 'The work of knowledge and the knowledge of women's work', in Mary Maynard and June Purvis (eds) *Researching Women's Lives from a Feminist Perspective*, pp. 149–165, London: Taylor and Francis.

Goddard, Ros (2001) 'Electronic fetal monitoring', *British Medical Journal*, 322: 1436–1437.

Goer, Henci (1999) *The Thinking Woman's Guide to a Better Birth*, New York: Perigree.

Goldbeck-Wood, Sandra (1997) 'Women's autonomy in childbirth', *British Medical Journal*, 314 (19 April): 1143.

Goldberger, Nancy Rule (1996) 'Cultural imperatives and diversity in ways of knowing', in Nancy Goldberger, Jill Tarule, Blythe Clinchy and Mary Belenky (eds) *Knowledge, Power, and Difference: Essays Inspired By Women's Ways of Knowing*, pp. 335–364, New York: Basic Books.

Coldberger, Nancy, Tarule, Jill, Clinchy, blythe, and Belenky, Mary (eds) (1996) *Knowledge, Power, and Difference: Essays Inspired by Women's Ways of Knowing*, New York: Basic Books.

Green, Jenny (1999) 'With woman', *Midwifery Matters*, 83: 8.

Green, Josephine, M., Curtis, Penny, Price, Helene, and Renfrew, Mary J. (1998a) *Continuing to Care: The Organization of Midwifery Services in the UK – a Structured Review of the Evidence*, Hale, Cheshire: Books for Midwives.

Green, Josephine, M., Coupland, Vanessa A., and Kitzinger, Jenny, V. (1998b) *Great Expectations: A Prospective Study of Women's Expectations and Experience of Childbirth*, 2nd edn, Hale, Cheshire: Books for Midwives.

Greenwood, Susan (1996) 'Feminist witchcraft: a transformatory politics', in Nickie Charles and Felicia Hughes-Freeland (eds) *Practising Feminism: Identity, Difference, Power*, pp. 109–134, London and New York: Routledge.

Gregg, Robin (1995) *Pregnancy in a High-Tech Age: Paradoxes of Choice*, New York and London: New York University Press.

Grieder, William (1992) 'Who will tell the people?', p. 54, New York: Simon and Schuster.

Griffiths, Morwenna (1995) *Feminisms and the Self: The Web of Identity*, London and New York: Routledge.

Grosz, Elizabeth (1993) 'Bodies and knowledge: feminism and the crisis of reason', in Linda Alcoff and Elizabeth Potter (eds) *Feminist Epistemologies*, pp. 187–215, New York and London: Routledge.

Guilliland, Karen, and Pairman, Sally (1995) *The Midwifery Partnership: A Model for Practice*, Wellington, NZ: Department of Nursing and Midwifery, Victoria University of Wellington.

Gyte, Gill (1994) 'Evaluation of the meta-analysis on the effects on both mother and baby, of the various components of "active management" of the third stage of labour', *Midwifery*, 10: 183–199.

Hadikin, Ruth, and O'Driscoll, Muriel (2000) *The Bullying Culture: Cause, Effect, Harm Reduction*, Oxford: Books for Midwives.

Hall, Jennifer (1999) 'Home birth: the midwife effect', *British Journal of Midwifery*, 7(4): 225–227.

Hall, Jenny, and Taylor, Meg (2004) 'Birth and spirituality', in Soo Downe (ed.) *Normal Childbirth: Evidence and Debate*, pp. 41–56, Edinburgh: Churchill Livingstone.

Halldorsdottir, Sigridur (1996) *Caring and Uncaring Encounters in Nursing and Health Care: Developing a Theory*, Linköping, Sweden: Department of Caring Sciences, Faculty of Health Sciences, Linköping University.

Halldorsdottir, Sigridur, and Karlsdottir, Sigfridur Inga (1996) 'Journeying through labour and delivery: perceptions of women who have given birth', *Midwifery*, 12: 48–61.

Haloob, R., and Thein, A. (1992) 'Born before arrival: a five year retrospective controlled study', *Journal of Obstetrics and Gynaecology*, 12: 100–104.

Hamer, Mary (1999) 'Listen to the voice: an interview with Carol Gilligan', *Women: A Cultural Review*, 10(2): 173–184.

Haraway, Donna (1988) 'Situated knowledges: the science question in feminism and the privilege of partial perspective', *Feminist Studies*, 14(3): 575–599.

Harding, Jennifer (1997) 'Bodies at risk: sex, surveillance and hormone replacement therapy', in Robin Brunton and Alan Petersen (eds) *Foucault, Health and Medicine*, pp. 134–149, London and New York: Routledge.

Harding, Sandra (1987) 'Is there feminist method?', in Sandra Harding (ed.) *Feminism and Methodology*, pp. 1–14, Milton Keynes: Open University Press and Bloomington, IN: Indiana University Press.

Harding, Sandra (1993) 'Rethinking standpoint epistemology: "What is strong objectivity?"', in Linda Alcoff and Elizabeth Potter (eds) *Feminist Epistemologies*, pp. 49–82, New York and London: Routledge.

Harding, Sandra (1996) 'Gendered ways of knowing and the "epistemological crisis" of the West', in Nancy Goldberger, Jill Tarule, Blythe Clinchy and Mary Belenky (eds) *Knowledge, Power, and Difference: Essays Inspired by Women's Ways of Knowing*, pp. 431–454, New York: Basic Books.

Harley, David (1993) 'Provincial midwives in England: Lancashire and Cheshire, 1660–1760', in Hilary Marland (ed.) *The Art of Midwifery*, pp. 27–48, London and New York: Routledge.

Hartsock, Nancy (1990) 'Foucault on power: a theory for women?', in Linda J. Nicholson (ed.) *Feminism/Postmodernism*, pp. 157–175, New York and London: Routledge.

Heagarty, Brooke V. (1997) 'Willing handmaidens of science? The struggle over the new midwife in early 20th century England', in Mavis J. Kirkham and Elizabeth R. Perkins (eds) *Reflections on Midwifery*, pp. 70–95, London: Balliere Tindall.

Health Education Board for Scotland (HEBS) (1998) *Ready Steady Baby: A Guide to Pregnancy, Birth and Early Parenthood*, Edinburgh: HEBS.

Health Policy and Public Health Directorate (1993) *Provision of Maternity Services in Britain: A Policy Review*, Scottish Home and Health Department: HMSO.

Hess, Ann Giardina (1993) 'Midwifery practice among the Quakers in southern rural England in the late seventeenth century', in Hilary Marland (ed.) *The Art of Midwifery*, pp. 49–76, London and New York: Routledge.

Hewson, Barbara (1994) 'Court-ordered caesarean: ethical triumph or surgical rape?', *AIMS Journal*, 6(2): 1–5.

Hewson, Barbara (2004) 'Is it murder to refuse a caesarean?' *AIMS Quarterly Journal*, 16(1).

Hodnett, Ellen D. (1989) 'Personal control and the birth environment: comparisons between home and hospital settings', *Journal of Environmental Psychology*, 9: 207–216.

Hodnett, E.D., Gates, S., Hofmeyr, G.J., and Sakala, C. (2004) 'Continuous support for women during childbirth', *The Cochrane Library, Issue 4*, Chichester: Wiley.

Hoff, Joan (1996) 'The pernicious effect of post-structuralism on women's history', in Diane Bell and Renate Klein (eds) *Radically Speaking: Feminism Reclaimed*, pp. 393–412, London: Zed Books.

Hogg, Christine (1999) *Patients, Power and Politics: From Patients to Citizens*, London: Sage Publications.

Holmwood, John (1995) 'Feminism and epistemology: what kind of successor science', *Sociology*, 29(3): 411–428.

hooks, bell (1990) *Yearning: Race, Gender and Cultural Politics*, Boston, MA: South End.

House of Commons (Health Committee) (1992) *Maternity Services Second Report Volume 1*, London: HMSO.

House of Commons (Social Services Committee) (1980) *Perinatal and Neonatal Mortality: Second Report from the Social Services Committee 1979–1980*, London: HMSO.

Howe, K.A. (1988) 'Home births in south-west Australia', *Medical Journal of Australia*, 149: 296–302.

Howson, Alexandra (1995) *The Female Body and Health Surveillance: Cervical Screening and the Social Production of Risk*, Edinburgh: Department of Sociology, University of Edinburgh.

Hundley, Vanora (2000) Paper given at the 8th International Conference of Care Researches, 6–8 September, Glasgow.

Hunt, Linda M., Jordan, Brigitte, Irwin, Susan, and Browner, C.H. (1989) 'Compliance and the patient's perspective', *Culture, Medicine and Psychiatry*, 13: 315–334.

Hunt, Sheila C., and Symonds, Andrea (1995) *The Social Meaning of Midwifery*, London: Macmillan.

Hutchinson, Sally A. (1990) 'Responsible subversion: a study of rule-bending among nurses', *Scholarly Inquiry for Nursing Practice*, 4(1): 3–17.

Illich, Ivan (1976) *Limits to Medicine: Medical Nemesis – The Expropriation of Health*, London and New York: Boyars.

Inch, Sally (1984) *Birthrights: A Parents' Guide to Modern Childbirth*, New York: Pantheon.

Inter-Departmental Committee (1904) *Report of the Inter-Departmental Committee on Physical Deterioration*, London: HMSO.

Irigaray, Luce (1985) *This Sex Which is Not One*, trans. C Porter, Ithaca, NY: Cornell University Press.

Jacobson, Bertil (1988) 'Obstetric pain medication and eventual amphetamine addiction in offspring', *Acta Obstetrica et Gynaecologica Scandinavica*, 67: 677–682.

Jacobson, Bertil, and Bygdeman, Marc (1998) 'Obstetric care and proneness of offspring to suicide as adults: case-control study', *British Medical Journal*, 317: 1346–1349.

Jacobson, Bertil, Nyberg, K., Gronbladh, L., Eklund, G., Bygdeman, M., and Rydberg, U. (1990) 'Opiate addiction in adult offspring through possible imprinting after obstetric treatment', *British Medical Journal*, 301: 1067–1070.

Jacoby, Ann, and Cartwright, Ann (1990) 'Finding out about the views and experiences of maternity-services users', in Jo Garcia, Robert Kilpatrick and Martin Richards (eds) *The Politics of Maternity Care: Services for Childbearing Women in Twentieth-Century Britain*, pp. 238–255, Oxford: Clarendon Press.

Jencks, Charles (1995) 'The origins of "postmodernism"', in Chris Garratt and Richard Appignanesi, *Postmodernism for Beginners*, Cambridge: Icon Books.

Jewell, David, Young, Gavin, and Zander, Luke (1992) *The Case for Community-Based Maternity Care*, 2nd edn. Available from Association for Community-Based Maternity Care, Barn Croft Surgery, Temple Sowerby, Penrith, Cumbria CA10 1RZ.

Johnson, K.C. (1997) 'Randomized controlled trials as authoritative knowledge: keeping an ally from becoming a threat to North American midwifery practice', in Robbie E. Davis-Floyd and Carolyn F. Sargent (eds) *Childbirth and Authoritative Knowledge: Cross-Cultural Perspectives*, pp. 350–365, Berkeley, CA: University of California Press.

Jones, Lyn (1991) *Maternity Services in Angus: A Survey of Mother's Opinions (Summary Report)*, Dundee: Tayside Health Board.

Jones, M.H., Barik, S., Mangune, H.H., Jones, P., Gregory, S.J., and Spring, J.E. (1998) 'Do birth plans adversely affect the outcome of labour', *British Journal of Midwifery*, 6(1): 38–41.

Jordan, Brigitte (1977) 'The self-diagnosis of early pregnancy: an investigation of lay competence', *Medical Anthropology*, 1(2): 20–35.

Jordan, Brigitte (1993) *Birth in Four Cultures: A Cross-cultural Investigation of Childbirth in Yucatan, Holland, Sweden and the United States*, 4th edn, Prospect Heights, IL: Waveland Press.

Jordan, Brigitte (1997) 'Authoritative knowledge and its construction', in Robbie E. Davis-Floyd and Carolyn F. Sargent (eds) *Childbirth and Authoritative Knowledge: Cross-Cultural Perspectives*, pp. 50–79, Berkeley, CA: University of California Press.

Kahn, Robbie Pfeufer (1996) *Bearing Meaning: The Language of Birth*, Urbana, IL: University of Illinois Press.

Kaufmann, Tara (2004) 'Introducing feminism', in Mary Stewart (ed.) *Pregnancy, Birth and Maternity Care: Feminist Perspectives*, pp. 1–10, Edinburgh: Books for Midwives.

Kennedy, Patricia (1998) 'Between the lines: mother and infant care in Ireland', in Patricia Kennedy and Jo Murphy-Lawless (eds) *Returning Birth to Women: Challenging Policies and Practices*, pp. 10–16, Dublin: Centre for Women's Studies, TCD/WERRC.

Kennedy, Patricia, and Murphy-Lawless, Jo (1998) 'Risk and safety in childbirth: who should decide', in Patricia Kennedy and Jo Murphy-Lawless (eds) *Returning Birth to Women: Challenging Policies and Practices*, pp. 2–9, Dublin: Centre for Women's Studies, TDC/WERRC.

King, Helen (1993) 'The politick midwife: models of midwifery in the work of Elizabeth Cellier', in Hilary Marland (ed.) *The Art of Midwifery*, pp. 115–130, London and New York: Routledge.

Kirby, Sandra L., and McKenna, Kate (1989*) Experience, Research, Social Change: Methods from the Margins*, Toronto: Garamond Press.

Kirkham, Mavis (1989) 'Midwives and information-giving during labour', in Sarah Robinson and Anne M. Thompson (eds) *Midwives, Research and Childbirth*, pp. 117–138, London: Chapman and Hall.

Kirkham, Mavis (1996) 'Professionalisation past and present: with women or with the powers that be?', in Debra Kroll (ed*.) Midwifery Care for the Future*, London: Bailliere Tindall.

Kirkham, Mavis (1999a) 'Bodily knowledge: the wisdom of nausea', *Midwifery Today*, 51: 15–16.

Kirkham, Mavis (1999b) 'The culture of midwifery in the National Health Service in England', *Journal of Advanced Nursing*, 30(3): 732–739.

Kirkham, Mavis (2000) 'How can we relate', in Mavis Kirkham (ed.) *The Midwife–Mother Relationship*, pp. 227–254, London: Macmillan.

Kirkham, Mavis (2003) *Birth Centres: A Social Model for Maternity Care*, Oxford: Butterworth-Heinemann.

Kirkham, Mavis (ed.) (2004) *Informed Choice in Maternity Care*, Basingstoke: Palgrave Macmillan.

Kirkham, Mavis, and Stapleton, Helen (2001) *Informed Choice in Maternity Care: An Evaluation of Evidence Based Leaflets*, Women's Informed Childbearing and Health Research Group, School of Nursing and Midwifery, University of Sheffield, and NHS Centre for Reviews and Dissemination, University of York.

Kirkham, Mavis, and Stapleton, Helen (2004) 'The culture of the maternity services in Wales and England as a barrier to informed choice', in Mavis Kirkham (ed.) *Informed Choice in Maternity Care*, Basingstoke: Palgrave Macmillan.

Kitzinger, Jenny (1990) 'Strategies of the early childbirth movement: a case-study of the National Childbirth Trust', in Jo Garcia, Robert Kilpatrick and Martin Richards (eds) *The Politics of Maternity Care: Services for Childbearing Women in Twentieth-Century Britain*, pp. 61–91, Oxford: Clarendon Press.

Kitzinger, Jenny (1992) 'Counteracting, not re-enacting, the violation of women's bodies: the challenge for perinatal caregivers', *Birth*, 19(4): 219–220.

Kitzinger, Sheila (1992) 'Birth and violence against women: generating hypotheses from women's accounts of unhappiness after childbirth', in Helen Roberts (ed.) *Women's Health Matters*, London: Routledge.

Kitzinger, Sheila (2000) *Rediscovering Birth*, Boston, MA: Little, Brown.

Kloosterman, G.J. (1984) 'The Dutch experience of domiciliary confinements', in Luke G. Zander and Geoffrey Chamberlain (eds) *Pregnancy Care for the 1980's*, London: Royal Society of Medicine and Macmillan Press.

Knipschild, P. (1994) 'Systematic reviews: some examples', *British Medical Journal*, 309: 719–721.

Knorr-Cetina, K.D. and Mulkay, M. (1983) 'Emerging principles in social studies', in K.D. Knorr-Cetina and M. Mulkay (eds) *Science Observed*, pp. 1–17, London: Sage.

Kuhn, Thomas S. (1970) *The Structure of Scientific Revolutions*, 2nd edn, Chicago: University of Chicago Press.

Lane, Karen (1993) 'The politics of home birth', in M. Mills (ed.) *Prevention, Health and British Politics*, Aldershot: Avebury.

Lane, Karen (1995) 'The medical model of the body as a site of risk: a case study of childbirth', in Jonathon Gabe (ed.) *Medicine Health and Risk: Sociological Approaches*, pp. 53–72, Oxford: Blackwell.

Lawson, Elaine (2000–2001) 'Diabetic birth without the drip', *AIMS Journal*, 12(4): 10–12.

Lazarus, Ellen (1997) 'What do women want? Issues of choice, control, and class in American pregnancy and childbirth', in Robbie E. Davis-Floyd and Carolyn F. Sargent (eds) *Childbirth and Authoritative Knowledge: Cross-Cultural Perspectives*, pp. 132–158, Berkeley, CA: University of California Press.

Leap, Nicky (1996) 'A midwifery perspective of pain in labour', MSc thesis, South Bank University, London.

Leap, Nicky (1997) 'Making sense of "horizontal violence" in midwifery', *British Journal of Midwifery*, 5(11): 689.

Leap, Nicky (2000) 'The less we do, the more we give', in Mavis Kirkham (ed.) *The Midwife–Mother Relationship*, pp. 1–18, London: Macmillan.

Leap, Nicky, and Anderson, T. (2004) 'The role of pain in normal birth and the empowerment of women', in Soo Downe (ed.) *Normal Childbirth: Evidence and Debate*, pp. 25–39, Edinburgh: Churchill Livingstone.

Leap, Nicky, and Hunter, Billie (1993) *The Midwife's Tale: An Oral History from Handywoman to Professional Midwife*, London: Scarlet Press.

Leatherbarrow, B., Winter, P., Macleod, L., Nicoll, A., McNicol, K., and Hoggins, K. (2004) 'From vision to reality: the development of a community maternity unit', *RCM Midwives Journal*, 7(5): 212–515.

Leboyer, Frederick (1977) *Birth without Violence*, London: Fontana.

Leder, Drew (1990) *The Absent Body*, Chicago: University of Chicago Press.

Lee, Gay (1997) 'The concept of "continuity": what does it mean?', in Mavis J. Kirkham and Elizabeth R. Perkins (eds) *Reflections on Midwifery*, pp. 1–25, London: Bailliere Tindall.

Lemay, Celine (1997) 'L'accouchement à la maison au Quebec: les voix du dedans', unpublished MSc thesis, University of Montreal.

Levy, Valerie (1998) 'Facilitating and making informed choices during pregnancy: a study of midwives and pregnant women', unpublished PhD thesis, University of Sheffield.

Levy, Valerie (1999a) 'Midwives, informed choice and power: part 1', *British Journal of Midwifery*, 7(9): 583–586.

Levy, Valerie (1999b) 'Protective steering: a grounded theory study of the processes by which midwives facilitate informed choices during pregnancy', *Journal of Advanced Nursing*, 29(1): 104–112.

Lewis, Jane (1990) 'Mothers and maternity policies in the twentieth century', in Jo Garcia, Robert Kilpatrick and Martin Richards (eds) *The Politics of Maternity Care: Services for Childbearing Women in Twentieth Century Britain*, pp. 15–29, Oxford: Clarendon Press.

Leyshon, Lynne (2004) 'Integrating caseloads across a whole service: the Torbay model', *MIDIRS 14*, Supplement 1, pp. S9–S11.

Lincoln, Marisa (2004) 'Changing childbirth and maternity services in Scotland', *AIMS Quarterly Journal*, 16(1): pp. 18–20.

Lindemann, Mary (1993) 'Professionals? Sisters? Rivals? Midwives in Braunschweig, 1750–1800', in Hilary Marland (ed.) *The Art of Midwifery*, pp. 176–191, London and New York: Routledge.

Longino, Helen (1993) 'Subjects, power and knowledge: description and prescription in feminist philosophies of science', in Linda Alcoff and Elizabeth Potter (eds) *Feminist Epistemologies*, pp. 101–120, New York and London: Routledge.

Lorde, Audre (1984) 'The master's tools will never dismantle the master's house', in Audre Lorde, *Sister/Outsider*, pp. 110–113, Freedom, CA: Crossing Press.

Lorde, Audre (1997) 'Uses of the erotic: the erotic as power', in Katie Conboy, Nadia Medina and Sarah Stanbury (eds) *Writing on the Body: Female Embodiment and Feminist Theory*, pp. 277–282, New York: Columbia University Press.

Lukes, Steven (1974) *Power: A Radical View*, London: Macmillan.

Lupton, Deborah (1997) 'Foucault and the medicalisation critique', in Alan Petersen and Robin Brunton (eds) *Foucault, Health and Medicine*, pp. 94–110, London and New York: Routledge.

Lyons, Suzanne (1998) 'Post-traumatic stress disorder following childbirth: causes, prevention and treatment, in Sarah Clement (ed.) *Psychological Perspectives on Pregnancy and Childbirth*, pp. 123–143, Edinburgh, London, New York, Philadelphia, San Francisco, Sydney, Toronto: Churchill Livingstone.

McAdam-O'Connell, Bridget (1998) 'Risk, responsibility and choice: the medical model of birth and alternatives', in Patricia Kennedy and Jo Murphy-Lawless (eds) *Returning Birth to Women: Challenging Policies and Practices*, pp. 21–29, Dublin: Centre for Women's Studies, TCD/WERRC.

MacArthur, Christine, Lewis, Margo, and Knox, George (1991) *Health after Childbirth*, London: HMSO.

McCourt, Christine (1998) 'Update on the future of one-to-one midwifery', *MIDIRS Midwifery Digest*, 8(1): 7–10.

McCourt, Christine, and Page, Lesley (1997) *One to One Midwifery Practice: Report on the Evaluation of One-to-One Midwifery*, Slough and London: Thames Valley University and The Hammersmith Hospital NHS Trust London.

McCrea, B. Hally, Wright, Marion E., and Murphy-Black, Tricia (1998) 'Differences in midwives' approaches to pain relief in labour', *Midwifery*, 14: 174–180.

Macfarlane, Alison (1997) 'Commentary: the safest place for birth – is there a better analysis than meta-analysis?' *Birth*, 24(1): 14–16.

Machin, David, and Scamell, Mandy (1997) 'The experience of labour using ethnography to explore the irresistible nature of the bio-medical metaphor during labour', *Midwifery*, 13, 78–84.

McKay, S. and Barrow, T. (1991) 'Holding back: maternal readiness to give birth', *American Journal of Maternal and Child Nursing*, 16(5): 250–254.

Mackenzie, Catriona (2000) 'Imagining oneself otherwise', in Catriona Mackenzie and Natalie Stoljar (eds) *Relational Autonomy: Feminist Perspectives on Autonomy, Agency, and the Social Self*, pp. 124–150, New York and Oxford: Oxford University Press.

Mackenzie, Catriona, and Stoljar, Natalie (eds) (2000) *Relational Autonomy: Feminist Perspectives on Autonomy, Agency, and the Social Self*, New York and Oxford: Oxford University Press.

McLain, Carol Shepherd (1987) 'Some social network differences between women choosing home and hospital birth', *Human Organisation*, 49(2): 146–152.

McLaren, Jane (1990) 'Defending choices in childbirth', in Shirley Henderson and Alison Mackay (eds) *Grit and Diamonds: Women in Scotland Making History 1980–1990*, pp. 171–174, Edinburgh: Stramullion.

McLennan, G. (1995) 'Feminism, epistemology and postmodernism: reflections on current ambivalence', *Sociology*, 29(2): 391–409.

McLeod, Caroline, and Sherwin, Susan (2000) 'Relational autonomy, self-trust, and health care for patients who are oppressed', in Catriona Mackenzie and Natalie Stoljar (eds) *Relational Autonomy: Feminist Perspective on Autonomy, Agency, and the Social Self*, pp. 259–279, New York and Oxford: Oxford University Press.

McNay, Lois (1992) *Foucault and Feminism: Power, Gender and the Self*, Cambridge: Polity Press.

MacVicar, J., Dobbie, J., Owen-Johnstone, L., Jagger, C., Hopkins, M., and Kennedy, J. (1993) 'Simulated home delivery in hospital: a randomised controlled trial', *British Journal of Obstetrics and Gynaecology*, 100: 316–323.

Madi, Banyana Cecilia, and Crow, Rosemary (2003) 'A qualitative study of information about available options for childbirth venue and pregnant women's preference for a place of delivery', *Midwifery*, 19(4): 328–336.

Mahoney, Emma (2004) 'I'll do it my way: a mother's perspective on giving birth to twins', *Birth and Beyond*, 22: 5–8, available from 40 Leamington Terrace, Edinburgh, EH10 4JL.

Maine, Deborah (1991) *Safe Motherhood Programmes: Options and Issues: Prevention of Maternal Mortality Programme. Centre for Population and Family Health*, New York: Columbia University Press.

Mair, J. Miller M. (1977) 'The community of self', in D. Bannister (ed.) *New Perspectives in Personal Construct Theory*, London: Academic Press.

Mander, Rosemary (1993) 'Who chooses the choices?', *Modern Midwife*, 3(1): 23–25.

Mander, Rosemary (1996) 'The childfree midwife: the significance of personal experience of childbearing', *Midwives*, 109(1302): 186–188.

Mander, Rosemary (1997) 'Choosing the choices in the USA: examples in the maternity area', *Journal of Advanced Nursing*, 25: 1192–1197.

Mander, Rosemary (2001) *Supportive Care and Midwifery*, Malden, MA: Blackwell Science.

Mann, Susan A., and Kelley, Lori R. (1997) 'Standing at the crossroads of modernist thought: Collins, Smith and new feminist epistemologies', *Gender and Society*, 11: 391–408.

Marland, Hilary (1993a) 'The "burgerlijke" midwife: the stadsvroedvrouw of eighteenth-century Holland', in Hilary Marland (ed.) *The Art of Midwifery*, pp. 192–213, London and New York: Routledge.

Marland, Hilary (ed.) (1993b) *The Art of Midwifery: Early Modern Midwives in Europe*, London and New York: Routledge.

Marshall, Helen (1996) 'Our bodies ourselves: why we should add old fashioned empirical phenomenology to the new theories of the body', *Women's Studies International Forum*, 19(3): 253–265.

Martin, Emily (1987) *The Woman in the Body: A Cultural Analysis of Reproduction*, Boston, MA: Beacon Press.

Martin, Emily (1990) 'Science and women's bodies: forms of anthropological knowledge', in Maey Jacobus, Evelyn Fox-Keller and Sally Shuttleworth (eds) *Body Politics: Women and the Discourse of Science*, pp. 69–82, New York and London: Routledge.

Mason, Margaret (1998) 'Hospital-based childbirth education: in whose interests?', in Patricia Kennedy and Jo Murphy-Lawless (eds) *Returning Birth to Women: Challenging Policies and Practices*, pp. 34–40, Dublin: Centre for Women's Studies, TCD/WERRC.

Maternity Services Advisory Committee (1982) *Report to the Secretaries of State for Social Services and for Wales Part I: Antenatal Care*, London: HMSO.

Maternity Services Advisory Committee (1984) *Report to the Secretaries of State for Social Services and for Wales Part II: Care during Childbirth*, London: HMSO.

Maternity Services Advisory Committee (1985) *Report to the Secretaries of State for Social Services and for Wales Part III: Care of the Mother and Baby*, London: HMSO.

Mauthner, Natasha, and Doucet, Andrea (1998) 'Reflections on a voice-centred relational method: analysing maternal and domestic voices', in Jane Ribbens and Rosalind Edwards (eds) *Feminist Dilemmas in Qualitative Research*, pp. 119–146, London: Sage.

Maynard, Mary (1994) 'Methods, practice and epistemology: the debate about feminism and research', in Mary Maynard, and June Purvis (eds) *Researching Women's Lives from a Feminist Perspective*, London: Taylor & Francis.

Maynard, Mary, and Purvis, June (eds) (1994) *Researching Women's Lives from a Feminist Perspective*, London: Taylor & Francis.

Mehl, L.E., Peterson, L.A., and Creevy, G.A. (1976) 'Home birth versus hospital birth: comparisons of outcomes of matched populations', in American Public Health Association Annual Meeting, Miami Beach, Florida.

Mercer, Judith, and Skovgaard, Rebecca (2004) 'Fetal to neonatal transition: first do no harm', in Soo Downe (ed.) *Normal Childbirth: Evidence and Debate*, pp. 141–160, Edinburgh: Churchill Livingstone.

Meyer, Diana T. (1992) 'The subversion of women's agency in psychoanalytic feminism: Chodorow, Flax, Kristeva', in Nancy Fraser and Sandra Lee Bartky (eds) *Revaluing French Feminism: Critical Essays on Difference, Agency, and Culture*, pp. 136–161, Bloomington, IN: Indiana University Press.

Meyer, Diana Tietjens (2000) 'Intersectional identity and the authentic self? Opposites attract!', in Catriona Mackenzie and Natalie Stoljar (eds) *Relational Autonomy: Feminist Perspectives on Autonomy, Agency, and the Social Self*, pp. 151–180, New York and Oxford: Oxford University Press.

Mikhailovich, Katja (1996) 'Post-modernism and its "contribution" to ending violence against women', in Diane Bell and Renate Klein (eds) *Radically Speaking: Feminism Reclaimed*, pp. 339–345, London: Zed Books.

Miller, Tina (1998) 'Shifting layers of professional, lay and personal narratives: longitudinal childbirth research', in Jane Ribbens, and Rosalind Edwards (eds) *Feminist Dilemmas in Qualitative Research*, pp. 58–71, London: Sage.

Ministry of Health (1930) *Interim Report of Departmental Committee on Maternal Mortality and Morbidity*, London: HMSO.

Ministry of Health (1932) *Final Report of Departmental Committee on Maternal Mortality and Morbidity*, London: HMSO.

Ministry of Health (1954) *Report for the Year Ended 31st December: Part II: On the State of the Public Health*, London: HMSO.

Ministry of Health (1956) *Report of the Committee of Enquiry into the Cost of the National Health Service*, London: HMSO.

Ministry of Health (1959) *Report of the Maternity Services Committee*, London: HMSO.

Ministry of Health (1961) *Human Relations in Obstetrics*, London: HMSO.

Ministry of Health (1970) *Domiciliary Midwifery and Maternity Bed Needs: The Report of the Standing Maternity and Midwifery Advisory Committee*, London: HMSO.

Ministry of Health (1979) *Royal Commission on the National Health Service*, London: HMSO.

Morgan, Mandy, and Coombes, Leigh (2001) 'Subjectivities and silences, mother and woman: theorizing an experience of silence as a speaking subject', *Feminism and Psychology*, 11(3): 361–375.

Murphy, J.F., Dauncey, M., Gray, O.P., and Chalmers, I. (1984) 'Planned and unplanned deliveries at home: implications of a changing ratio', *British Medical Journal*, 288: 1429–1432.

Murphy-Black, Tricia (1993) I*dentifying the Key Features of Continuity of Care in Midwifery*, Edinburgh: Department of Nursing Studies, University of Edinburgh.

Murphy-Black, Tricia (1994a) 'The research process: a mind map', *British Journal of Midwifery*, 2(11): 545–548.

Murphy-Black, Tricia (1994b) 'Searching the midwifery literature', *British Journal of Midwifery*, 2(9): 441–443.

Murphy-Lawless, Jo (1991) 'Piggy in the middle: the midwife's role in achieving woman-controlled childbirth', *Irish Journal of Psychology*, 12(2): 198–215.

Murphy-Lawless, Jo (1998a) *Reading Birth and Death: A History of Obstetric Thinking*, Cork: Cork University Press.

Murphy-Lawless, Jo (1998b) 'Women dying in childbirth: "Safe Motherhood in the International Context", in Patricia Kennedy and Jo Murphy-Lawless (eds) *Returning Birth to Women: Challenging Policies and Practices*, pp. 41–55, Dublin: Centre for Women's Studies, TCD/WERRC.

Murphy-Lawless, Jo (2000) 'Reinstating women's time in childbirth', *AIMS Journal*, 12(1): 5–7.

Murphy-Lawless, Jo (2003) 'How will the world be born: the critical importance of indigenous midwifery', *Midwives*, 6(10): 432–436.

Myles, Margaret, F. (1981) *Textbook for Midwives with modern concepts of Obstetric and Neonatal Care*, p.2, Edinburgh: Churchill Livingstone.

Nash, Kate (1994) 'The feminist production of knowledge: is deconstruction a practice for women?', *Feminist Review*, 47: 65–77.

National Childbirth Trust (NCT) (1999) 'Totness the tops', *New Generation*, December; 18–19.

Nelkin, Dorothy (1982) 'Controversy as a political challenge', in B. Barnes and D. Edge (eds) *Science in Context: Readings in the Sociology of Science*, pp. 276–281, Milton Keynes: Open University Press.

Nelson, Lynn H. (1993) 'Epistemological communities', in Linda Alcoff and Elizabeth Potter (eds) *Feminist Epistemologies*, pp. 121–160, New York and London: Routledge.

Nettleton, Sarah (1997) 'Governing the risky self: how to become healthy, wealthy and wise', in Alan Petersen and Robin Bunton (eds) *Foucault, Health and Medicine*, pp. 207–222, London and New York: Routledge.

Nicholson, Linda (1990) *Feminism/Postmodernism*, New York and London: Routledge.

Nicholson, Linda (1999) *The Play of Reason: From the Modern to the Postmodern*, Buckingham: Open University Press.

Nicoll, A. (2004a) 'Keeping MUM: reflections on a campaign to save a maternity unit', *AIMS Journal*, 16(3): 20.

Noble, Carolyn (2001) *Birth Storie*, Charnwood, ACT: Ginninderra Press.

Noddings, Nel (1984) *Caring*, Berkeley, CA: University of California Press.

Northern Regional Perinatal Mortality Survey Coordinating Group (1996) 'Collaborative survey of perinatal loss in planned and unplanned home births', *British Medical Journal*, 313: 1306–1309.

North West Surrey Community Health Council (1992) 'Having your baby at home: a local issue', Available from NW Surrey CHC, St Peter's Hospital, Chertsey, Surrey KT16 0PZ.

Nursing and Midwifery Council (NMC) (2002) 'Practitioner–client relationships and the prevention of abuse', www.nmc-uk.org.

Nursing and Midwifery Council (NMC) (2004) 'Midwives rules and standards', www.nmc-uk.org

Oakley, Ann (1984) *The Captured Womb: A History of the Medical Care of Pregnant Women*, Oxford: Basil Blackwell.

Oakley, Ann (1992) *Social Support and Motherhood*, Oxford and Cambridge, MA: Blackwell.

Oakley, Ann (2000) *Experiments in Knowing: Gender and Method in the Social Sciences*, Cambridge: Polity Press.

Oakley, A., and Houd, Susanne (1990) *Helpers in Childbirth: Midwifery Today*, Basingstoke: Hemisphere.

Oakley, Ann, Hichet, D., Rajan, L., and Rigby, A.S. (1996) 'Social support in pregnancy: does it have long term effects?', *Journal of Reproductive and Infant Psychology*, 14(1): 7–22.

O'Brien, Maureen (1978) 'Home and hospital: a comparison of the experiences of mothers having home and hospital confinements', *General Practitioner Obstetrics 2, Journal of the Royal College of General Practitioners*, 28: 460–466.

O'Connor, Marie (1992) *Women and Birth: A National Study of Intentional Home Births in Ireland*, Dublin: Coombe Lying-in Hospital.

O'Connor, Marie (1998) 'Redefining risk: life, death and home birth', in Patricia Kennedy and Jo Murphy-Lawless (eds) *Returning Birth to Women: Challenging Policies and Practices*, pp. 56–62, Dublin: Centre for Women's Studies, TCD/WERRC.

Odent, Michel (1999) *The Scientification of Love*, London and New York: Free Association Books.

O'Driscoll, Kieran, Meagher, Declan, and Boylan, Peter (1993) *Active Management of Labor*, 3rd edn, London: Mosby.

Ogden, Jane, Shaw, Adrienne, and Zander, Luke (1997a) 'Part 1 Women's memories of homebirth 3–5 years on', *British Journal of Midwifery*, 5(4): 208–211.

Ogden, Jane, Shaw, Adrienne, and Zander, Luke (1997b) 'Part 2 Deciding on a homebirth: help and hindrances', *British Journal of Midwifery*, 5(4): 212–215.

Ogden, Jane, Shaw, Adrienne, and Zander, Luke (1997c) 'Part 3 A decision with a lasting effect', *British Journal of Midwifery*, 5(4): 216–218.

Ogden, Jane (1998) 'Having a homebirth: decisions, experiences and long-term consequences, in Sarah Clement (ed.) *Psychological Perspectives on Pregnancy and Childbirth*, pp. 101–121, Edinburgh, London, New York, Philadelphia, San Francisco, Sydney, Toronto: Churchill Livingstone.

Okely, Judith (1994) 'Thinking through fieldwork', in Alan Bryman, and Robert G. Burgess (eds) *Analyzing Qualitative Data*, pp. 18–34, London and New York: Routledge.

Oleson, Virginia (1994) 'Feminisms and models of qualitative research', in Norman K. Denzin and Yvonna S. Lincoln (eds) *Handbook of Qualitative Research*, pp. 158–174, Thousand Oaks, CA: Sage.

Olsen, O. (1997) 'Meta-analysis of the safety of home birth', *Birth*, 24(1): 4–13.

Olsen, O., and Jewell, M.D. (2001) 'Home versus hospital birth (Cochrane Review)', *The Cochrane Library, Issue 4*, Oxford: Update Software.

O'Neill, Eileen (1998) 'Disappearing ink: early modern women philosophers and their fate in history', in Janet A. Kourany (ed.) *Philosophy in a Feminist Voice: Critiques and Reconstructions*, pp. 17–62, Princeton, NJ: Princeton University Press.

Opie, Anne (1992) 'Qualitative research, appropriation of the "Other" and empowerment', *Feminist Review*, 40 (spring): 52–69.

Ortiz, Teresa (1993) 'From hegemony to subordination: midwives in early modern Spain', in Hilary Marland (ed.) *The Art of Midwifery*, pp. 95–114, London and New York: Routledge.

Ortner, S.B. and Whitehead, H. (1981) *Sexual Meanings: The Cultural Construction of Gender and Sexuality*, London: Cambridge University Press.

Oswin, J. (1993) *Home Deliveries: How Mothers who Planned to Have their Baby at Home Found the Experience*, Bristol: MIDRS, www.midirs.org.

Page, Lesley (1992) 'Choice, control and continuity: the 3 "C"s', *Modern Midwife*, 2(4): 8–10.

Page, Lesley (ed.) (2000) *The New Midwifery: Science and Sensitivity in Practice*, London: Churchill Livingstone.

Pairman, Sally (2000) 'Women-centred midwifery: partnerships or professional friendships', in Mavis Kirkham (ed.) *The Midwife–Mother Relationship*, pp. 207–226, London: Macmillan.

Pasveer, Bernike, and Akrich, Madeleine (2001) 'Obstetrical trajectories: on training women/bodies for (home) birth', in Raymond DeVries, Cecilia Benoit, Edwin R. van Teijlingen and Sirpa Wrede (eds) *Birth by Design: Pregnancy, Maternity Care, and Midwifery in North America and Europe*, pp. 229–242, New York and London: Routledge.

Pateman, Carol (1989) *The Disorder of Women*, Cambridge: Polity Press.

Peretz, Elizabeth (1990) 'A maternity service for England and Wales: local authority maternity care in the inter-war period in Oxfordshire and Tottenham', in Jo Garcia, Robert Kilpatrick and Martin Richards (eds) *The Politics of Maternity Care: Services for Childbearing Women in Twentieth-Century Britain*, pp. 15–29, Oxford: Clarendon Press.

Perkins, Elizabeth R., and Unell, Judith (1997) 'Continuity and choice in practice: a study of a community-based team midwifery practice', in Mavis J. Kirkham and Elizabeth R. Perkins (eds) *Reflections on Midwifery*, pp. 26–46, London: Bailliere Tindall.

Petersen, Alan (1997) 'Risk, governance and the new public health', in Alan Petersen and Robin Bunton (eds) *Foucault, Health and Medicine*, pp. 189–206, London and New York: Routledge.

Phillips, Ann (1992) 'Universal pretensions in political thought', in Michele Barratt and Ann Phillips (eds) *Destabilizing Theory: Contemporary Feminist Debates*, pp. 10–30, Cambridge: Polity Press.

Pitt, Susan (1999) 'Midwifery and medicine: gendered knowledge in the practice of delivery', in Hilary Marland and Anne Marie Rafferty (eds) *Midwives, Society and Childbirth: Debates and Controversies in the Modern Period*, pp. 218–231, London and New York: Routledge.

Pizzini, Franca (1992) 'Women's time, institutional time', in Ronald Frankenberg (ed.) *Time, Health and Medicine*, pp. 68–74, London: Sage.

Potter, Elizabeth (1993) 'Gender and epistemic negotiation', in Linda Alcoff and Elizabeth Potter (eds) *Feminist Epistemologies*, pp. 161–186, New York and London: Routledge.

Price, Sian, and Williams, Elizabeth (1998) 'Intrapartum continuity of care in a Welsh rural community', *British Journal of Midwifery*, 6(1), 43–46.

Pritchard, K., O'Boyle, A., and Hogden, J. (1995) 'Third stage of labour: outcomes of physiological third stage of labour care in the homebirth setting', *New Zealand College of Midwives Journal*, April: 8–10.

Priya, Jaqueline Vincent (1992) *Birth Traditions: Modern Pregnancy Care*, Shaftesbury, Dorset and Rockport, MA: Element.

Rabuzzi, Kathryn Allen (1994) *Mother with Child: Transformations through Childbirth*, Bloomington, IN: Indiana University Press.

Reiger, Kerreen (2000) 'Reconceiving citizenship: the challenge of mothers as political activists', *Feminist Theory*, 1(3): 309–327.

Reinharz, Shulamit (1992) *Feminist Methods in Social Research*, New York and Oxford: Oxford University Press.

Ribbens, Jane (1998) 'Hearing my feeling voice? An autobiographical discussion of motherhood', in Jane Ribbens and Rosalind Edwards (eds) *Feminist Dilemmas in Qualitative Research*, pp. 24–38, London: Sage.

Roberts, Helen (1981) 'Women and their doctors: power and powerlessness', in Helen Roberts (ed.) *Doing Feminist Research*, pp. 7–29, London: Routledge.

Robinson, Jean (1982) 'Complaints confined to childbirth', *Nursing Mirror*, 8 September.

Robinson, Jean (1995) 'How we lost home births', *British Journal of Midwifery*, 3(12): 669–670.

Robinson, Jean (1998) 'Birth after multiple miscarriages: emotional needs', *British Journal of Midwifery*, 6(2): 93.

Robinson, Jean (1999) 'Home birth: the midwife effect', *British Journal of Midwifery*, 7(4): 225–227.

Robinson, Jean (2004a) 'Whose baby? Complaints about neonatal care', *British Journal of Midwifery*, 12(3): 175.

Robinson, Jean (2004b) 'Cot deaths: still blaming the mother', *British Journal of Midwifery*, 12(2): 86.

Robinson, Jean (2004c) 'Memories are made of this: the midwife effect', *British Journal of Midwifery*, 12(8): 515.

Robinson, Sarah (1990) 'Maintaining the independence of the midwifery profession: a continuing struggle', in Jo Garcia, Robert Kilpatrick and Martin Richards (eds) *The Politics of Maternity Care: Services for Childbearing Women in Twentieth-Century Britain*, pp. 47–60, Oxford: Clarendon Press.

Robson, S. Elizabeth E. (1992) 'Variation of cervical dilation estimation by midwives, doctors, student midwives and medical students in 1985: a small study using cervical simulation models', in *Research and the Midwife Conference Proceedings 1991*, pp. 26–33, University of Manchester.

Romalis, Shelly (1985) 'Struggle between providers and the recipients: the case of birth practices', in E. Lewin and V. Olesen (eds) *Women, Health and Healing: Toward a New Perspective*, pp. 174–208, London: Tavistock.

Roncalli, Lucia (1997) 'Standing by process: a midwife's notes on storytelling: passage and intuition', in Robbie Davis-Floyd and P. Sven-Arvidson (eds) *Intuition: The Inside Story – Interdisciplinary Perspectives*, pp. 177–200, New York and London: Routledge.

Rooks, Judith (1997) *Midwifery and Childbirth in America*, Philadelphia, PA: Temple University Press.

Rorty, Richard (1991) 'Feminism and pragmatism', *Radical Philosophy*, 59(autumn): 3–14.

Rosenblatt, Louise M. (1978) *The Reader, the Text, the Poem: The Transactional Theory of the Literary Work*, London: Feffer & Simons.

Roseneil, Sasha (1996) 'Transgressions and transformations: experience, consciousness and identity at Greenham', in Nickie Charles and Felicia Hughes-Freeland (eds) *Practising Feminism: Identity, Difference, Power*, pp. 86–108, London and New York: Routledge.

Rosser, Jilly (1998) 'Home birth: where does the buck stop?', *The Practising Midwife*, 1(12): 4–5.

Rosser, Jilly, and Anderson, Tricia (2000) 'What next? Taking normal birth out of the labour ward', *The Practising Midwife*, 3(4): 4–5.

Rothman, Barbara Katz (1986) *The Tentative Pregnancy: Prenatal Diagnosis and the Future of Motherhood*, New York: Viking Press.

Rothman, Barbara Katz (1993) 'Going Dutch: lessons for Americans', in E.A. Vandermaark (ed.) *Successful Homebirth and Midwifery: The Dutch Model*, Westport, CT: Bergin & Garvey.

Rothman, Barbara Katz (2001) 'Spoiling the pregnancy: prenatal diagnosis in the Netherlands', in Raymond DeVries, Cecilia Benoit, Edwin R. van Teijlingen and Sirpa Wrede (eds) *Birth by Design: Pregnancy, Maternity Care, and Midwifery in North America and Europe*, pp. 180–198, New York and London: Routledge.

Rouf, Khaoji (1999) 'Child sexual abuse and pregnancy', *The Practising Midwife*, 2(6): 29–31.

Royal College of Ostetricians and Gynaecologists (RCOG) (2001) *The Use of Electronic Fetal Monitoring: the Use and Interpretation of Cardiotocography in Intrapartum Fetal Surveillance*, London: RCOG.

Ruddick, Sara (1989) *Maternal Thinking: Towards a Politics of Peace*, London: The Women's Press.

Rutanen, E.M., Ylikorkala, O. (1998) 'Raskaus ja snnytys suomessa – onko valtalkunnassa kaikki hyvin?' *Duodecim*, 114: 2209–2211.

Saks, Mike (1992) *Alternative Medicine in Britain*, Oxford: Clarendon Paperbacks.

Sandall, Jane (1995) 'Choice, continuity and control: changing midwifery towards a sociological perspective', *Midwifery*, 11: 201–209.

Sandall, Jane (1997) 'Midwives' burnout and continuity of care', *British Journal of Midwifery*, 5(2): 106–111.

Sandall, Jane, Bourgeault, Ivy Lynn, Meijer, Wouter J., and Schuecking, Beate A. (2001a) 'Deciding who cares: winners and losers in the late twentieth century', in Raymond DeVries, Cecilia Benoit, Edwin R. van Teijlingen and Sirpa Wrede (eds) *Birth by Design: Pregnancy, Maternity Care and Midwifery in North America and Europe*, pp. 117–138, New York and London: Routledge.

Sandall, Jane, Davies, Jacqueline, and Warwick, Cathy (2001b) *Evaluation of the Albany Midwifery Practice*, London: King's College Hospital.

Sandroff, Ronni (1994) 'Beware of the phallic drift, on the issues', *The Progressive Woman's Quaterly 3*, 2: 2.

Saunders, Dawn, Boulton, Mary, Chapple, Jean, Ratcliffe, Julie, and Levitan, Judith (2000) *Evaluation of the Edgware Birth Centre*, Harrow: North Thames Perinatal Public Health.

Savage, Wendy (1990) 'How obstetrics might change: Wendy Savage talks to Robert Kilpatrick', in Jo Garcia, Robert Kilpatrick and Martin Richards (eds) *The Politics of Maternity Care: Services for Childbearing Women in Twentieth-Century Britain*, pp. 325–340, Oxford: Clarendon Press.

Sbisa, Marina (1996) 'The feminine subject and female body in discourse about childbirth', *European Journal of Women's Studies*, 3: 363–376.

Scambler, Graham (1987) 'Habermas and the power of medical expertise', in Graham Scambler (ed.) *Sociological Theory and Medical Sociology*, pp. 165–193, London: Tavistock.

Schlenzka, Peter F. (1999) 'Safety of alternative approaches to childbirth', unpublished PhD thesis, Stanford University, CA: USA.

Schmid, Verena (2003) Birth Centres in Italy, in Mavis Kirkham (ed.) *Birth Centres: A Social Model of Maternity Care*, pp. 161–172, Books for Midwives.

Schrader, Catharina, with Lieburg, M.J. and Kloosterman, G.L. (1987) *'Mother and Child Were Saved': The Memoirs (1693–1740) of the Frisian Midwife Catharina Schrader*, trans. Hilary Marland, Amsterdam: Rodopi.

Schwarz, Eckart W. (1990) 'The engineering of childbirth: a new obstetrics programme as reflected in British textbooks, 1960–1980', in Jo Garcia, Robert Kilpatrick and Martin Richards (eds) *The Politics of Maternity Care: Services for Childbearing Women in Twentieth-Century Britain*, pp. 30–46, Oxford: Clarendon Press.

Scott, Joan W. (1992) '"Experience"', in Judith Butler and Joan W. Scott (eds) *Feminists Theorize the Political*, pp. 22–40, New York and London: Routledge.

Scottish Health Feedback (1993) *Lothian Maternity Survey 1992: A Report to Lothian Health Council*, Edinburgh: Lothian Health Council.

Scottish Home and Health Department (SHHD) (1965) *The Staffing of the Midwifery Services in Scotland: Scottish Home and Health Services Report by a Committee of the Council*, Edinburgh: HMSO.

Scottish Home and Health Department (1973a) *Community Medicine in Scotland: Report by the Joint Working Party on the Integration of Medical Work*, Edinburgh: HMSO.

Scottish Home and Health Department (1973b) *Maternity Services: Integration of Maternity Work*, Edinburgh: HMSO.

Scottish Home and Health Department (1980) *Scottish Health Authorities Priorities for the Eighties: A Report by the Scottish Health Services Planning Council*, Edinburgh: HMSO.

Scottish Home and Health Department (1988) *Scottish Health Authorities Review of Priorities for the Eighties and Nineties: A Report by the Scottish Health Services Planning Council*, Edinburgh: HMSO.

Scottish Office Home and Health Department (1994) *Report on Maternal and Perinatal Deaths in Scotland 1986–1990*, Edinburgh: HMSO.

Scully, Diana (1994) *Men Who Control Women's Health*, New York and London: Teachers College Press.

Searles, C. (1981) 'The impetus towards home birth', *Journal of Nurse-Midwifery*, 26(3): 51–56.

Shallow, Helen (1999) An exploration of midwives' experience of becoming integrated within teams: with an emphasis on their experience of providing continuity of care', unpublished M.Med.Sci thesis, University of Sheffield.

Shallow, Helen (2003) 'The birth centre project', in Mavis Kirkham (ed.) *Birth Centres: A Social Model for Maternity Care*, pp. 11–24, Oxford: Butterworth-Heinemann.

Shanley, Laura (1994) *Unassisted Childbirth*, Westport, CT: Bergin & Garvey.

Shapiro, M.C., Najam, J.M., Chang, A., Keeping, D., Morrison, J., and Western, J.S. (1983) 'Information control and the exercise of power in the obstetrical encounter', *Social Science and Medicine*, 17(3): 139–146.

Shearer, J.M.L. (1985) 'Five year survey of risk of booking for a home birth in Essex', *British Medical Journal*, 291: 1478–1480.

Shildrick, Margrit (1997) *Leaky Bodies and Boundaries: Feminism, Postmodernism and (Bio)Ethics*, London and New York: Routledge.

Shipman, Martin (1988) *The Limitations of Social Research*, 3rd edn, London: Longman.

Siddiqui, Jeanne (1999) 'The therapeutic relationship in midwifery', *British Journal of Midwifery*, 7(2): 111–114.

Simkin, Penny (1991) 'Just another day in a woman's life? Part 1: Women's long-term perceptions of their first birth experience', *Birth*, 18(4): 203–210.

Simkin, Penny (1992) 'Just another day in a woman's life? Part 2: Nature and consistence of women's long-term memories of their first birth experiences', *Birth*, 19(2): 64–81.

Simpson, Julia (2004) 'Negotiating elective caesarean section: an obstetric team perspective', in Mavis Kirkham (ed.) *Informed Choice in Maternity Care*, pp. 211–36, Basingstoke: Palgrave Macmillan.

Sleep, J., Grant, A., Garcia, J., Elbourne, D., Spencer, J., and Chalmers, I. (1984) 'West Berkshire perineal management trial', *British Medical Journal*, 289: 587–590.

Smethurst, Gill (1997) 'Extending choices', *MIDIRS Midwifery Digest*, 7(3), 376–377.

Smith, Dorothy E. (1987) 'Women's perspective as a radical critique of sociology', in Sandra Harding (ed.) *Feminism and Methodology*, pp. 84–96, Milton Keynes: Open University Press and Bloomington, IN: Indiana University Press.

Smulders, Beatrijs, and Limburg, Astrid (1988) 'Obstetrics and midwifery in the Netherlands', in Sheila Kitzinger (ed.) *The Midwife Challenge*, pp. 235–249, London: Pandora.

Smythe, Elizabeth (1998) '"Being safe" in childbirth: a hermeneutic interpretation of the narratives of women and practitioners', unpublished PhD thesis, Massey University, New Zealand.

Soper, Kate (1990) 'Feminism, humanism and postmodernism', *Radical Philosophy*, 55: 11–17.

Spacks, Patricia (1982) 'In praise of gossip', *Hudson Review*, p. 24.

Spender, Dale (1980) *Man Made Language*, London: Routledge and Kegan Paul.

Spivak, Gayatri Chakravorty (1982) 'Displacement and the discourse of woman', in Mary Krupnick (ed.) *Displacement, Derrida and After*, pp. 185–186, Bloomfield: Indiana University Press.

Spretnak, Charlene (1999) The Resurgence of the Real: Body, Nature, and Place in a Hypermodern World, New York: Routledge.

Spurrett, B. (1988) 'Home births and the women's perspective in Australia', *Medical Journal of Australia*, 149: 289–290.

Stacey, Judith (1991) 'Can there be a feminist ethnography?,' in Sherna Berger Gluck and Daphne Patai (eds) *Women's Words: The Feminist Practice of Oral History*, pp. 111–119, New York and London: Routledge.

Stanko, Elizabeth A. (1994) 'Dancing with denial: researching women and questioning men', in Mary Maynard and June Purvis (eds) *Researching Women's Lives from a Feminist Perspective*, pp. 93–105, London: Taylor & Francis.

Stanley, Liz, and Wise, Sue (1990) 'Method, methodology and epistemology in feminist research processes', in Liz Stanley (ed.) *Feminist Praxis: Research, Theory and Epistemology in Feminist Sociology*, pp. 20–60, London and New York: Routledge.

Stanley, Liz, and Wise, Sue (1993) *Breaking Out Again*, London and New York: Routledge.

Stanley, Liz, and Wise, Sue (2000) 'But the empress has no clothes! Some awkward questions about the "missing revolution" in feminist theory', *Feminist Theory*, 1(3): 261–288.

Stanton, Ann (1996) 'Reconfiguring teaching and knowing in the college classroom', in Nancy Goldberger, Jill Tarule, Blythe Clinchy and Mary Belenky (eds) *Knowledge, Difference, and Power: Essays Inspired by Women's Ways of Knowing*, pp. 25–56, New York: Basic Books.

Stapleton, Helen (1997) 'Choice in the face of uncertainty', in Mavis J. Kirkham and Elizabeth R. Perkins (eds) *Reflections on Midwifery*, pp. 47–69, London: Bailliere Tindall.

Stapleton, Helen (2004) 'Is there a difference between a free gift and a planned purchase? The use of evidence-based leaflets in maternity care', in Mavis Kirkham (ed.) *Informed Choice in Maternity Care*, Basingstoke: Palgrave Macmillan.

Stapleton, Helen, Duerden, Jean, and Kirkham, Mavis (1998) *Evaluation of the Impact of the Supervision of Midwives on Professional Practice and the Quality of Midwifery Care*, English National Board for Nursing, Midwifery and Health Visiting and the University of Sheffield.

Starhawk (1990) *Truth or Dare: Encounters with Power, Authority, and Mystery*, San Francisco, CA: Harper Collins.

Stewart, Mary (ed.) (2004a) *Pregnancy, Birth and Maternity Care: Feminist Perspectives*, Edinburgh, London, New York, Oxford, Philadelphia, St Louis, Sydney, Toronto: Books for Midwives.

Stewart, Mary (2004b) 'Feminisms and the body', in Mary Stewart (ed.) *Pregnancy, Birth and Maternity Care: Feminist Perspectives*, pp. 25–40, Edinburgh, London, New York, Oxford, Philadelphia, St Louis, Sydney, Toronto: Books for Midwives.

Stoljar, Natalie (2000) 'Autonomy and the feminist intuition', in Catriona Mackenzie and Natalie Stoljar (eds) *Relational Autonomy: Feminist Perspectives on Autonomy, Agency, and the Social Self*, pp. 94–111, New York and Oxford: Oxford University Press.

Strong, Thomas H. (2000) *Expecting Trouble: The Myth of Prenatal Care in America*, New York and London: New York University Press.

Sumpter, Yasmin (2001) 'Water birth mother accused of illegal birth and child neglect', *AIMS Journal*, 13(1): 7–9.

Sutton, Jean (2001) *Let Birth be Born Again: Rediscovering and Reclaiming our Midwifery Heritage*. Available from Birth Concepts UK, 95 Beech Road, Bedfont, Middx TW14 8AJ.

Teixeira, Jeronima M.A, Fisk, Nicholas M., and Glover, Vibette (1999) 'Association between maternal anxiety in pregnancy and increased uterine artery resistance index: cohort based study', *British Medical Journal*, 318: 153–157.

Tew, Marjorie (1985) 'Place of birth and perinatal mortality', *Journal of the Royal College of General Practitioners*, 35: 390–394.

Tew, Marjorie (1995) *Safer Childbirth? A Critical History of Maternity Care*, London: Chapman and Hall.

Tew, Marjorie (1998) *Safer Childbirth? A Critical History of Maternity Care*, 3rd edn, London and New York: Free Association Books.

Tew, Marjorie, and Damstra-Wijmenga, Sonja M.I. (1991) 'Safest birth attendants: recent Dutch evidence', *Midwifery*, 7: 55–63.

Thomas, Hilary (1992) 'Time and the cervix', in R. Frankenberg (ed.) *Time, Health and Medicine*, pp. 56–67, London: Sage.

Thomas, Pat (1994) 'Accountable for what? New thoughts on the midwife/mother relationship', *AIMS Journal*, 6(3): 1–5.

Thomas, Pat (1997) *Every Birth is Different*, London: Headline Press.

Thomas, Pat (1998) *Choosing a Home Birth*, Association for Improvements in Maternity Services, 5 Ann's Court, Grove Road, Surbiton, Surrey KT6 4BE.

Thompson, Faye E. (2004) *Mothers and Midwives: The Ethical Journey*, Edinburgh: Books for Midwives.

Thornton, J.G. and Lilford, R.J. (1994) 'Active management of labour: current knowledge and research issues', *British Medical Journal*, 309: 366–368.

Tilley, Jo (2000) 'Sexual assault and flashbacks in the labour ward', *The Practising Midwife*, 3(4): 18–19.

Torres, A., and Reich, M.R. (1989) 'The shift from home to institutional childbirth: a comparative study of the United Kingdom and the Netherlands', *International Journal of Health Services*, 19(3): 405–419.

Towler, Jean and Bramall, Joan (1986) *Midwives in History and Society*, London: Croom Helm.

Townsend, Peter, Davidson, Nick, and Whitehead, Margaret (1992) *Inequalities in Health: The Black Report and The Health Divide*, London: Penguin.

Treffers, P.E., and Laan, R. (1986) 'Regional perinatal mortality and regional hospitalization at delivery in the Netherlands', *British Journal of Obstetrics and Gynaecology*, 93: 690–693.

Treffers, P.E., Eskes, M., Kleiverda, G., and van Alten, D. (1990) 'Letter from Amsterdam: home births and minimal medical interventions', *Journal of the American Medical Association*, 264: 17.

Treichler, Paula (1990) 'Feminism, medicine and the meaning of childbirth', in Mary Jacobus, Evelyn Fox-Keller and Sally Shuttleworth (eds) *Body/Politics: Women and the Discourse of Science*, pp. 113–138, New York and London: Routledge.

Trevathan, Wendy (1997) 'An evolutionary perspective on authoritative knowledge about birth', in Robbie E. Davis-Floyd and Carolyn F. Sargent (eds) *Childbirth and Authoritative Knowledge: Cross-Cultural Perspectives*, pp. 80–88, Berkeley, CA: University of California Press.

Turner, Bryan S. (1987) *Medical Power and Social Knowledge*, London: Sage.

Turner, Bryan S. (1991) 'Recent developments in the theory of the body', in M. Featherstone, M. Hepworth and B.S. Turner (eds) *The Body: Social Process and Cultural Theory*, pp. 1–35, London: Sage.

Tyson, Holliday (1991) 'Outcomes of 1001 midwife-attended home births in Toronto 1983–1988', *Birth*, 18(1): 14–19.

UKCC (2000) *UKCC Position Statement: 'Supporting Women who wish to have a Home Birth'*, UKCC.

van Alten, Dirk, Eskes, Martine, and Treffers, Pieter E. (1989) 'Midwifery in the Netherlands: the Wormeveer study selection mode of delivery, perinatal mortality and infant morbidity', *British Journal of Obstetrics and Gynaecology*, 96: 656–662.

van der Hulst, Leonie, and van Teijlingen, Edwin R. (2001) 'Telling stories of midwives', in Raymond DeVries, Cecilia Benoit, Edwin R. van Teijlingen and Sirpa Wrede (eds) *Birth by Design: Pregnancy, Maternity Care, and Midwifery in North America and Europe*, pp. 166–179, New York and London: Routledge.

van der Hulst, Leonie, van Teijlingen, Edwin R., Bonsei, Gouke J., Eskes, Martine, and Bleker, Otto P. (2004) 'Does a pregnant woman's intended of birth influence her attitude toward and occurrence of obstetric interventions?', *Birth*, 31(1): 28–33.

van Lieburg, M.J. and Marland, H. (1989) 'Midwife regulation, education and practice in the Netherlands during the nineteenth century', *Medical History*, 33: 296–317.

van Manen, Max (1990) *Researching Lived Experience: Human Sciences for an Action Sensitive Pedagogy*, London, Ont.: Althouse Press.

van Olphen Fehr, Juliana (1999) 'The lived experience of being in a caring relationship with a midwife during childbirth', unpublished PhD thesis, George Mason University, Fairfax, Virginia.

van Teijlingen, Edwin R. (1990) 'The profession of maternity home care assistant and it's significance for the Dutch midwifery profession', *International Journal of Nursing Studies*, 27(4): 355–366.

van Teijlingen, Edwin R. (1992) 'The organisation of maternity care in the Netherlands', *Association for Community Based Maternity Care*, 5: 2–4.

van Teijlingen, Edwin (1994) 'Dutch maternity services from a social or medical model of childbirth? Comparing the arguments in Grampian (Scotland) and the Netherlands', unpublished PhD thesis, University of Aberdeen.

van Teijlingen, Edwin, and van der Hulst, Leonie (1995) 'Midwifery in the Netherlands: more than a semi-profession?', in T. Johnston, G. Larkin and M. Saks (eds) *Health Professions and the State in Europe*, pp. 178–186, London: Routledge.

van Teijlingen, Edwin, R., Hundley, Vanora, Rennie, Ann-Marie, Graham, Wendy, Fitzmaurice, Ann (2003) 'Maternity satisfaction studies and their limitations: "What is must still be best"', *Birth*, 30(2): 75–82.

Viisainen, Kirsi (2000a) *Choices in Birth Care: The Place of Birth*, Research Report 115, Helsinki: STAKES National Research and Development Centre for Welfare and Health, Department of Public Health, Faculty of Medicine, Helsinki University.

Viisainen, Kirsi (2000b) 'The moral dangers of home birth: parents' perceptions of risks in home birth in Finland', *Sociology of Health and Illness*, 22(6): 792–814.

Viisainen, Kirsi (2001) 'Negotiating control and meaning: home birth as a self-constructed choice in Finland', *Social Science and Medicine*, 52(7): 1109–1121.

Viisainen, Kirsi, Gissler, Mika, Hartikainen, Anna-Liisa, and Hemminki, Elina (1999) 'Accidental out-of-hospital births in Finland: incidence and geographical distribution', *Acta Obstetrica et Gynaecologica Scandinavica*, 79: 372–378.

Wagner, Marsden (1994) *Pursuing the Birth Machine: The Search for Appropriate Birth Technology*, Camperdown, NSW: Ace Graphics.

Wagner, Marsden (1995) 'A global witch-hunt', *Lancet*, 346: 1020–1022.

Wagner, Marsden (2001) 'Fish can't see water: the need to humanize birth', *Journal of Gynecology and Obstetrics*, 75(suppl. 1): S25–S37.

Waldenstrom, Ulla (2004) 'Why do some women change their opinions about childbirth over time', *Birth*, 31(2): 102–107.

Waldenstrom, Ulla, Hildingsson, Ingegerd, and Christie, Radestrad Ingela (2004) 'A negative birth experience: prevalence and risk factors in a national sample', *Birth*, 31(1): 17–27.

Walker, Jane (2000) 'Women's experiences of transfer from a midwifery-led to a consultant-led maternity unit in the UK during late pregnancy and labour', *Journal of Midwifery and Women's Health*, 45(2): 161–168.

Walsh, Dennis (2003) 'We should go with the rhythm of labour', *British Journal of Midwifery*, 11(11): 656.

Warren, Chris (1999a) 'Invaders of privacy', *Midwifery Matters*, 81: 8–9.

Warren, Chris (1999b) 'Why should I do vaginal examinations?', *The Practising Midwife*, 2(6): 12–13.

Waterstone, Mark, Bewley, Susan, and Wolfe, Charles (2001) 'Incidence and predictors of severe obstetric morbidity: case-control study', *British Medical Journal*, 322: 1089–1093.

Wayne, F., Schramm, M.A., Barnes, D.E., and Bakewell, J.M. (1987) 'Neonatal mortality in Missouri home births 1978–84', *American Journal of Public Health*, 77(8): 930–935.

Weiner, Carolyn, Strauss, Anselm, Fagerhaugh, Shzuko, and Suczek, Barbara (1997) 'Trajectories, biographies, and the evolving medical technology scene', in Anselm Strauss and Juliet Corbin (eds) *Grounded Theory in Practice*, Thousand Oaks, CA: Sage.

Welsh Assembly (2002) 'Delivering the future in Wales: a framework for realizing the potential of midwives in Wales', Briefing Paper 4, Key principle 1.3, Cardiff: National Assembly.

Wesson, Nicky (1990) *Home Birth: A Practical Guide*, 2nd edn, London: Optima.

Which? Way to Health (1990) 'Are hospitals the worst place to get well?', in *Which? Way to Health*, London: Which?

Wickham, Sara (2004) 'Feminism and ways of knowing', in Mary Stewart (ed.) *Pregnancy, Birth and Maternity Care: Feminist Perspectives*, pp. 157–68, Edinburgh: Books for Midwives.

Wiegers, T.A., Keirse, M.J.N.C., van der Zee, J., and Berghs, G.A.H. (1996) 'Outcome of planned home and planned hospital births in low risk pregnancies: prospective study in midwifery practices in the Netherlands', *British Medical Journal*, 313: 1309–1313.

Wiesner, Merry E. (1993) 'The Midwives of South Germany and the public/private dichotomy, in Hilary Marland (ed.) *The Art of Midwifery*, pp. 77–94, London and New York: Routledge.

Wilkins, Ruth (2000) 'Poor relations: the paucity of the professional paradigm', in Mavis Kirkham (ed.) *The Midwife–Mother Relationship*, pp. 28–54, London: Macmillan.

Williamson, Charlotte (1988) 'Dominant, challenging interests in the NHS', *Health Services Management*, December: 170–174.

Williamson, Charlotte (1992) *Whose standards? Consumer and Professional Standards in Health Care*. Oxford University Press.

Wilson, Adrian (1995) *The making of the man-midwife: childbirth in England*, pp. 1660–1770, Cambridge, MA: Harvard University Press.

Witz, Anne (1992) *Professions and Patriarchy*, London and New York: Routledge.

Wolford, M.C. (1997) 'First do no harm', *Midwifery Today*, 15–17.

Women's Health Information Collective (WHIC) (2000) *Pregnancy and Birth: In Support of Autonomy*, Glasgow: WHIC Publications.

Woodcock, H.C., Read, A.W., Bower, C., Stanley, F.J., and Moore, D.J. (1994) 'A matched cohort study of planned home and hospital births in Western Australia 1981–1987', *Midwifery*, 10: 125–135.

Wright, Carol (1992) *Birth – Hospital or Home*, Hinchingbrooke, UK: Hinchingbrooke Health Care Trust Obsteric Unit.

Wright, Erna (1964) *The New Childbirth*, London: Tandem.

Young, Iris Marion (1990a) 'Pregnant embodiment: subjectivity and alienation', in Iris Marion Young, *Throwing like a Girl, and Other Essays in Feminist Philosophy and Social Theory*, pp. 160–174, Bloomington, IN: Indiana University Press.

Young, Iris Marion (1990b) *Throwing like a Girl and Other Essays in Feminist Philosophy and Social Theory*, Bloomington, IN: Indiana University Press.

Young, Iris Marion (1997a) *Intersecting Voices*, Princeton, NJ: Princeton University Press.

Index